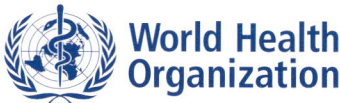

Geneva 2008

ANTI-TUBERCULOSIS DRUG RESISTANCE IN THE WORLD

Fourth Global Report

The World Health Organization/International Union Against Tuberculosis
and Lung Disease (WHO/UNION) Global Project on
Anti-Tuberculosis Drug Resistance Surveillance
2002–2007

WHO Library Cataloguing-in-Publication Data

Anti-tuberculosis drug resistance in the world : fourth global report.

«WHO/HTM/TB/2008.394»

1.Tuberculosis, Multidrug-resistant - epidemiology. 2.Drug resistance, Bacterial - statistics. 3.Bacteriological techniques. 4.Data collection - methods. 5.Cross-sectional studies. I.WHO/IUATLD Global Project on Anti-Tuberculosis Drug Resistance Surveillance.

ISBN 978 92 4 156361 1   (NLM classification: WF 360)

© **World Health Organization 2008**
All rights reserved. Publications of the World Health Organization can be obtained from WHO Press, World Health Organization, 20 Avenue Appia, 1211 Geneva 27, Switzerland (tel.: +41 22 791 3264; fax: +41 22 791 4857; e-mail: bookorders@who.int). Requests for permission to reproduce or translate WHO publications – whether for sale or for noncommercial distribution – should be addressed to WHO Press, at the above address (fax: +41 22 791 4806; e-mail: permissions@who.int).
The designations employed and the presentation of the material in this publication do not imply the expression of any opinion whatsoever on the part of the World Health Organization concerning the legal status of any country, territory, city or area or of its authorities, or concerning the delimitation of its frontiers or boundaries. Dotted lines on maps represent approximate border lines for which there may not yet be full agreement.

The mention of specific companies or of certain manufacturers' products does not imply that they are endorsed or recommended by the World Health Organization in preference to others of a similar nature that are not mentioned. Errors and omissions excepted, the names of proprietary products are distinguished by initial capital letters.

All reasonable precautions have been taken by the World Health Organization to verify the information contained in this publication. However, the published material is being distributed without warranty of any kind, either expressed or implied. The responsibility for the interpretation and use of the material lies with the reader. In no event shall the World Health Organization be liable for damages arising from its use.

Designed and typeset in Italy
Printed in Italy

WRITING COMMITTEE

The report was written by:
Abigail Wright, Matteo Zignol

The following WHO staff assisted in compiling, analysing and editing information:
WHO Headquarters, Geneva
Abigail Wright, Matteo Zignol, Christopher Dye, Brian Williams, Mehran Hosseini Ana Bierrenbach, Salah Ottmani, Mohamed Aziz, Ernesto Jaramillo, Mario Raviglione, Paul Nunn, Kathrin Thomas, Rosalie Edma, Fabio Scano, Karin Weyer Louise Baker, Diana Weil.
WHO African Region Office (AFRO)
Oumou Bah-Sow (AFRO), Bah Keita (AFRO, West Africa), Daniel Kibuga (AFRO), Motseng Makhetha (South Africa), Vainess Mfungwe (AFRO), Wilfred Nkhoma (AFRO), Tom Sukwa (AFRO).
WHO Region of the Americas Office (AMRO)
Raimond Armengol (AMRO), Mirtha del Granado (AMRO), Rafael Lopez Olarte (AMRO), Pilar Ramon-Pardo (AMRO), Rodolfo Rodriguez-Cruz (Brazil), Matías Villatoro (Brazil).
WHO Eastern Mediterranean Region Office (EMRO)
Samiha Baghdadi (EMRO), Ghada Muhjazi (EMRO), Akihiro Seita (EMRO).
WHO European Region Office (EURO)
Evgeny Belilovsky (Russian Federation), Andrei Dadu (EURO), Pierpaolo de Colombani (EURO), Irina Danilova (Russian Federation), Jean de Dieu Iragena (Russian Federation), Lucica Ditiu (EURO), Wieslaw Jakubowiak (Russian Federation), Kestutis Miskinis (Ukraine), Gombogaram Tsogt (Central Asia), Richard Zaleskis (EURO).
WHO South-East Asia Region Office (SEARO)
Mohammed Akhtar (Nepal), Erwin Cooreman (Bangladesh), Puneet Dewan (SEARO), Hans Kluge (Myanmar), Nani Nair (SEARO), Suvanand Sahu (India), Chawalit Tantinimitkul (Thailand), Fraser Wares (India), Supriya Weerusavithana (Sri Lanka).
WHO Western Pacific Region Office (WPRO)
Daniel Chin (China), Philippe Glaziou (WPRO), Cornelia Hennig (China), Liu Yuhong (China), Pieter van Maaren (WPRO), Masaki Ota (WPRO), Michael Voniatis (Philippines).
International Union Against TB and Lung Disease (UNION), Paris, France
Hans Rieder, Armand Van Deun, Sang Jae Kim
EuroTB, Paris, France
Fatima Aït-Belghiti, Hedwidge Bousquié, Isabelle Devaux, Dennis Falzon, Yao Kudjawu.

GLOBAL NETWORK OF SUPRANATIONAL REFERENCE LABORATORIES

- Laboratoire de la Tuberculose, Institut Pasteur d'Algérie, *Alger, ALGERIA* (Prof. Fadila Boulahbal)
- Mycobacteria Laboratory, National Institute of Infectious Diseases, ANLIS (Dr Carlos G Malbran), *Buenos Aires, ARGENTINA* (Dr Lucia Barrera)
- Mycobacterium Reference Laboratory, Institute of Medical and Veterinary Science, *Adelaide, AUSTRALIA* (Dr Ivan Bastian, Dr Richard Lumb)
- Queensland Mycobacterium Reference Laboratory, *Brisbane, AUSTRALIA* (Dr Chris Coulter, Dr Chris Gilpin)
- Département de Microbiologie Unité de Mycobactériologie, Institut de Médecine Tropicale, *Antwerp, BELGIUM* (Prof. Françoise Portaels, Dr Armand Van Deun)
- Instituto de Salud Publica de Chile, *Santiago, CHILE* (Dr. María Cecilia Riquelme Jaqke)
- National Institute of Public Health, *Prague, CZECH REPUBLIC* (Dr Marta Havelková)
- Central Health Laboratory, Ministry of Health and Population, *Cairo, EGYPT* (Dr Mushira Ismail)
- Institut Pasteur, Centre National de Référence des Mycobacteries, *Paris, FRANCE* (Dr Véronique Vincent)
- Institute of Microbiology and Laboratory Medicine (IML) IML Diagnostik MVZ GmbH c/o Asklepios *Fachkliniken-Muenchen-Gauting, GERMANY* (Prof Knut Feldman, Dr med Harald Hoffmann)
- National Reference Center for Mycobacteria, *Borstel, GERMANY* (Dr Sabine Rüsch-Gerdes)
- TB Reference Laboratory Department of Health, *Hong Kong SAR, CHINA* (Dr Kai Man Kam)
- TB Research Centre (TRC), Indian Council of Medical Research, *Chennai, INDIA* (Dr Selvakumar, Dr Ranjani Ramachandran)
- Istituto Superiore di Sanità Dipartimento di Malattie Infettive, Parassitarie e Immunomediate, *Rome, ITALY* and Laboratory of Bacteriology & Medical Mycology and San Raffaele del Monte Tabor Foundation (hSR), *Milan, ITALY* (Dr Lanfranco Fattorini, Dr Daniela Cirillo)
- Research Institute of Tuberculosis, Japan Anti-Tuberculosis Association, *Tokyo, JAPAN* (Dr Satoshi Mitarai)
- Korean Institute of Tuberculosis, *Seoul, REPUBLIC OF KOREA* (Dr Woojin Lew)
- Departamento de Micobacterias, Instituto de Diagnostico y, Referencia Epidemiologicos (INDRE), *MEXICO* (Dr Susana Balandrano)
- National Institute of Public Health and the Environment (RIVM), *Bilthoven, NETHERLANDS* (Dr Dick van Soolingen)
- Centro de Tuberculose e Micobacterias (CTM), Instituto Nacional de Saude, *Porto, PORTUGAL* (Dr Maria Filomena Rodrigues)
- The Medical Research Council, TB Research Lead Programme, *Pretoria, SOUTH AFRICA* (Dr Karin Weyer)
- Servicio de Microbiologia Hospital Universitaris, Vall d'Hebron, *Barcelona, SPAIN* (Dr Nuria Martin-Casabona)
- Swedish Institute for Infectious Disease Control (SIDC), *Solna, SWEDEN* (Dr Sven Hoffner)

- National TB Reference Laboratory Center Tuberculosis Cluster, *Bangkok, THAILAND* (Somsak Rienthong, Dhanida Rienthong)
- Health Protection Agency, National Mycobacterium Reference Unit, Department of Infectious Diseases, *UNITED KINGDOM* (Dr Francis Drobniewski)
- Centers for Disease Control and Prevention, Mycobacteriology/Tuberculosis Laboratory, *Georgia, UNITED STATES OF AMERICA* (Dr Tom Shinnick, Dr Beverly Metchock)
- Massachusetts State Laboratory, *Massachusetts, UNITED STATES* (Dr Alexander Sloutsky)

CONTRIBUTORS

WHO African Region
Côte d'Ivoire: Jacquemin Kouakou, **Ethiopia:** Daniel Demisse, Getachew Eyob, Mekedes Gebeyehu, Wenimagene Getachew, Feven Girmachew, Eshetu Lemma, Zerihun Taddesew, Jan van den Hombergh, Dick van Soolingen, **Madagascar:** Rarivoson Benjamin, Ramarokoto Herimanana, **Rwanda:** Michel Gasana, John Gatabazi, Leen Rigouts, Alaine Umubyeyi, Greet Vandebriel, **Senegal:** Fatoumata Ba, Henriette Cécile Diop, **United Republic of Tanzania:** Saidi Egwaga, Fred Lwilla, Martin Chonde, Basra E. Doulla, Sayonki Mfinanga, Saidi Mfaume.

WHO Region of the Americas
Argentina: Lucía Barrera, Maria Delfina Sequeira, Elsa Zerbini **Canada:** Edward Ellis, Victor Gallant, Melissa Phypers, Derek Scholten, Joyce Wolfe, **Costa Rica:** Zeidy Mata A, Maria Cecilia Matamoros, **Cuba:** María Josefa Llanes Cordero, Miguel Echemendía, Ernesto Montoro, Dihadenys Lemus Molina, **Guatemala:** Licda Nancy Ayala Contreras, Edwin Antonio Quiñonez Villatoro, **Nicaragua:** Luis Alberto Chacón, Alejandro A. Tardencilla Gutiérrez, **Paraguay:** Juan Carlos Jara Rodríguez, Nilda Jimenez de Romero, **Peru:** Cesar Antonio Bonilla Asalde, Luis Asencios Solis, **Puerto Rico:** Ada S. Martinez, Beverly Metchock, Valerie Robinson, **Uruguay:** Carlos María Rivas-Chetto, Jorge Rodriguez-De Marco, **United States of America:** Sandy Althomsons, Kenneth G Castro, Beverly Metchock, Valerie Robison, Ryan Wallace.

WHO Eastern Mediterranean Region
Jordan: Said Abu Nadi, Khaled Yusra Rihani, Abu Rumman, **Lebanon:** Georges Aaraj, Mtanios Saade, **Morocco:** Naima Ben Cheikh, Quafae Lahlou, **Oman:** Hassan Al Tuhami, **Qatar:** Abdul Latif Al Khal, **Syrian Arab Republic:** Roula Hammoud, Fadia Maamari, **Yemen:** Amin N Al-Absi,

WHO European Region
Andorra: Margarita Coll Armangue, **Armenia**: Alvard Mirzoyan, Andrei Mosneaga, Vahan Poghosyah, **Austria:** Alexandra Indra, Jean-Paul Klein, **Azerbaijan:** Rafik Abuzarov, Faik Agayev, Ogtay Gozalov, Andrei Mosneaga, **Belgium:** Maryse Fauville-Dufaux, Francoise Portaels, Leen Rigouts, Greet Vankersschaever, Maryse Wanlin, **Bosnia & Herzegovina:** Zehra Dizdarevic, Mladen Duronjic, Hasan Zutic, **Croatia:** Aleksandar Simunovic, Vera Katalinic-Jankovic, **Czech Republic:** Martha Havelkova, Ludek Trnka, Jiri Wallenfels, **Denmark:** Peter Henrik Andersen, Zaza Kamper-Jorgensen, **Estonia:** Kai Kliiman, Tiina Kummik, **Finland:** Merja Marjamäki, Petri Ruutu, **France:** Delphine Antoine, Marie Claire Paty, Jérome Robert, **Georgia:** Archil Salakaia, Nino Lomtadze, Marina Janjgava, Rusudan Aspindzelashvili, Maia Kipiani, Ucha Nanava, **Germany:** Bonita Brodhun, Walter Haas, Sabine Rüsch-Gerdes, **Iceland:** Thorsteinn Blondal, Ingibjörg Hilmarsdotttir, **Ireland:** Noel Gibbons, Joan O'Donnell, **Israel:** Daniel Chemtob, **Italy:** Daniela Cirillo, F Piana, Maria Grazia Pompa, **Latvia:** Janis Leimans, Girts Skenders, **Lithuania:** Edita Davidaviciene, Anaida Sosnovska, **Luxembourg:** Pierrette HUberty-Krau, François Schneider, **Malta:** Analita Pace Asciak, **Netherlands:** Connie Erkens, Vincent Kuyvenhoven, Dick van Soolingen, **Norway:** Brita Askleand Winje, Turid Mannsaker, **Poland:** Kazimierz Roszkowski, Maria Korzeniewska-Kosela, Zofia Zwolska, **Republic of Moldova:** Valeriu Crudu, Nicolae Moraru, Dimitrii Sain, Silviu Sofronie, **Romania:** Domnica Chiotan, Daniela Homorodean, Ioan Paul Stoicescu, **Russian Federation:** Michael V Nikiforov, Yekaterina Kakorina, **Serbia:** Gordana

Radosavljevic Asic, Rukije Mehmeti, **Slovakia:** Ivan Solovic, Juraj Trenkler, **Slovenia:** Manca Žolnir Dovc, Damjan Erzen, Jurij Sorli, **Spain:** Odorina Tello Anchuela, Nuria Martín Casabona, Fernando Alcaide Fernandez de la Vega, Elena Cruz Ferro, Luisa Pérez del Molino Bernal, Soledad Jimenez, Antonia Lezcano, Julia Gonzalez Martin, Elena Rodriguez Valin, Asunción Vitoria, **Sweden:** Sven Hoffner, Victoria Romanus, **Switzerland:** Peter Helbling, **Ukraine:** Iryna Dubrovina, Mykhailo Golubchykov, Svetlana Lyepshina, Igor Raykhert, Yelena Yann, **United Kingdom:** Francis Drobniewski, Jim McMenamin, Roland Salmon, Brian Smyth, John Watson, **Uzbekistan:** Dilrabo Ulmasova.

WHO South-East Asia Region
India: LS Chauhan, PR Narayanan, Ranjani Ramachandran, MR Joseph, CN Paramasivan, B Mahadev, P Kumar, Nalini Sundarmohan, **Indonesia:** Carmelia Basri, Paul Kelly, **Myanmar:** Win Maung, Ti Ti, CN Paramasivan **Nepal:** Pushpa Malla, SS Jha, Niraj Tuladar, Bhagawan Maharjan, Bhabna Shrestha, **Sri Lanka:** Chandra Sarukkali, **Thailand:** Sriprapa Nateniyom, Dhanida Rienthong, Somsak Rienthong.

WHO Western Pacific Region
Australia: Ivan Bastian, Krissa O'Neil, Richard Lumb, John Walker, Sandra Gebbie **China:** Wang Lixia, Liu Jianjun, Zhao Yanlin, Mei Jian, An Yansheng, Ren Yulin, Xie Yanguang, **China, Hong Kong Special Administrative Region (SAR):** Kai Man Kam, Cheuk-ming Tam, **Macao SAR, China:** Chou Kuok Hei, Lao U Lei, **Fiji:** William B. Kaitani, **Guam:** Cecilia Teresa T. Arciaga, **Japan:** Satoru Miyake, Satoshi Mitarai, **New Caledonia:** Bernard Rouchon, **New Zealand:** Kathryn Coley, Helen Heffernan, Leo McKnight, Alison Roberts, Ross Vaughan, Northern Mariana **Island:** Richard Brostrom, Susan Schorr, **Philippines:** Nora Cruz, Noel Macalalad, Remingo Olveda, Rosalind Vianzon, **Republic of Korea:** Hwa Hyun Kim, Woojin Lew, **Singapore:** Gary Ong, Raymond Lin Tzer Pin, Khin Mar Kyi Win, Wang Yee Tang, Sng Li Hwei, **Solomon Islands:** Noel Itogo, **Vanuatu:** Russel Tamata, **Viet Nam:** Dinh Ngoc Sy.

The primary aim of this report is to share survey and surveillance data on drug resistance in tuberculosis (TB). The data presented here are supplied largely by the programme managers who have led the work on surveys, but also by heads of reference laboratories and by principal investigators who may have been hired to assist the national TB programmes with the study. We thank all of them, and their staff, for their contributions. The World Health Organization/International Union Against Tuberculosis and Lung Disease (WHO/UNION) Global Project on Anti-Tuberculosis Drug Resistance Surveillance is carried out with the financial backing of United States Agency for International Development (USAID) and Eli Lilly and Company as part of the Lilly multidrug resistant (MDR)-TB Partnership. Drug resistance surveys were supported financially by the Dutch Government, the Global Fund, Japan International Cooperation Agency (JICA), Kreditanstalt für Wiederaufbau (KfW Entwicklungsbank), national TB programmes and USAID). The Supranational Reference Laboratory Network provided the external quality assurance, as well as technical support to many of the countries reporting. Technical support for surveys was provided by the Centers for Disease Control and Prevention (CDC), JICA, the Royal Netherlands Tuberculosis Association (KNCV), and WHO. Data for the WHO European Region were collected and validated jointly with EuroTB (Paris) — a European TB surveillance network funded by the European Commission.

CONTENTS

Executive summary 13

    Background and methods 13

    Results 14

        Magnitude of drug-resistant TB 14
        Survey coverage and population-weighted means 15
        Global estimates 15
        Trends 16
        Extensively drug-resistant TB 16
        HIV and multidrug-resistant TB 17
        Multidrug-resistant TB treatment programmes 17

    Conclusions 18

        Magnitude of drug-resistant TB 18
        Trends 19
        Coverage and methods 20
        TB control and drug-resistant TB [4] 21

Chapter 1: Introduction 23

Chapter 2: Methods 25

    Definitions of drug resistance 25

        Drug resistance among new cases 25
        Drug resistance among previously treated cases 25
        Combined proportion of drug resistance 26
        Extensively drug-resistant TB 26

    Survey areas and sampling strategies 26

        Terminology 27
        Survey areas 27
        Calculation of sample size 27
        Sampling methods 28
        Survey protocols 28

Collection of data **28**
    Patient eligibility and registration 28
    Resistance to second-line anti-TB drugs 28
    HIV 28
    Age and sex 29
    Accuracy of information on prior TB treatment 29
    Data management in individual countries 29
    Bacteriological methods 29
    Quality assurance of laboratories 30
    HIV testing 31

Statistical procedures — data collection, entry, checking and cleaning..31
    Statistical analysis 31
    Global data using the last data point from all reporting countries 32
    HIV, resistance to second-line anti-TB drugs, age group and sex 32
    Dynamics of resistance over time 32

Estimates **33**
Validity of the findings **33**

Chapter 3: Results 35

Phase 4 of the global project 2002–2007 ....**35**
    Types of data 35
    Proportion of drug resistance among new TB cases 36
    Any resistance among new cases 36
    Multidrug-resistant TB among new cases 37
    Any isoniazid resistance among new cases 37
    Drug resistance among previously treated TB cases 38
    Any resistance among previously treated cases 38
    Multidrug-resistant TB among previously treated cases 39
    Any isoniazid resistance among previously treated cases 40
    Drug resistance among all TB cases 41
    Multidrug-resistant TB among new and previously treated cases
    by region 42
    Drug-resistant TB by age and sex 47
    Drug resistance and HIV 47
    Extensively drug-resistant TB 48

**Data reported to the global project 1994–2007, and estimated
global and regional means of resistance** **51**
    Correlation between multidrug-resistant TB cases in national
    registers and survey data 58
    Dynamics of drug resistance over time, 1994–2007 59
    Declining trends in resistance 59
    Stable trends in resistance 62
    Increasing trends in resistance 65

Global estimates of multidrug-resistant TB	**68**
New cases	69
Previously treated cases	69
Total cases	69
Supranational Reference Laboratory Network	69

Chapter 4: Discussion ... 73

Overview	**73**
Survey methods	**73**
Magnitude and trends	**76**
Extensively drug-resistant TB	**77**
Drug resistance and HIV	**78**
Global estimates	**80**
Supranational Reference Laboratory Network	**80**
WHO regions	**82**
WHO African Region	82
WHO Region of the Americas	84
WHO Eastern Mediterranean Region	85
WHO European Region	86
WHO South-East Asia Region	90
WHO Western Pacific region	93

References ... 97
Annexes ... 101

EXECUTIVE SUMMARY

BACKGROUND AND METHODS

This is the fourth report of the World Health Organization/International Union Against Tuberculosis and Lung Disease (WHO/UNION) Global Project on Anti-Tuberculosis Drug Resistance Surveillance. The three previous reports were published in 1997, 2000 and 2004, and included data from 35, 58 and 77 countries, respectively. This report includes drug susceptibility test (DST) results from 91 577 patients from 93 settings in 81 countries and 2 special administrative regions (SARs) of China (i.e. Hong Kong and Macau). The data were collected between 2002 and 2007, and represent more than 35% of the global total of notified new smear-positive tuberculosis (TB) cases.

Data from 33 countries that have never previously reported are included in this report. New data are available from the following high TB burden countries[1]: China, Ethiopia, India, Indonesia, Myanmar, the Philippines, the Russian Federation, the United Republic (UR) of Tanzania, Thailand and Viet Nam. Between 1994 and 2007, data were reported to the global project from a total of 138 settings in 114 countries and 2 SARs of China.

Trend data (three or more data points) are available from 47 countries. Most trend data are reported from settings with a low TB prevalence; however, this report includes trend data from five settings where prevalence is high – three Baltic countries and two Russian oblasts[2]. Trend data were also available from six countries conducting periodic or sentinel surveys (Cuba, Republic of Korea, Nepal, Peru, Thailand and Uruguay).

For the first time, 36 countries reported data on age and sex of cases stratified by any resistance or by multidrug resistant (MDR) TB[3]. Seven countries reported data disaggregated by human immunodeficiency virus (HIV) status and drug resistance pattern (Cuba, Donetsk Oblast [Ukraine], Honduras, Latvia, Spain, Tomsk Oblast [Russian Federation] and Uruguay). A total of 34 countries and 2 SARs of China reported data on second-line anti-TB drug resistance among patient isolates identified as MDR-TB. This report focuses on MDR-TB because patients with this type of TB have significantly poorer outcomes than patients with drug-susceptible TB.

Data were included if they were consistent with the principles of the global project, which require accurate representation of the population under evaluation and external quality assurance conducted by a supranational reference

---

[1] The 22 high TB burden countries account for approximately 80% of the estimated number of new TB cases (all forms) arising each year.
[2] An oblast is a type of administrative division.
[3] MDR-TB is defined as TB with resistance to isoniazid and rifampicin, the two most powerful first-line drugs.

laboratory (SRL). Although differentiation by treatment history is required for data interpretation, the report also includes data from some countries where such differentiation is not possible. Data were obtained through routine or continuous surveillance of all TB cases (48 countries) or from specific surveys of sampled patients, as outlined in approved protocols (35 countries). Data were reported on a standard reporting form, either annually or at the completion of the survey. Data on resistance to second-line anti-TB drugs were included if drug-susceptibility testing was conducted at an SRL, or if the national reference laboratory (NRL) was participating in a quality-assurance programme for first-line anti-TB drugs. Currently, there is no established system for international external quality assurance for second-line anti-TB drugs.

The Supranational Reference Laboratory Network (SRLN) was formed in 1994 to ensure optimal performance of the laboratories participating in the global project. The network has expanded since 2004; it now includes 26 laboratories in 6 WHO regions, and is coordinated by the Prince Léopold Institute of Tropical Medicine in Antwerp, Belgium. A panel of 30 pretested and coded isolates is exchanged annually within the network for proficiency testing (with each annual exchange referred to as a 'round' of testing). The 14th round, initiated in 2007, includes isolates with resistance to second-line anti-TB drugs. Results will be available in 2008.

RESULTS

Magnitude of drug-resistant TB

New cases

Data on new cases in the most recent phase of the global project (i.e. Phase 4, which covers the period 2002–2007) were available for 72 countries and 2 SARs of China. DST results were available for 62 746 patients. The proportion of resistance to at least one anti-TB drug (any resistance) ranged from 0% in two Western European countries to 56.3% in Baku City, Azerbaijan. The proportion of MDR-TB ranged from 0% in eight countries to 19.4% in the Republic of Moldova and 22.3% in Baku City, Azerbaijan. Twenty of the settings surveyed had the highest proportion of MDR-TB among new cases in the history of the project. Of these 20 settings, 14 are located in countries of the former Soviet Union and 4 are in China.

Of the 20 settings with the highest prevalence of resistance ever recorded, 15 have been reported in Phase 4 of the project. Data from countries of the Eastern Mediterranean showed that MDR-TB among new cases was higher than previously estimated, with the exception of Morocco (0.5%) and Lebanon (1.1%). MDR-TB among new cases was 2.9% in Yemen and 5.4% in Jordan. The Americas, Central Europe and Africa reported the lowest proportions of MDR-TB among new cases, with the notable exceptions of Guatemala (3.0%), Rwanda (3.9%) and Peru (5.3%).

Previously treated cases

Data on previously treated cases were available for 66 countries and 2

SARs of China. DST results were available for 12 977 patients. Resistance to at least one anti-TB drug (any resistance) ranged from 0% in three European countries to 85.9% in Tashkent, Uzbekistan. The highest proportions of MDR-TB were reported in Baku City, Azerbaijan (55.8%) and Tashkent, Uzbekistan (60.0%). New data from Gujarat State, India are the first reliable source of data on previously treated cases in India; they show 17.2% MDR-TB among this group.

Unknown and combined cases

A total of 36 countries reported data on cases with unknown treatment history. In most countries, this group of cases represented a small proportion of total cases; however, in eight countries (Australia, Fiji, Guam, New Caledonia, Puerto Rico, Qatar, Solomon Islands and the United States of America), and one city in Spain (Barcelona), this was either the main or the only group reported.

Survey coverage and population-weighted means

Based on information gathered throughout the global project, the most recent data available from 114 countries and 2 SARs of China was weighted by the population in areas surveyed. The data represent 2 509 545 TB cases, and gave the following results for global population weighted proportion of resistance among[4]:
- new cases
  any resistance 17.0% (95% confidence levels, CLs, 13.6–20.4)
  isoniazid resistance 10.3% (95% CLs, 8.4–12.1)
  MDR 2.9% (95% CLs, 2.2–3.6)
- previously treated cases
  any resistance 35.0% (95% CLs, 24.1–45.8)
  isoniazid resistance 27.7% (95% CLs, 18.7–36.7)
  MDR-TB 15.3% (95% CLs, 9.6–21.1)
- all TB cases
  any resistance 20.0% (95% CLs, 16.1–23.9)
  isoniazid resistance 13.3% (95% CLs, 10.9–15.8)
  MDR-TB 5.3% (95% CLs, 3.9–6.6).

Global estimates

Based on drug-resistance information from 114 countries and 2 SARs of China reporting to this project, combined with 9 epidemiological factors, the proportion of MDR-TB among new, previously treated and combined cases was estimated for countries with no survey information available. The estimated proportion of MDR-TB for all countries was then applied to estimated new (incident) TB cases. Based on this approach, it is estimated that 489 139 (95% CLs; 455 093–614 215) cases emerged in 2006, and that the global proportion of resistance among all cases is 4.8% (95% CLs; 4.6–6.0). China, India and the Russian Federation are estimated to carry the highest number of MDR-TB cases. China and India carry approximately 50% of the global burden, and the Russian Federation a further 7%.

---

[4] Population figures are based on data reported in 2005.

Trends

Trends were evaluated in 47 countries with three or more data points. In low TB prevalence countries conducting continuous surveillance, trends were determined in the group of total cases reported. In countries conducting surveys, or where population of previously treated cases tested changed over time[5], trends were determined in new cases only.

In the United States and Hong Kong SAR, significant reduction of the burden of MDR-TB in the population continues. In these two settings, both TB notifications and MDR-TB are declining, but MDR-TB is declining at a faster rate. In most central and western European countries — where TB (particularly drug-resistant forms of TB) is imported — absolute numbers as well as proportions of MDR-TB among all cases are relatively stable. Both Peru and the Republic of Korea are showing increases in MDR-TB among new cases. Both countries showed steady declines in TB notification rates, followed by recent levelling off. In countries of the former Soviet Union, there are two scenarios: two Baltic countries — Estonia and Latvia — are showing a stable and flat trend in proportions of MDR-TB among new cases; Lithuania shows a gradual and significant increase, but at a slow rate. All three countries are showing a decreasing TB notification rate (5–8% reduction per year). This is in contrast to two oblasts in the Russian Federation (Orel and Tomsk) which are showing an increase in the proportion of MDR-TB among new cases, as well as increases in absolute numbers. Notification rates are declining in both regions, but at a slower rate than in the Baltic countries.

Extensively drug-resistant TB

Thirty five countries and two special administrative regions (SARS) were able to report data on extensively drug resistant (XDR) TB[6], either through routine surveillance data or through drug resistance surveys. Quality assurance for laboratory testing was variable across reporting countries[7]. Twenty five countries reported routine surveillance data, while ten countries reported from periodic surveys. Some countries reported data aggregated over a three-year period; other countries reported over a one-year period. The numbers of MDR-TB cases tested for the appropriate second-line anti-TB drugs are used as a denominator. In total, data were reported on 4012 MDR-TB cases, among which 301 (7.0%) XDR-TB cases were detected. Twenty five countries that reported were European; however, three countries from the WHO Region of the Americas and seven settings from the WHO Western Pacific Region also reported data. Survey data were available from two African countries — Rwanda and UR Tanzania (preliminary data) — and no XDR-TB was found in either country. No data were reported from the WHO Eastern Mediterranean Region or from the WHO South-East Asia Region, although surveys that include second-line anti-TB drug-susceptibility testing are ongoing in both regions.

---

[5] Proportion of resistance among new cases is considered a more robust indicator of recent transmission. Additional information regarding the previous history of treatment is required to determine trends of resistance in this population.

[6] XDR-TB is defined as TB with resistance to at least isoniazid and rifampicin, and resistance to a fluoroquinolone and a second-line injectable agent.

[7] Previous reported data from South Africa following a different methodology are included in the maps and discussions, but not in the analysis.

In general, absolute numbers of XDR-TB cases were low in Central and Western Europe, the Americas and in the Asian countries that reported data. The proportion of XDR-TB among MDR-TB in these settings varied from 0% in 11 countries to 30.0% in Japan. These countries have a relatively low MDR-TB burden, so the figure represents few absolute cases. A more significant problem lies in the countries of the former Soviet Union. Of the nine countries that reported, approximately 10% of all MDR-TB cases were XDR, ranging from 4.0% in Armenia to almost 24.0% in Estonia; however, these proportions represent a much larger absolute number of cases. Data recently released from South Africa showed that 996 (5.6%) of 17 615 MDR isolates collected from 2004 through to October of 2007 were XDR-TB. Proportions varied across provinces, with KwaZulu-Natal reporting 656 (4%) of 4701 MDR-TB cases as XDR-TB. Selection and testing practices varied across the country and over time; however, all isolates correspond to individual cases[8]. Since 2002, a total of 45 countries have reported at least one case globally. Several other countries are in the process of completing DST.

HIV and multidrug-resistant TB

Of the seven countries that reported data on drug resistance stratified by HIV status, only Latvia and Donetsk Oblast, Ukraine reported numbers sufficiently high to examine the relationship between the two epidemics. Any resistance and MDR were significantly associated with HIV in both Latvia and in Donetsk Oblast; however, HIV negative and HIV unknown were not distinguished in Latvia. From the data reported in Latvia, the proportion of MDR-TB among HIV-positive cases was shown to be stable over time.

Multidrug-resistant TB treatment programmes

By the end of 2007, 67 projects in 51 countries had been provided with second-line anti-TB drugs through the Green Light Committee (GLC)[9], for a cumulative total of more than 30 000 MDR-TB patients. A total of 23 256 cases of MDR-TB were notified in 2006 (8.7% of these cases were reported from GLC projects) representing less than 5% of the global number of MDR-TB cases estimated to have emerged in 2006. The average treatment success rate within GLC projects was 62%[10], with Latvia reporting the best treatment success rate (69%). Globally, both the number of MDR-TB patients treated, as well as the projected numbers for MDR-TB cases to be treated in 2007 and 2008, as reported by national TB programmes (NTPs)[1], are far below targets set out in the Global MDR-TB & XDR-TB Response Plan 2007–2008.[2]

---

[8] Data from a retrospective review of the National Health Laboratory Service of South Africa were presented at the 38th World Conference on Lung Health. 8–12 November 2007, Cape Town, South Africa.

[9] The GLC is committee of partners that provides access to reduced priced, quality assured second line drugs, as well as monitoring support for the implementation of MDR-TB programmes. (see http://www.who.int/tb/challenges/mdr/greenlightcommittee/en/index.html)

[10] Mirzayev F, Treatment outcomes from nine projects approved by the Green Light Committee between 2000 and 2003. 38th World Conference on Lung Health. 8–12 November 2007. Cape Town, South Africa.

CONCLUSIONS

Magnitude of drug-resistant TB

The population-weighted mean of MDR-TB among all TB cases from the 114 countries and 2 SARs of China that have reported to the global project is 5.3% (95% CLs, 3.9–6.6), but ranges from 0% in some western European countries to more than 35% in some countries of the former Soviet Union. In terms of proportion, the countries of the former Soviet Union are facing a serious and widespread epidemic, where the population-weighted average of countries reporting indicates that almost half of all TB cases are resistant to at least one drug, and every fifth case of TB will have MDR-TB. In these countries, MDR-TB cases have more extensive resistance patterns, including some of the highest proportions of XDR-TB.

Provinces in China reported the next highest proportions of resistance after countries of the former Soviet Union; Western Europe, followed by countries in Africa, reported the lowest proportions of MDR-TB. At least one country in all six WHO regions has reported more than 3.0% MDR-TB among new cases.

Recent survey data from 114 countries and 2 SARs of China was combined with 9 epidemiological factors to estimate the burden of incident MDR-TB for a further 69 countries. The aim was to develop a global estimate and to better establish the incident global burden of MDR-TB cases. We estimate that 489 139 (95% CLs, 455 093–614 215) MDR-TB cases emerged in 2006, and the global proportion of resistance among all TB cases is 4.6% (95% CLs, 4.6–6.0). China and India are estimated to carry 50% of the global burden of cases, and the Russian Federation is estimated to carry a further 7%.

Data from surveys in 10 of 31 provinces in China over a 10-year period indicate that drug resistance is widespread. In terms of proportion, China ranks second to countries of the former Soviet Union; however, in absolute numbers, China has the highest burden of cases in the world. It is estimated that 130 548 (95% CLs, 97 633–164 900) MDR-TB cases emerged in 2006, or more than 25% of the global burden. The high proportion of drug-resistant TB among new cases in China suggests a concerning level of transmission of drug-resistant strains. More than 1 in 10 cases of MDR-TB that emerged in 2006 globally are estimated to have occurred in patients in China without a history of prior anti-TB treatment. Now that China has reached the global targets for case detection and treatment success, the rapid implementation of services for the diagnosis and treatment of MDR-TB is necessary to ensure success of the TB control programme and to control transmission of drug-resistant strains. Careful monitoring of the trends of resistance in China should remain a priority.

Data from nine sites in India show that drug resistance among new cases is relatively low; however, new data from Gujarat indicate that, at 17.2%, MDR-TB among re-treatment cases is higher than previously anticipated. Also, it is estimated that 110 132 (95% CLs, 79 975–142 386) MDR-TB cases emerged in India in 2006, representing more than 20% of the global burden. Although plans have been developed for management of 5000 MDR-TB cases annually by 2010, insufficient laboratory capacity is the main factor limiting the implementation of these plans.

Trends

Multidrug-resistant TB

Trend data show a range of scenarios. Most low TB burden countries reporting surveillance data showed stable proportions of both resistance and absolute numbers of cases. Trends in resistance in Hong Kong SAR represent the best-case scenario, where MDR-TB is falling faster than TB. Countries such as Peru and the Republic of Korea showed increasing proportions in MDR-TB. Although both countries have shown a decline in overall TB notifications, the decline has slowed in recent years. In Peru, this may reflect weakening in basic TB control, including management of MDR-TB. The Republic of Korea has recently integrated the private sector into a national surveillance network, which may explain the recent levelling of the TB notification rate. The reason for the increase in proportion of MDR-TB among new cases is not yet clear.

The most important findings of this report, however, are the trend data reported from the Baltic countries and the Russian Federation, where the MDR-TB epidemic is widespread. The Baltic countries are showing a decline in TB notification rates, with the proportion of MDR-TB held relatively stable. The Baltic countries probably represent the best scenario for this region. The surveyed oblasts of the Russian Federation show a different picture – one in which TB notifications are falling but at a much slower rate, and in which both the proportion and absolute numbers of MDR-TB are significantly increasing, especially among new cases. The declining notifications in these oblasts suggest that TB control is improving, and susceptible TB cases are being successfully treated, but it is likely that a large pool of chronic cases continues to fuel the epidemic, reflected in the growing proportion of MDR-TB cases. The two oblasts that reported are some of the best performing regions in the country. Commitment to TB control seen in recent years indicates positive momentum; evidence of commitment is seen in new legislation updating the TB strategy, and the nationwide implementation of TB control activities, including management of MDR-TB cases and the upgrade of diagnostic services (financed by the Global Fund and the World Bank). However, efforts will have to be accelerated to have an impact on what appears to be a growing epidemic of drug-resistant TB.

Extensively drug-resistant TB

XDR-TB is more expensive and difficult to treat than MDR-TB, and outcomes for patients are much worse[11]; therefore, it is important to understand the magnitude and distribution of XDR-TB. Despite limitations in the quality assurance applied to laboratory testing, data from this report indicate that XDR-TB is widespread, with 45 countries having reported at least one case. The high proportion of XDR-TB among MDR-TB, as well as the large overall burden, suggests a significant problem within the countries of the former Soviet Union. Japan (and the Republic of Korea in a previous study) has also shown a high proportion of

---

[11] Leimane V (2006) MDR-TB and XDR-TB: Management and treatment outcomes in Latvia [presentation]. 37th Union World Conference on Lung Health; 31 October-4 November 2006; Paris, France.

XDR-TB among MDR. South Africa reported a moderate proportion of XDR-TB among MDR-TB cases; however, the underlying burden of MDR-TB is considerable, with 44% of TB patients estimated to be coinfected with HIV. Few representative data from Africa are available, with the exception of Rwanda and preliminary data from UR Tanzania, which showed no XDR-TB and very little second-line resistance among MDR-TB cases, suggesting that second-line anti-TB drugs have not been widely used in these two countries; however, high-risk populations should continue to be monitored. XDR-TB is likely to emerge where second-line anti-TB drugs are widely and inappropriately used; however, transmission is not limited to these settings. Data were largely reported from high-income countries or with the assistance of an SRL, indicating that countries require strengthened capacity to monitor second-line resistance if we are to develop an accurate understanding of the global magnitude and distribution of XDR-TB.

Multidrug-resistant TB and HIV

Despite the expansion of HIV testing and treatment globally, only seven countries were able to report drug-resistance data disaggregated by HIV status. The two countries with the most robust data both showed a significant association between HIV and MDR-TB. Both of these countries are situated in the former Soviet Union, where diagnostic networks for both TB and HIV are relatively well developed. This population-level association is a great concern for countries without accessible diagnostic networks in place, indicating that HIV-positive TB patients will not receive appropriate diagnosis and therapy quickly enough to avert mortality. The association between HIV and MDR-TB may be more closely related to environmental factors, such as transmission in congregate settings, than to biological factors[3]. Although this finding requires further investigation, it indicates that improving infection control in congregate settings, including health-care facilities and prisons, may be one of the most critical components in addressing dual infection. The development of laboratory networks to provide rapid diagnosis of resistance using molecular methods, particularly for HIV-positive TB patients, is vital.

Coverage and methods

Survey coverage continues to expand, with data reported from several additional high-burden countries, and the reliability of surveillance data continues to improve; however, there are major gaps in populations covered and epidemiological questions answered. Laboratory capacity remains the largest obstacle, but other survey components also strain the capacity of most NTPs, making it difficult to determine trends in most high-burden countries. HIV testing continues to scale up, but has proven difficult to incorporate where testing is not already a component of routine care. Second-line testing is not available in most countries. Newly available policy guidance will assist in the development of this capacity in countries. However, SRLs will continue to play an important role in providing this service in the meantime. As part of the Global Plan to Stop TB, 2006–2015, all countries are committed to scaling up diagnostic networks, but until culture and drug-susceptibility testing are the standard of diagnosis everywhere, surveys will continue to be important for monitoring resistance. Currently, molecular methods are being piloted to expand coverage and increase trends, but new survey methods — such as continuous sentinel surveillance — must also be considered. Special studies must supplement surveys to answer questions about risk factors for acquisition and transmission dynamics of drug resistance, which routine surveillance cannot answer.

TB control and drug-resistant TB

Preventing the development of drug-resistant TB through optimal implementations of DOTS should continue to be the top priority for all countries; however, managing the MDR-TB cases that emerge is part of the Stop TB Strategy and should be a component of all TB programmes. Developing rapid detection and management of drug-resistant cases is of great urgency for countries facing high proportions of drug resistance, high-burden countries carrying the largest absolute burden of MDR-TB, and countries with a population heavily coinfected with HIV. By 2006, basic TB control had expanded to 184 countries globally, yet the targets for the number of MDR-TB cases detected and treated have not been reached, and the latest information reported indicates that, at the current pace, few countries will reach the targets outlined in the Global Plan to Stop TB, 2006–2015.

If targets are to be achieved, coordinated global efforts will be required to roll out the full package of TB services as outlined by the Stop TB Strategy[12] to prevent the further emergence of MDR-TB. Areas that need more attention are improvement of infection-control measures to prevent transmission, expansion of high-quality diagnostic services for timely detection of cases and expansion of community involvement to improve adherence. However, perhaps the most fundamental area for attention is the development of treatment programmes into which patients can be enrolled and treated successfully.

In the two countries with the highest TB burden, China and India, 8% and 5% of TB cases respectively are estimated to have MDR-TB and are unlikely to respond to the treatment they currently receive. In countries of Eastern Europe, 1 in 5 cases will have MDR-TB, signalling that new drugs are urgently needed. Unfortunately, there are few new drugs in the pipeline, making it unlikely that new compounds will be available to respond to the pressing need.

---

[12] http://www.who.int/tb/strategy/stop_tb_strategy/en/index.html

INTRODUCTION

This document — the fourth report of the World Health Organization/International Union Against Tuberculosis and Lung Disease (WHO/UNION) Global Project on Anti-Tuberculosis Drug Resistance Surveillance — provides the latest data on the magnitude of drug resistance in 81 countries and 2 special administrative regions (SARs) of China (Hong Kong and Macao), collected between 2002 and 2007. The report also provides the most up-to-date trends from 47 countries, collected over a 13-year period.

The global project was initiated in 1994, with the aim of estimating the global burden of drug-resistant TB worldwide using standardized methodologies, so that data could be compared across and within regions. Further aims were to monitor trends in resistance, evaluate the performance of TB control programmes and advise on drug regimens. A report is published every three years because most countries require 12–18 months to complete a drug-resistance survey.

Until 2000, very few national TB programmes (NTPs) globally were managing drug-resistant TB cases in the public sector and — with the exception of high-income countries and countries of the former Soviet Union — diagnosis of drug resistance in TB was largely unavailable. Between 2000 and 2005, "DOTS-Plus" (which refers to DOTS programmes that add components for diagnosis of multidrug-resistant (MDR) TB) — were implemented in five settings, and then expanded. Following evaluation and successful results from these projects, a new Stop TB Strategy[13] was launched in 2006; the new strategy includes diagnosis and management of drug-resistant TB. The launch of the Stop TB Strategy was followed by the Global Plan to Stop TB, 2006–2015, which provided targets for scale up and the budgets required for the implementation of the strategy. Now, through the Global Fund to fight AIDS, Tuberculosis and Malaria, and with the help of the Green Light Committee (GLC)[14], most countries are initiating or scaling up the diagnosis and management of drug-resistant TB. Until diagnosis of drug resistance is routine, surveys or surveillance systems will play an important role in determining the magnitude and trends in drug-resistant TB.

In terms of the initial goals of the global project, considerable progress has been made in expanding coverage, estimating the global burden of MDR-TB and strengthening laboratories. However, the project has not met several of its initial goals, suggesting that it may be time to review some of the project methods. There are still major geographical gaps in information on the burden of drug-resistant TB.

---

[13] http://www.who.int/tb/strategy/stop_tb_strategy/en/index.html
[14] The GLC is a WHO initiative that promotes implementation of the Stop TB Strategy (see http://www.who.int/tb/challenges/mdr/greenlightcommittee/en/index.html)

Trend data from high-burden countries are few. Adjustment of regimens is limited not by lack of data but by the lack of availability of new drugs and treatments. There is also a need for the monitoring of resistance to some of the key second-line anti-TB drugs, and a better understanding of the epidemiological relationship between drug resistance and human immunodeficiency virus (HIV). Interim drug-resistance surveillance guidelines were published in 2007, and a meeting planned for 2008 to review current methods in drug resistance surveillance will provide key input for revising these technical guidelines.

This report is based on the analysis of 250 000 isolates collected since 1994, in 114 countries and 2 SARs of China, representing half of all notified TB cases. The report addresses the following areas:
- the most recent profile of anti-TB drug resistance, looking at the latest data available for the period 2002–2007
- dynamics of anti-TB drug resistance over time, or trends
- HIV and drug resistance
- extensively drug resistant (XDR) TB
- the global means and distribution of resistance across and within regions, looking at the most recent data for each country or geographical setting surveyed since 1994
- estimates of the burden of MDR-TB by country and region
- results of proficiency testing of laboratories over time.

METHODS

The methodology for surveillance of drug resistance in the global project was developed by a WHO/UNION working group in 1994. The group published guidelines for surveillance of resistance in TB in 1994, and these guidelines were updated in 1997 and 2003[5]. Further interim guidelines have been published in 2007[6]. The methodology operates on three main principles:
- the survey must be based on a sample of TB patients representative of all cases in the geographical setting under evaluation
- drug resistance must be clearly distinguished according to the treatment history of the patient (i.e. never treated or previously treated), to allow correct interpretation of the data
- optimal laboratory performance of each participating laboratory must be attained through engaging in a quality-assurance programme, including the international exchange of isolates of Mycobacterium tuberculosis.

DEFINITIONS OF DRUG RESISTANCE

Drug resistance among new cases

Resistance among new cases is defined as the presence of resistant isolates of *M. tuberculosis* in patients who fit the following criteria:
- in response to direct questioning, the patient denies having had any prior anti-TB treatment (for up to one month)
- in countries where adequate documentation is available, there is no evidence of a history of anti-TB treatment.

Drug resistance among new cases is used to evaluate recent transmission.

Drug resistance among previously treated cases

Resistance among previously treated cases is defined as the presence of resistant isolates of *M. tuberculosis* in patients who fit one of the following criteria:
- in response to direct questioning, the patient admits having been treated for TB for one month or more
- in countries where adequate documentation is available, there is evidence of such a history.

In previous reports, resistance among previously treated patients was used as a proxy for acquired resistance; however, this patient category is now known to comprise patients who have:

- acquired resistance
- been primarily infected with a resistant strain, and subsequently failed therapy
- been reinfected.

Therefore resistance among previously treated cases is not a useful proxy for truly acquired resistance[7, 8].

Combined proportion of drug resistance

"Combined proportion of drug resistance" is the proportion of drug resistance in the population surveyed, regardless of prior treatment. Despite the importance of the distinction between drug resistance among new and previously treated cases, 36 countries reported data on cases with unknown treatment history. In most countries, this group of cases represented a small proportion of total cases; however, in eight countries (Australia, Fiji, Guam, New Caledonia, Puerto Rico, Qatar, Solomon Islands and the United States of America), and in one city in Spain (Barcelona), this was the only group reported or represented in most cases.

Given the risk of misclassification due to reporting bias by patients or health staff, the combined proportion of anti-TB drug resistance represents a better approximation to the level of drug resistance in the community than the separate data for new and previously treated patients. Combined figures represent data collected on new and previously treated cases, and on all cases with an unknown treatment history.

Extensively drug-resistant TB

XDR-TB is defined as TB with resistance to at least isoniazid and rifampicin, and resistance to a fluroquinolone and a second line injectable agent (i.e. amikacin, kanamycin or capreomycin).

SURVEY AREAS AND SAMPLING STRATEGIES

New surveillance or survey projects presented in this report were carried out between 2002 and 2007, with the exception of two surveys in India (carried out in the districts of Hoogli in West Bengal State, and Mayhurbhanj in Orissa State) in 2001, and a nationwide survey in Paraguay in 2001. Since 1999, the United Kingdom has submitted data to EuroTB (a project funded by the European Commission and based in Paris, France) in two ways — for England, Wales and Northern Ireland together, either with or without Scotland. In this report, Scotland is included in data reported from the United Kingdom. The countries Cuba, France, Italy and Japan operate sentinel networks for surveillance. All, with the exception of Italy, can be considered nationally representative.

Trend data from Germany and from the United Kingdom are evaluated from 2001 because surveillance methods changed in that year. Final data from the United Republic (UR) of Tanzania and Madagascar were not available at the time of analysis for this report, and results should be considered preliminary. Data from Senegal were still undergoing quality control.

Terminology

For the purposes of this report, it is important to distinguish between surveys and surveillance:
- "Surveillance" is used here to refer to either continuous or sentinel surveillance. Continuous surveillance is based on routine TB diagnosis, including drug-susceptibility testing, provided to all TB cases in the coverage area. Thus, it reflects the entire TB population — smear-positive, smear-negative and extrapulmonary — regardless of treatment status.
- "Sentinel surveillance" of drug resistance, in the context of this report, comprises reporting of drug susceptibility test (DST) results from all TB cases from a (random or non-random) sample of sites. Sentinel surveillance reports annual data from the same sites, with the exception of Japan, which conducts sentinel surveys every three years.

Surveys are periodic, and reflect the population of registered pulmonary smear-positive cases. Depending on the area surveyed, a cluster-sampling technique may be adopted, or all diagnostic units may be included. While some countries, such as Botswana, repeat surveys every 3–5 years, for the purposes of this report they are considered as repeated surveys and not surveillance.

Survey areas

In both survey and surveillance settings, the coverage area is usually the entire country, but in some cases, subnational units are surveyed. Large countries, such as Brazil, China, India, Indonesia, the Russian Federation and South Africa, tend to survey large administrative units (e.g. province, state, district or oblast). Some countries have opted to limit surveys or surveillance to metropolitan areas, as in the case of Azerbaijan, China and Uzbekistan. Several countries (e.g. Cuba, France, Italy and Japan) conduct sentinel surveillance, and some other countries have restricted surveys to subnational areas, either because of the remoteness of certain provinces or to avoid conflict areas. Data for Denmark do not include Greenland and the Faroe Islands.

Calculation of sample size

Calculation of sample size for surveys follows the principles outlined in the WHO/UNION guidelines for the surveillance of resistance in TB[5]. Briefly, sample sizes are calculated on the basis of the number of new sputum smear-positive cases registered in the previous year and the expected proportion of rifampicin resistance in new TB cases, based on previous studies or data available from the NTP. Separate sample sizes should be calculated for new cases and previously treated cases. However, the number of sputum-positive previously treated cases reported per year is usually small, meaning that a long intake period needed to achieve a statistically adequate sample size. Therefore, most countries have obtained an estimate of the drug-resistance level among previously treated cases by including all previously treated cases who present at centres during the intake period. While this may not provide a statistically adequate sample size, it can nevertheless give a reasonable estimate of drug resistance among previously treated cases. Surveys in Armenia, Baku City (Azerbaijan), Georgia, Gujarat state (India) were designed with separate sample sizes for re-treatment cases. In efforts to scale up diagnosis and treatment of MDR-TB, many countries plan to expand routine culture and DST to all re-treatment cases. Once fully implemented, these routine data will provide estimates of drug resistance in these populations.

Sampling methods

Sampling strategies for monitoring of drug resistance include:
- nationwide, continuous surveillance of the population
- surveys with
  - sampling of all diagnostic centres during a specified period
  - randomly selected clusters of patients
  - cluster sampling, proportional to the number of cases notified by the diagnostic centre.

Survey protocols

The quality of survey protocols has improved over the last 10 years. Most protocols reviewed in Phase 4 of the project were complete, and included detailed budgets, timelines and plans for quality assurance at several levels. Most of the protocols reviewed were submitted through a local ethics review board or through the ethics review board of a technical partner supporting the project.

COLLECTION OF DATA

Patient eligibility and registration

For surveys, all newly registered patients with smear-positive TB were eligible for inclusion, including children and foreign-born persons. In surveillance settings, all TB patients were included. As in previous phases of the global project, HIV testing was not a mandatory component of these surveys; however, it has increasingly been incorporated in survey settings. Geographical settings that performed HIV testing as part of the survey were advised to follow international guidelines on counselling and confidentiality. This report includes data from 93 settings in 81 countries and 2 SARs of China. Survey data were reported from 35 countries or geographical settings, and surveillance data from 48 countries or geographical settings.

Resistance to second-line anti-TB drugs

Thirty five countries and two SARs reported data on second-line anti-TB drug resistance among confirmed MDR-TB isolates identified in routine surveillance or in surveys. A further five countries reported data on cohorts of known MDR-TB patients. Data from laboratory registers from South Africa were reported but not included in any analyses.

HIV

Eight settings in seven countries reported data on drug resistance stratified by HIV status. These settings were Cuba, Honduras, Latvia, the Russian Federation (Tomsk Oblast), Spain (Barcelona and Galicia), Ukraine (Donetsk Oblast) and Uruguay. Data were reported stratified by positive and unknown HIV status from Latvia and Galicia, Spain, and were disaggregated by positive, negative and unknown HIV status from the remaining settings. Four countries were unable to discriminate between negative and unknown HIV status.

Age and sex
Data on drug resistance stratified by sex and age groups was reported by 43 settings in 36 countries from all the 6 WHO regions. Among these settings, seven were able to report information for more than one year.

Accuracy of information on prior TB treatment
It was recommended that re-interview and double-checking of patient histories be undertaken in survey settings, to reduce the possibility of misclassification of previously treated cases. Most countries cross-checked patient history collected in the survey with medical records, but fewer countries re-interviewed a percentage of patients.

Data management in individual countries
Since 1998, EuroTB has continuously collected and verified drug resistance surveillance data in Western Europe and much of Central Europe. Since 2001, WHO and EuroTB have used a common collection form. All the data for Western Europe, and much of that for Central Europe included in the present report, were provided by EuroTB and conform to the standards of the global project. Other countries conducting surveillance have provided data either directly to WHO Headquarters or via WHO regional offices. All new data reported have been returned to countries for verification before publication. In this phase of the global project, a fourth version of WHO software — *Surveillance of Drug Resistance in Tuberculosis* (SDRTB 4.0) — was used for data entry, management and analysis of survey data by many countries conducting surveys[15]. However, most countries conducting continuous surveillance of drug resistance in all TB cases use their own software. The global project requests that survey protocols include a description of methods used for the quality assurance of data collection, entry and analysis.

Bacteriological methods
In survey settings, sputum smear microscopy using the Ziehl–Neelsen technique was used for diagnosis of TB and subsequent enrolment in the survey. In surveillance settings, a combination of smear and culture was used for initial diagnosis. Most laboratories used Löwenstein–Jensen (L–J) culture medium on which the specimen was inoculated after decontamination with sodium hydroxide (2–4%) or 1% cetyl-pyridium chloride (CPC). Some laboratories inoculated sodium hydroxide decontaminated specimen directly onto Ogawa medium without centrifugation. Laboratories in high-income countries generally used liquid medium or agar-based medium. Identification of isolates was based on the following tests:
- niacin production
- nitrate reduction
- para-nitrobenzoic (PNB) acid (500 mg/l) test[9]
- thiophene-2-carboxylic acid hydrazide (TCH) (2 mg/l) resistance test[10].

---

[15] Brenner E. *Surveillance of drug resistance in tuberculosis software*: SDRTB3. Geneva, World Health Organization Geneva. 2000.

Some countries also used molecular hybridization probes. Mycobacteria other than *M. tuberculosis* complex were excluded from the analysis.

DSTs were performed using the simplified variant of the indirect proportion method on L–J medium, the absolute concentration method, the resistance ratio method[11, 12], or the radiometric Bactec 460 or MGIT 960 method[16]. The proportion method was most frequently used in all phases of the global project. Resistance was expressed as the percentage of colonies that grew on recommended critical concentrations of the drugs tested; that is, 0.2 mg/l for isoniazid, 2 mg/l for ethambutol, 4 mg/l for dihydrostreptomycin sulfate and 40 mg/l for rifampicin when L–J medium is used. The criterion used for drug resistance was growth of 1% or more of the bacterial population on media containing the critical concentration of each drug. The results of the tests were recorded on standardized forms.

Quality assurance of laboratories

Proficiency testing and retesting of a proportion of survey strains are two components of external quality assurance of laboratories[17]. Briefly, proficiency testing requires the exchange of a panel of 20 (or more) pretested isolates between the supranational reference laboratory (SRL) and the national reference laboratory (NRL). Results of this round of testing determine, in part, whether the performance of the laboratory is of a sufficiently high standard to conduct DST for the survey, or whether additional training is necessary. For retesting of survey strains, the laboratory conducting the survey sends a percentage of both resistant and susceptible isolates to the SRL for checking. The percentage of isolates sent for checking is determined before the beginning of the survey. Adequate performance is defined as no more than one false-positive or false-negative result for rifampicin or isoniazid, and no more than two for streptomycin or ethambutol. To date, the results of NRL proficiency testing have been evaluated by the corresponding SRL, and interventions have been based on the judgement of the SRL. In several instances, testing has been repeated to ensure acceptable performance; in exceptional instances, surveys have been interrupted and data excluded because there was significant discordance between the results obtained by the SRL and an NRL.

Susceptibility testing for second-line anti-TB drugs was performed using a range of methods and concentrations. Until 2007, there was limited international consensus on susceptibility testing for second-line anti-TB drugs. At the time of this report, WHO has published policy recommendations for second-line DST[13], and full technical guidelines are under development. External quality assurance for second-line anti-TB drugs was not available during the period of data collection. Starting in 2007, isolates with resistance to second-line anti-TB drugs have been included in the panels exchanged within the network of SRLs, and extended to a few selected NRLs. Data on second-line drug resistance were included if the country was participating in annual external quality assurance for first-line anti-TB drugs, or if isolates were tested for second-line resistance at an SRL. In general, countries conducting surveys sent MDR-TB isolates to SRLs for retesting and for DST for second-line anti-TB drugs. Several Pacific island countries used a

---

[16] Siddiqi SH. *BACTEC 460TB System. Product and Procedure Manual, 1996.* Becton Dickinson and Company, 1996.
[17] In most cases, external quality control is international, because often the SRL is located outside of the country.

laboratory network that is supported by the Supranational Reference Laboratory Network (SRLN). Fiji and Vanuatu are supported by Queensland Mycobacterium Reference Laboratory, Brisbane, Australia. The Solomon Islands are supported by the Mycobacterium Reference Laboratory, Institute of Medical and Veterinary Science, Adelaide, Australia. The Commonwealth of the Northern Marianas Island is supported by the Hawaii State Laboratory, Honolulu, Hawaii, United States. Guam is supported by the Microbial Diseases Laboratory, San Francisco, California, United States.

HIV testing

All countries that reported information on HIV status, except Ukraine, reported routine HIV testing information used for patient care. Information on methods used and quality assurance were not collected for this report. In Donetsk Oblast, Ukraine, a locally produced HIV enzyme-linked immunosorbent assay (ELISA) test detecting HIV-1 and HIV-2 antibodies (Diaprof Med, Kiev, Ukraine) was used for screening. All positive results were confirmed by the Genscreen Plus HIV Ag-Ab test (Bio-Rad Laboratories, Steenvoorde, France).

STATISTICAL PROCEDURES — DATA COLLECTION, ENTRY, CHECKING AND CLEANING

With the exception of Central and Western European countries, all settings reported data and other information about survey and surveillance methods through a standard data collection form, which was used to compile aggregated survey results. Completed forms were collected and reviewed at all levels of WHO, by country offices, regional offices and at WHO headquarters. All data (in the form of annexed tables) were returned to the country for a final review before publication, and were then entered into a Microsoft Access database.

Statistical analysis

Drug-resistance data for new, previously treated and combined cases were analysed. The following patterns of drug resistance were highlighted:
- resistance to any TB drug
- MDR-TB
- any resistance to isoniazid, rifampicin, streptomycin and ethambutol.
- non-MDR rifampicin resistance.

XDR-TB was also highlighted where data were available. Descriptive statistics were calculated in Stata (version 9.0; StataCorp). Arithmetic means, medians and ranges were determined as summary statistics for new, previously treated and combined cases; for individual drugs; and for pertinent combinations. For geographical settings reporting more than a single data point since the third report, only the latest data point was used for the estimation of point proportion. All tests of significance were two-tailed, and the alpha-error was kept at the 0.05 level in all inference procedures. Ninety-five per cent confidence levels (CLs) were calculated around the proportions and the means. Box plots were developed to illustrate the distribution of the data reported in WHO regions. Population-weighted means from the last data point of all countries reporting to the project were calculated to reflect the mean proportion of resistance by region, based on countries within the region reporting data to the project. In the past, unweighted medians were reported by regions; however, as expansion of surveys takes place within countries, and increasing numbers of low TB prevalence countries report data to the project, a population-weighted mean was considered more valuable for estimating proportions of resistance (see below).

Global data using the last data point from all reporting countries

For maps, means and global project coverage estimates, the last data point from all settings ever reporting to the project were included. Global and regional means of resistance were weighted as follows:
- for new cases — by new smear-positive cases notified in 2005
- for previously treated cases — by re-treatment cases notified in 2005
- for all TB cases — by all TB cases notified in the area surveyed in 2005[1].

For surveys carried out on a subnational level (states, provinces, oblasts), information representing only the population surveyed is included where appropriate.

HIV, resistance to second-line anti-TB drugs, age group and sex

If data on HIV, second-line DST, age group and sex from a given setting were available from more than one survey and one year, the information was combined for the analysis. Information from new and previously treated cases was also combined for analysis.

The association between HIV and drug-resistant TB was evaluated by calculating an odds ratio, to compare the proportion of drug resistance in HIV-positive and uninfected patients. Statistical significance was tested using a Fisher's exact test.

For analysis of resistance to second-line anti-TB drugs, the denominator used was MDR isolates tested for resistance to at least one fluroquinolone and one injectable second-line anti-TB drug (which is required to establish XDR-TB). XDR-TB and fluroquinolone resistance are the two categories reported.

The association between MDR-TB and the two variables "sex" and "age group" was studied in a multivariate logistic regression analysis. Statistical analyses were performed using Stata (version 9.0; StataCorp).

Dynamics of resistance over time

A proportion of drug resistance among new cases was analysed in survey settings among new and combined cases in settings conducting routine surveillance. Only countries and settings with three or more data points were included in this exercise. The patterns of drug resistance highlighted were any drug resistance, MDR and any isoniazid resistance. For settings that reported at least three data points, the trend was determined visually as ascending, descending, flat or indeterminate. The relative increase or decrease was expressed as a proportion, and statistical significance of trends was determined through a logistic regression.

ESTIMATES

A total of 183 countries and 2 SARs of China that account for nearly 100% of the world's population were included in the present analysis, which used data from the most recent national surveys. For Brazil, the Central African Republic, Kenya, Sierra Leone and Zimbabwe, the surveys covered most of the area of each country. For China, India, Italy, Malaysia, Mexico, the Russian Federation, Spain, Turkmenistan, Uganda, Ukraine and Uzbekistan, the surveys were subnational. For these countries, the proportion of MDR-TB cases was estimated as the mean of the results obtained from surveys conducted at the subnational level weighted by the population of patients with TB, as described above. For countries for which data from repeated surveys were available, only the most recent data were included. MDR-TB rates among new cases were available from 104 countries and 2 SARs of China. Among these, 97 also reported data on MDR-TB rates among previously treated cases. A total of 10 countries reported data on combined cases only. The estimated number of new TB cases globally, and by country, was used to calculate the number of MDR-TB cases that occurred among new cases. To estimate the number of previously treated cases, we multiplied the ratio of notified previously treated cases to notified new cases in 2006 by the total number of new cases estimated to have occurred in the same year for each country; therefore, the total number of estimated cases includes estimated re-treatment cases. Estimates were developed using a logistic regression model described in detail elsewhere[14].

VALIDITY OF THE FINDINGS

Surveillance and survey data are prone to errors that may to some extent invalidate the findings. Errors, or biases, may be related to selection of subjects, laboratory testing, data gathering or data analysis. Where cases are sampled only for a short period or in a restricted geographical area, the sample may not be fully representative of the total eligible population. Selection bias may also occur when only a particular subgroup of TB patients is included in the sample.

Distinguishing accurately between new and previously treated cases is not always possible, because this depends on a patient's willingness to disclose a history of prior anti-TB treatment, and on the training and motivation of the staff. For various reasons, patients may be unaware of their treatment antecedents, or prefer to conceal this information. Consequently, in some survey settings, a certain number of previously treated cases may have been misclassified as new cases. Any misclassification of re-treatment cases as new cases may lead to overestimation of the resistance rates among new cases, although it is difficult to estimate the magnitude of this bias unless all patients are re-interviewed. However, the proportion of resistance will be biased only if the correctly classified and misclassified TB patients have different risks for drug resistance.

Another bias, which is often not addressed in field studies, is the difference between the true prevalence and the observed or "test" prevalence. That difference depends on the magnitude of the true prevalence in the population, and the performance of the test under study conditions (i.e. its sensitivity and specificity). In practice, no test is completely accurate. Therefore, reported prevalence will either overestimate or underestimate the true prevalence in the population. In general, the sensitivity and specificity of tests for resistance to isoniazid and rifampicin tend to be high. Errors are more likely to be found in tests for ethambutol and streptomycin. This is particularly true for the evaluation of second-line anti-TB drugs, where external quality assurance does not exist and resistance to these drugs is relatively rare.

Some settings reported a small number of resistant cases, and a few settings reported a small number of total cases examined. Possible reasons for these small denominators in various participating geographical settings ranged from small absolute populations in some surveillance settings to feasibility problems in survey settings. This was particularly true for previously treated cases. The resulting reported prevalences thus lack stability, and important variations are seen over time, although most of these are not statistically significant. Where there were serious doubts about the representativeness of the sample of previously treated cases, the data were not included in the final database.

Re-treatment cases are a heterogeneous group, comprising patients who have relapsed, defaulted, been treated in the private sector, failed treatment once or several times, or been re-infected. Thus, for optimal interpretation of survey results, patient data need to be disaggregated by treatment history as accurately as possible. Few settings have been able to do this, due to the complexity of the interviews and the review of medical history required.

RESULTS

PHASE 4 OF THE GLOBAL PROJECT 2002–2007

Phase 4 of the global project provides the most recent data on anti-TB drug resistance, from 93 geographical settings in 81 countries and 2 SARs of China. Of these settings, 33 provided national or subnational data that have never previously been reported.

Subnational surveys — that is, surveys at the provincial, district, or city level — account for the discrepancy between the number of geographical settings and the number of countries. Eight countries provided results for 20 subnational areas (including 2 SARS), as follows:
- Azerbaijan reported data from Baku City
- China reported data from
    - one province (Heilongjiang)
    - one autonomous region (Inner Mongolia)
    - two municipalities (Beijing and Shanghai)
    - two SARs (Hong Kong and Macao)
- India reported data from
    - one state (Gujarat)
    - three districts (Ernakulam, which is within Kerala State; Hoogli, which is within West Bengal State; and Mayhurbhanj, which is within Orissa State)
- Indonesia reported data from Mimika district, in the Papua Province
- the Russian Federation reported data from 3 of 89 oblasts (Mary El, Orel and Tomsk)
- Spain reported data from
    - two regions (Aragon and Galicia)
    - one city (Barcelona)
- Ukraine reported data from Donetsk Oblast
- Uzbekistan reported data from Tashkent city.

Types of data
The most recent anti-TB drug resistance profile contains data from 93 settings in 81 countries and 2 SARs of China:
- 66 countries and 2 SARs of China provided information on drug resistance among new, previously treated and combined cases
- 6 countries reported drug resistance information on new cases only
- Andorra, Luxembourg and Malta did not detect any previously treated cases.

A total of 36 countries reported on cases with unknown treatment history. In most countries, this group of cases represented a small proportion of total cases;

however, in eight countries (Australia, Fiji, Guam, New Caledonia, Puerto Rico, Qatar, Solomon Islands and the United States) and one region in Spain (Barcelona), this represented the majority or the only group reported.

Proportion of drug resistance among new TB cases

Full details of the proportion of drug resistance among new cases for the period 1994-2007 are given in Annex 1. This section of the report covers the latest data from countries reporting from 2002 to 2007. The median number of cases tested per setting in survey settings was 547, and ranged from 101 new cases in Mimika district in the Papua province of Indonesia to 1619 new cases in Viet Nam. The median number of new cases tested among the settings conducting surveillance was 485, and ranged from 7 cases in Iceland to 3379 in the United Kingdom.

Any resistance among new cases

Data on the prevalence of any drug resistance among new cases of TB were provided by 72 countries and 2 SARs of China. The overall drug resistance ranged from 0% (Iceland[18]), 1.4% (95% CLs, 0.6-2.9) in Bosnia and Herzegovina, and 1.5% (95% CLs, 0.6-2.9) in Sri Lanka, to 49.2 (95% CLs, 44.4-54.3) in Georgia, 51.2 (95% CLs, 44.1-58.3) in Tashkent (Uzbekistan), and 56.3 (95% CLs, 50.2-62.9) in Baku City (Azerbaijan). Thirteen settings reported prevalence of resistance to any drug of 30% or higher (Figure 1).

Figure 1: Countries or settings with prevalence of any resistance higher than 30% among new cases, 2002-2007.

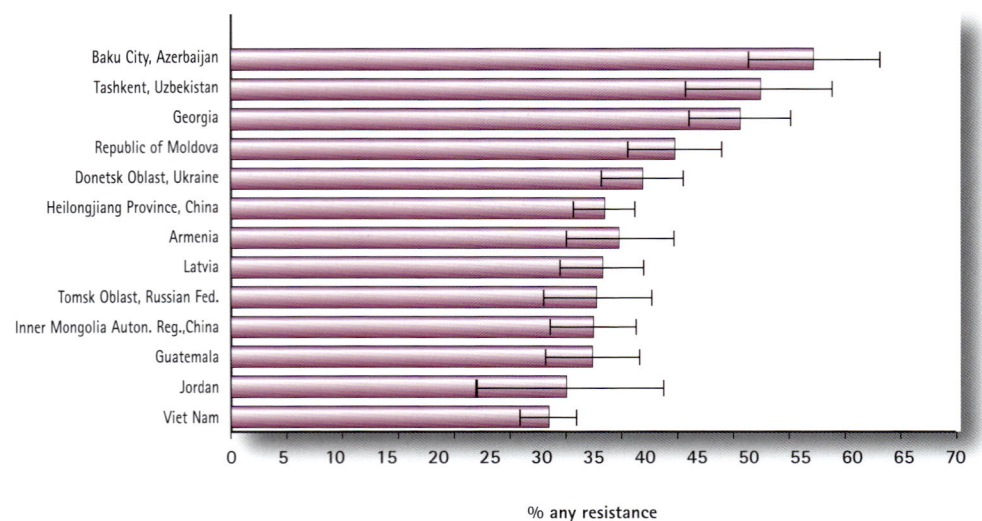

[18] Iceland has been excluded from further analyses because no resistance was detected in the latest data reported.

Multidrug-resistant TB among new cases

Prevalence of MDR-TB ranged from 0% (Andorra, Cuba, Luxembourg, Malta, Slovenia, Aragon, Spain and Uruguay) to 19.4% (95% CLs, 16.5–22.6) in the Republic of Moldova, and 22.3% (95% CLs, 18.5–26.6) in Baku City, Azerbaijan. Fourteen settings reported a prevalence of MDR-TB among new cases higher than 6.0% (Figure 2).

Figure 2: Countries or settings with multidrug-resistant TB prevalence higher than 6.0% among new cases, 2002–2007.

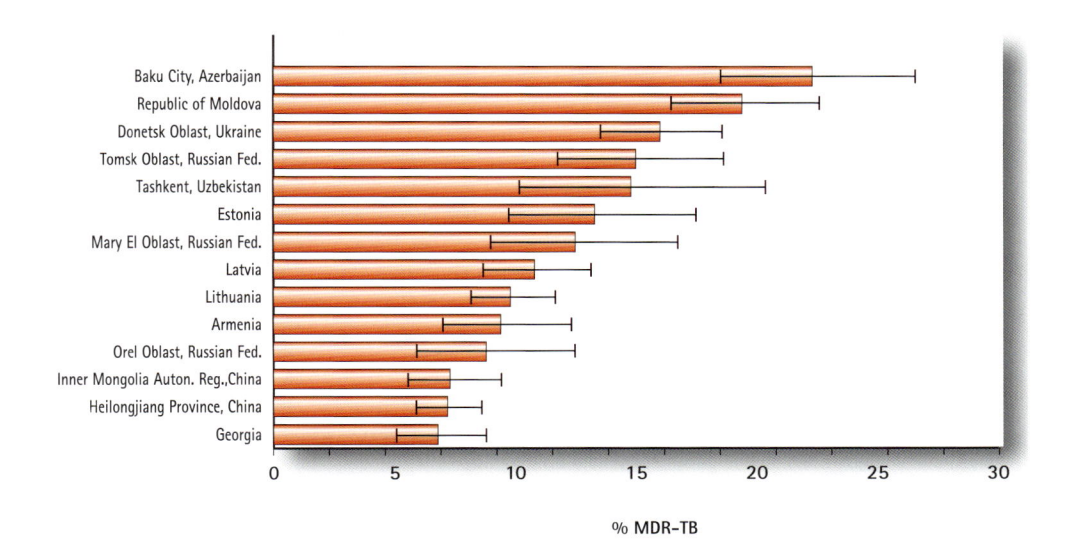

Any isoniazid resistance among new cases

Prevalence of isoniazid resistance ranged from 0% in Malta and Iceland, 0.6% (95% CLs, 0.0–3.3) in Cuba and 0.7% (95% CLs, 0.2–1.9) in Sri Lanka to 40.8% (95% CLs, 35.7–46.5) in Baku City (Azerbaijan) and 42.4% (95% CLs, 35.5–49.5) in Tashkent (Uzbekistan). Sixteen settings reported a prevalence of isoniazid resistance 15% or higher among new cases (Figure 3).

Figure 3: Prevalence of any resistance to isoniazid among new cases, 2002–2007.

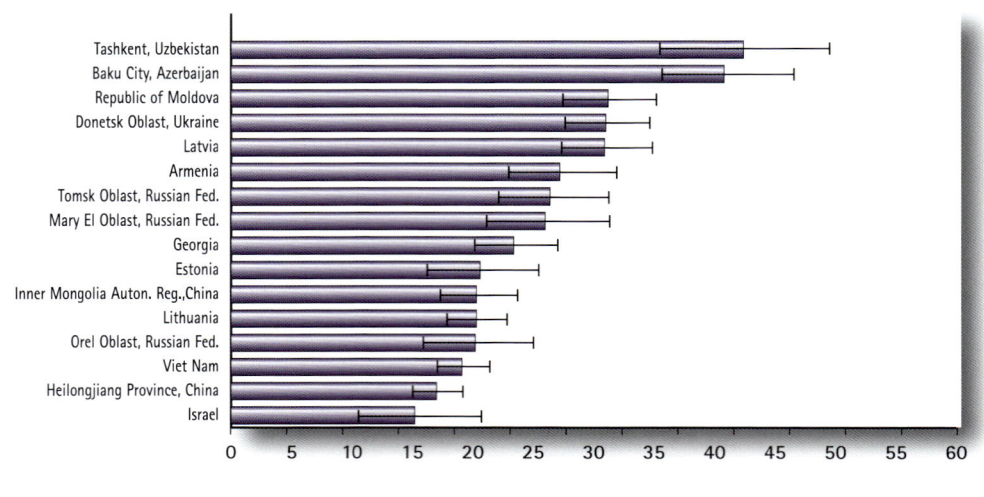

[Bar chart showing % resistance to isoniazid for the following settings, from highest to lowest:
Tashkent, Uzbekistan; Baku City, Azerbaijan; Republic of Moldova; Donetsk Oblast, Ukraine; Latvia; Armenia; Tomsk Oblast, Russian Fed.; Mary El Oblast, Russian Fed.; Georgia; Estonia; Inner Mongolia Auton. Reg., China; Lithuania; Orel Oblast, Russian Fed.; Viet Nam; Heilongjiang Province, China; Israel. X-axis: 0 to 60, % resistance to isoniazid.]

Drug resistance among previously treated TB cases

Data on the prevalence of drug resistance among previously treated cases were available for 66 countries and 2 SARs of China (Annex 2). The number of cases tested in settings conducting routine surveillance ranged from 1 (Iceland) to 522 (Poland), with a median of 58 cases per setting. The number of cases tested in settings conducting surveys ranged from 16 (Lebanon) to 1047 (Gujarat State, India) and 2054 cases in the Republic of Moldova[19], with a median of 110.

Any resistance among previously treated cases

No resistance was reported in Iceland, Israel or Norway, where the number of previously treated cases was very small. In contrast, high prevalence of any resistance was seen in Baku City, Azerbaijan (84.4%; 95% CLs, 76.9–92.4) and Tashkent, Uzbekistan (85.9%; 95% CLs, 76.6–92.5). In 16 settings, prevalence of any resistance was reported as 50% or higher (Figure 4).

---

[19] The sample of previously treated cases included in the survey from the Republic of Moldova includes a large proportion of cases that had been on treatment for more than month but were not classified as re-treatment cases in the TB register.

Figure 4: Countries or settings with a prevalence of any resistance higher than 50% among previously treated cases, 2002–2007.

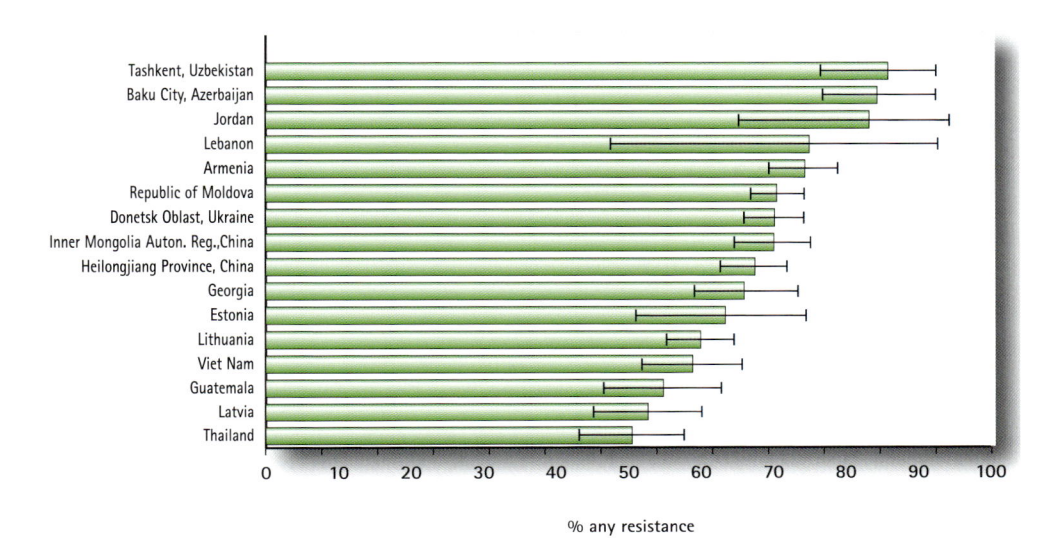

% any resistance

Multidrug-resistant TB among previously treated cases

No MDR-TB was reported in Denmark, New Zealand, Sri Lanka, or among the preliminary data from UR Tanzania. Estonia reported 52.1% (95%CLs, 39.9–64.1%) MDR-TB among previously treated cases; Baku City, Azerbaijan reported 55.8% (95% CLs, 49.7–62.4%); and Tashkent, Uzbekistan reported 60.0% (95% CLs, 48.8–70.5). Lebanon reported 62.5% (95% CLs, 35.4–84.8); however, only 16 cases were included in the sample. The Russian Federation reported data on re-treatment cases in Orel Oblast only. Sixteen settings reported MDR-TB of 25% or higher among previously treated cases (Figure 5).

Figure 5: Countries or settings with prevalence of multidrug-resistant TB higher than 30% among previously treated cases, 2002–2007.

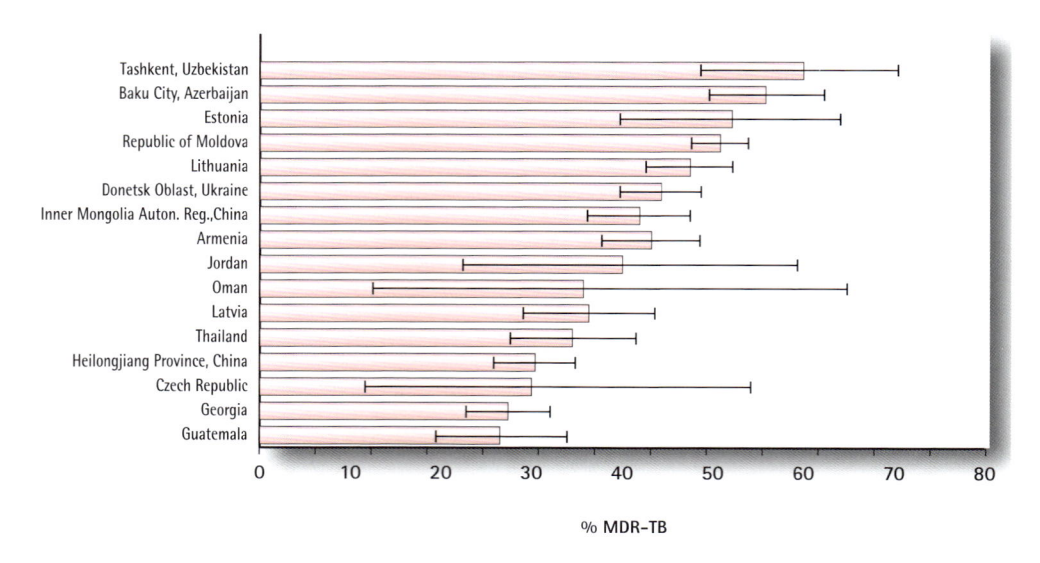

% MDR-TB

Any isoniazid resistance among previously treated cases

Prevalence of isoniazid resistance ranged from 0% in Iceland, Israel, and Norway, 3.8% (95% CLs, 1.0–9.5) in Singapore and 4.5% (95% CLs, 0.1–22.8) in Finland to 79.7% (95% CLs, 72.4–87.5) in Baku City, Azerbaijan, and 81.2 (95% CLs, 71.2–88.8) in Tashkent, Uzbekistan. Fifteen settings reported a prevalence of isoniazid resistance 30% or higher among previously treated cases (Figure 6).

Figure 6: Prevalence of any resistance to isoniazid among previously treated cases, 2002–2007.

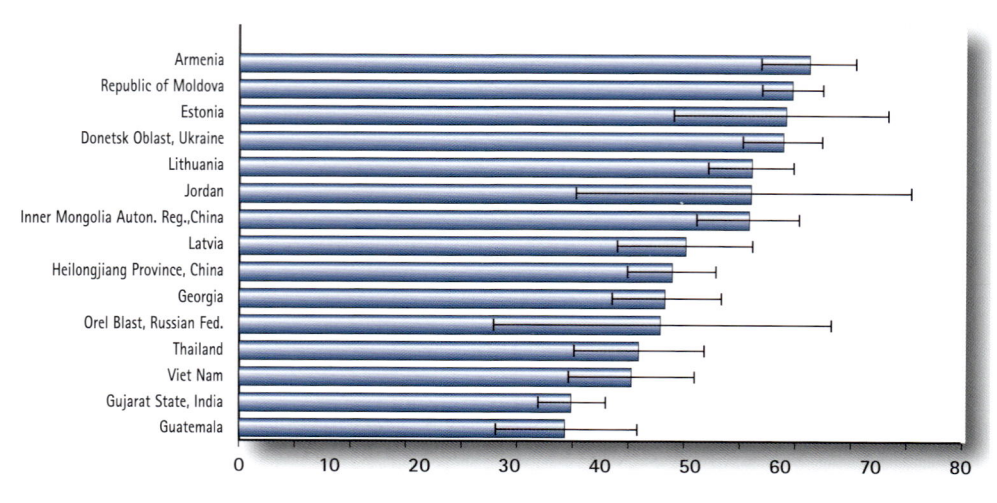

% isoniazid resistance

Drug resistance among all TB cases

Drug resistance among all TB cases is examined in detail in the trends section of this report for countries conducting routine surveillance, and all data are available in Annex 3. In many survey settings, the number of previously treated cases is small and does not reflect the proportion of re-treatment cases within the TB programme. Therefore, when estimating proportions of resistance among combined cases, proportions must be weighted by their population within the programme; this generates wide confidence levels. Hence, the only proportion examined without distinguishing by treatment history is the proportion of non-MDR rifampicin resistance.

Non-MDR rifampicin resistance is an important indicator (in terms of programmes) that should be known if screening for MDR-TB on the basis of rifampicin testing alone. Rifampicin resistance unaccompanied by isoniazid resistance is rare, and may thus also be a good laboratory indicator. If non-MDR-TB rifampicin resistance is greater than 3%, this should be considered unusual — it may suggest errors in either rifampicin or isoniazid testing. Of the 93 settings that reported, 80% reported less than 1% non-MDR rifampicin resistance; only three settings reported non-MDR rifampicin resistance above 3% (Table 1).

Table 1: Prevalence of non-MDR rifampicin resistance among all TB cases, 2002–2007[20]

Prevalence of non-MDR rifampicin resistance (%)	Number and location of settings
0.0	30 settings
0.1–1.0	47 settings
1.1–3.0	13 settings: • Armenia • Beijing Municipality, China • Donetsk Oblask, Ukraine • Ernakulam District, Kerala State, India • Ethiopia • Guatemala • Lebanon • Paraguay • Republic of Korea • Republic of Moldova • Romania • Shanghai Municipality, China • Tomsk Oblast, Russian Federation
>3.0	3 settings: • Heilongjiang Province, China • Inner Mongolia Autonomous Region, China • Jordan

non-MDR rifampicin resistance = TB with resistance to rifampicin but susceptibility to isoniazid.

---

[20] Data from countries and settings only reporting on new cases were also included in this analysis.

Multidrug-resistant TB among new and previously treated cases by region

WHO African Region

Six countries reported from the WHO African Region (Figure 7). The median sample size was 471 new cases and 46 previously treated cases. MDR-TB among new cases ranged from 0.7% (95% CLs, 0.2–1.8) in Madagascar to 3.9% (95% CLs, 2.5–5.8) in Rwanda. Côte d'Ivoire did not survey previously treated cases, and the preliminary data from UR Tanzania showed no MDR-TB among previously treated cases[21].

Figure 7: Prevalence of multidrug-resistant TB among new and previously treated cases in the WHO African Region, 2002–2007.

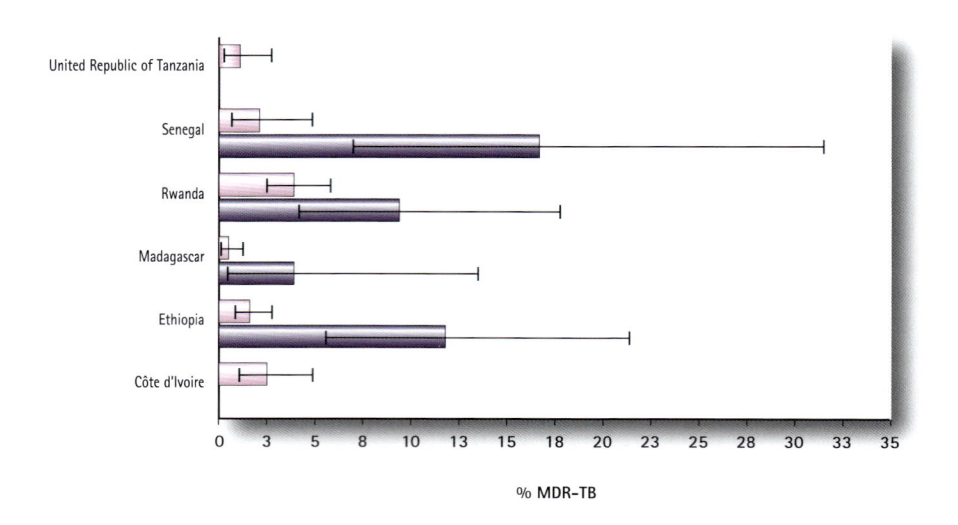

UR Tanzania = United Republic of Tanzania

WHO Region of the Americas

Eleven countries reported from the WHO Region of the Americas[22] (Figure 8). The median sample size was 335 for new cases, and ranged from 169 new cases in Cuba to 1809 in Peru. The median sample size for previously treated cases was 80. No MDR-TB was found among new cases in Cuba or Uruguay. The highest proportion of MDR-TB among new cases was seen in Guatemala (3.0%; 95% CLs, 1.8–4.6) and Peru (5.3%; 95% CLs, 4.2–6.4).

---

[21] Data from Madagascar and UR Tanzania are preliminary; external quality assurance of laboratory testing was not complete at the time of this report.
[22] The United States and Puerto Rico reported on combined cases only and are excluded from this analysis.

Figure 8: Prevalence of multidrug-resistant TB among new and previously treated cases in the WHO Region of the Americas, 2002-2007.

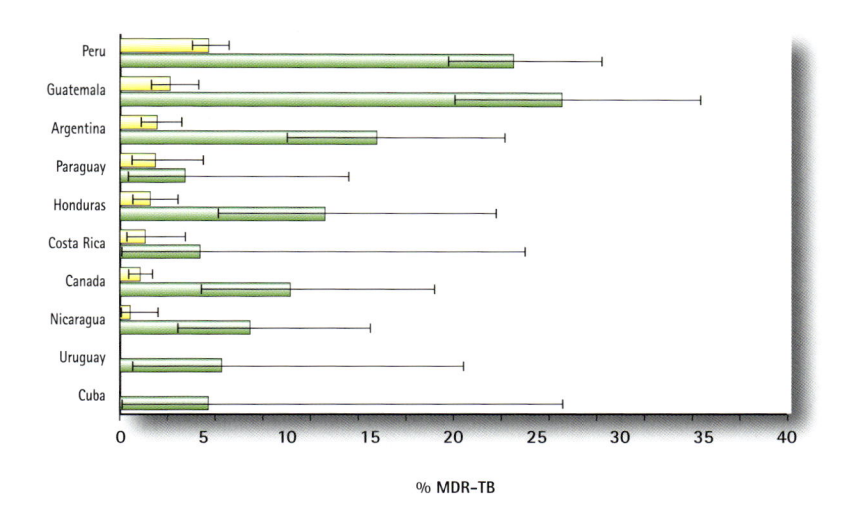

% MDR-TB

WHO Eastern Mediterranean Region

Five countries reported from the WHO Eastern Mediterranean Region (Figure 9). The median sample size was 264 for new cases, and ranged from 111 new cases in Jordan to 1049 in Morocco. The median sample size for previously treated cases was 42. MDR-TB among new cases ranged from 0.5% (95% CLs, 0.2–1.1) in Morocco to 5.4 (95% CLs, 2.0–11.4), in Jordan.

Figure 9: Prevalence of multidrug-resistant TB among new and previously treated cases in the WHO Eastern Mediterranean Region, 2002-2007.

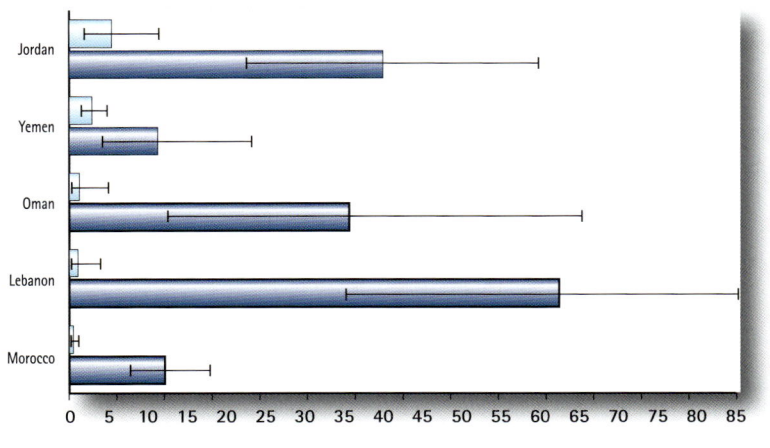

% UDR-TB

WHO European Region

Thirty eight countries reported data from the WHO European Region (Figure 10). A total of 30 countries conducted routine nationwide surveillance, with three settings in Spain. The median of combined cases tested was 483, and ranged from 8 in Iceland to 4800 in the United Kingdom. Both absolute numbers and proportion of MDR-TB were highest in the Baltic countries.

Figure 10: Total number of multidrug-resistant (MDR) TB cases reported in European countries and settings conducting routine surveillance, and percentage of multidrug-resistant TB among all TB cases reported.

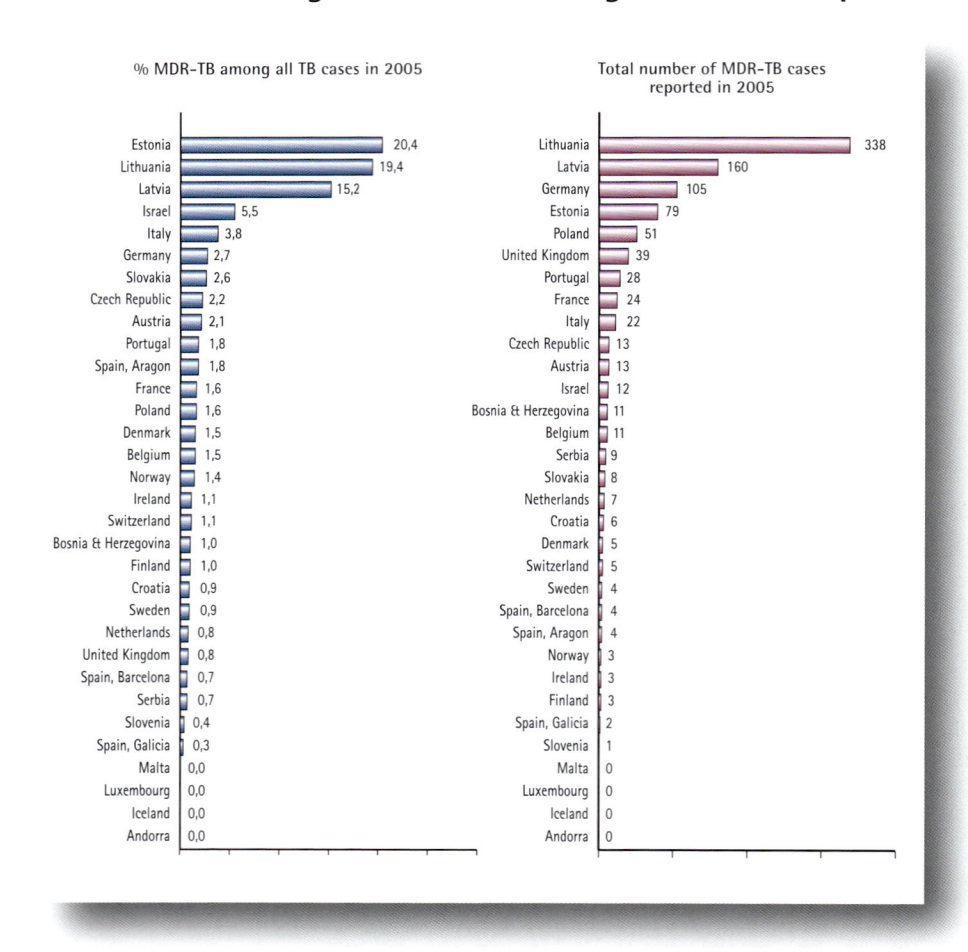

% MDR-TB among all TB cases in 2005

Country	%
Estonia	20,4
Lithuania	19,4
Latvia	15,2
Israel	5,5
Italy	3,8
Germany	2,7
Slovakia	2,6
Czech Republic	2,2
Austria	2,1
Portugal	1,8
Spain, Aragon	1,8
France	1,6
Poland	1,6
Denmark	1,5
Belgium	1,5
Norway	1,4
Ireland	1,1
Switzerland	1,1
Bosnia & Herzegovina	1,0
Finland	1,0
Croatia	0,9
Sweden	0,9
Netherlands	0,8
United Kingdom	0,8
Spain, Barcelona	0,7
Serbia	0,7
Slovenia	0,4
Spain, Galicia	0,3
Malta	0,0
Luxembourg	0,0
Iceland	0,0
Andorra	0,0

Total number of MDR-TB cases reported in 2005

Lithuania	338
Latvia	160
Germany	105
Estonia	79
Poland	51
United Kingdom	39
Portugal	28
France	24
Italy	22
Czech Republic	13
Austria	13
Israel	12
Bosnia & Herzegovina	11
Belgium	11
Serbia	9
Slovakia	8
Netherlands	7
Croatia	6
Denmark	5
Switzerland	5
Sweden	4
Spain, Barcelona	4
Spain, Aragon	4
Norway	3
Ireland	3
Finland	3
Spain, Galicia	2
Slovenia	1
Malta	0
Luxembourg	0
Iceland	0
Andorra	0

Of the eight countries conducting surveys or reporting subnational data, seven were countries of the former Soviet Union (Figure 11). The prevalence of MDR-TB among new cases ranged from 2.8% (95% CLs, 1.8–4.2) in Romania to 22.3% (95% CLs, 18.5–26.6) in Baku City, Azerbaijan, 28.6%. Data on previously treated cases were not included from the Mary El or Tomsk oblasts of the Russian Federation.

Figure 11: Prevalence of multidrug-resistant TB among new and previously treated cases among countries or settings conducting surveys in the WHO European Region, 2002–2007.

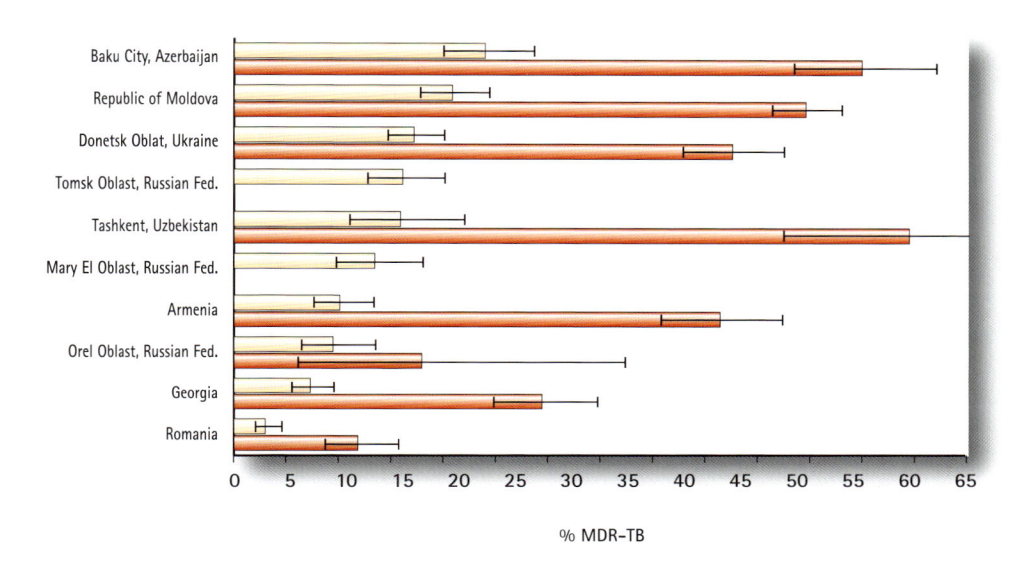

WHO South-East Asia Region

Six countries (including four settings in India) reported data from the WHO South-East Asia Region (Figure 12). Of the six countries, the median number of new cases tested was 547, and ranged from 101 in Mimika district in the Papua province of Indonesia to 1571 in Gujarat, India. The median number of previously treated cases tested was 162. MDR-TB among new cases ranged from 0.2% (95% CLs, 0.0–1.0) in Sri Lanka and 0.7% (95% CLs, 0.1–2.5) in Mayhurbhanj District, Orissa State, India to 4.0% (95% CLs, 2.6–5.7) in Myanmar. India, Nepal and Myanmar showed similar proportions of resistance among re-treatment cases. Sri Lanka showed no resistance and Thailand showed 34.5% (95% CLs, 27.9–41.7) MDR-TB among previously treated cases.

Figure 12: Prevalence of multidrug-resistant TB among new and previously treated cases in the WHO South-East Asia Region, 2002–2007.

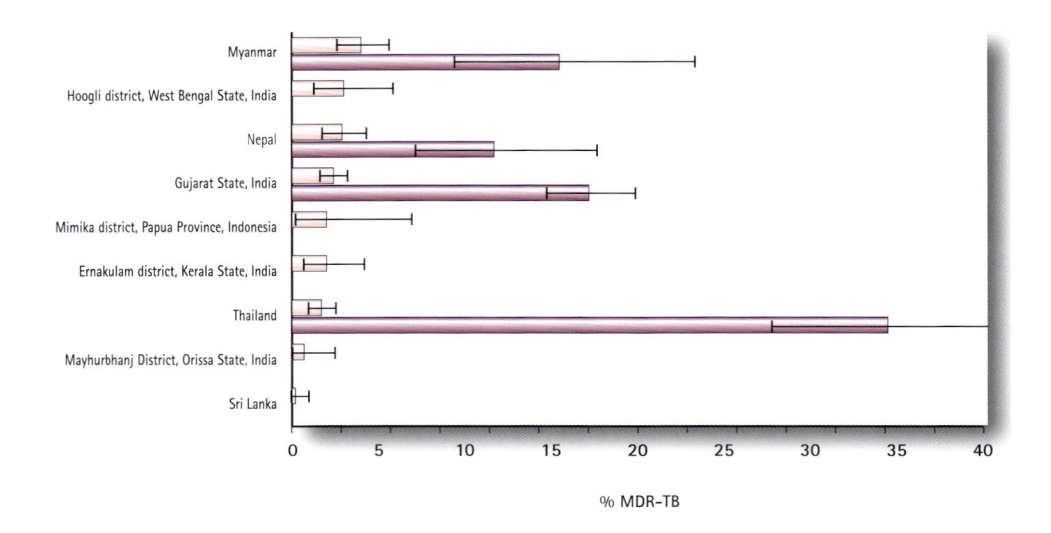

WHO Western Pacific Region

Seven countries and two SARs of China[23] reported drug-resistance data from the WHO Western Pacific Region (Figure 13). Six countries reported data distinguished by treatment history, including four settings in mainland China. For these six countries, the median number of new cases tested was 1004, and ranged from 250 in New Zealand to 3271 in Hong Kong SAR, both of which conduct routine surveillance of all TB cases. The median number of previously treated cases tested was 182. MDR-TB among new cases ranged from less than 1.0% in Hong Kong SAR, Japan, New Zealand and Singapore to 7.2% (95% CLs, 5.9–8.6) in Heilongjiang Province and 7.3% (95% CLs, 5.6–9.4) in Inner Mongolia Autonomous Region of China.

---

[23] Australia, Guam, Fiji, New Caledonia and the Solomon Islands reported on combined cases only and are excluded from this analysis.

Figure 13: Prevalence of multidrug-resistant TB among new and previously treated cases in the WHO Western Pacific Region, 2002–2007

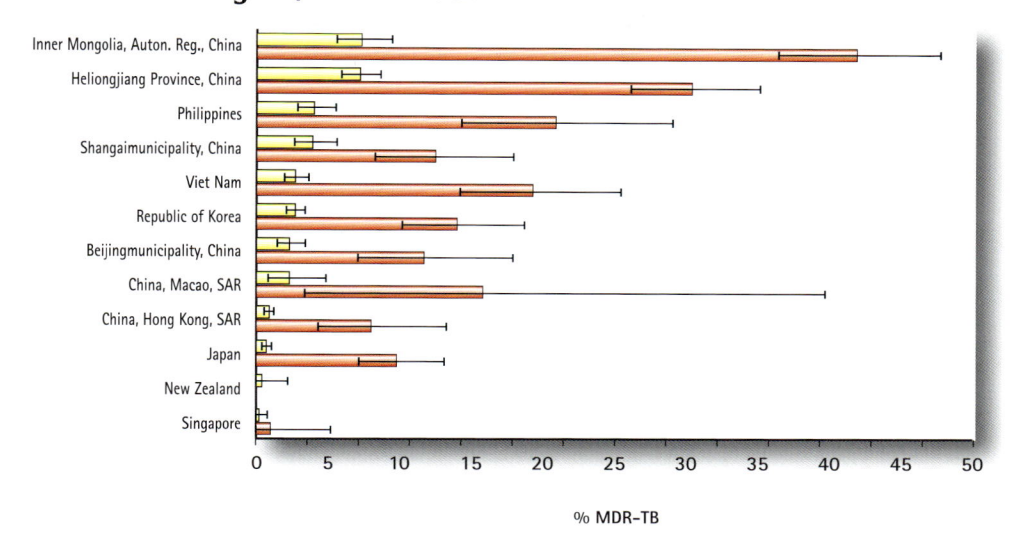

Drug-resistant TB by age and sex

Data on drug resistance stratified by sex and age groups was reported by 42 settings in 36 countries from all the six WHO regions. Among these settings, seven were able to report information for more than one year. MDR-TB among combined cases was found to be associated with male sex and with younger age groups (25–44 years old) in most of the WHO regions.

Drug resistance and HIV

A total of eight settings in seven countries reported data on drug resistance stratified by HIV status. The settings that reported were Cuba, Honduras, Latvia, Tomsk Oblast (Russian Federation), Barcelona and Galicia (Spain), Donetsk Oblast (Ukraine) and Uruguay. Data were reported:
- stratified by positive and unknown HIV status from Latvia and from Galicia
- disaggregated by positive, negative and unknown HIV status from the remaining settings.

The analysis was weakened by lack of differentiation between HIV unknown and HIV negative. Where data on drug resistance stratified by HIV status from a given setting were available from more than one survey and one year, the information was combined for the analysis. Information from new and previously treated cases was also combined for analysis.

Due to the low number of HIV-positive cases diagnosed with MDR-TB or with resistance to any TB drug in most settings, the data were not sufficiently powerful to examine an association between HIV and drug-resistant TB. The only two settings with sufficiently large numbers of cases to be able to examine the relationship between the two epidemics were Latvia and Donetsk Oblast, Ukraine, where HIV infection was found to be significantly associated to both MDR-TB and any anti-TB drug resistance (Table 2).

Table 2: Prevalence of multidrug-resistant TB and any resistance among HIV-positive TB cases and TB cases with unknown HIV status in Latvia, 2001–2005

	Multidrug resistance	Any resistance
Drug resistance in HIV-unknown TB cases (%)	765/5,162 (14.8)	1,782/5,162 (34.5)
Drug resistance in HIV-positive TB cases (%)	39/148 (26.4)	66/148 (44.6)
Odds ratio (95% confidence level)	2.1 (1.4–3.0)	1.5 (1.1–2.1)
P value	<0.01	<0.05

TB = tuberculosis; HIV = human immunodeficiency virus

In Donetsk Oblast, Ukraine, the drug resistance survey was linked to a TB/HIV survey. In this study, positive HIV status was found to be an independent predictor for MDR-TB, as were history of previous anti-TB treatment and history of imprisonment[24] (Table 3).

Table 3: Prevalence of multidrug-resistant TB and any resistance among HIV-positive and HIV-negative TB cases in Donetsk Oblast, Ukraine, 2006.

	Multidrug resistance	Any resistance
Drug resistance in HIV-negative TB cases (%)	272/1,143 (23.8)	551/1,143 (48.2)
Drug resistance in HIV-positive TB cases (%)	97/307 (31.6)	173/307 (56.4)
Odds ratio (95% confidence level)	1.5 (1.1–2.0)	1.4 (1.1–1.8)
P value	<0.01	<0.05

TB = tuberculosis; HIV = human immunodeficiency virus

Extensively drug-resistant TB

Thirty-five countries and two SARs were able to report data on XDR-TB, either through routine surveillance data or through drug-resistance surveys. Twenty-five countries and two SARs reported routine surveillance data, and ten countries reported from periodic surveys. Data on new and previously treated cases were combined; data from multiple years were also combined if available. The denominator used was MDR-TB cases tested for second-line anti-TB drugs that would allow the definition of XDR-TB. Data from the national laboratory registers in South Africa are included in the table, although these data are not considered nationally representative. A further five countries reported data from risk groups. Nineteen countries have reported at least one case since 2001, although no

---

[24] Lyepshina S. *Association between Multidrug-Resistant Tuberculosis and HIV Status in the Civilian and Penitentiary Sectors of Donetsk Oblast, Ukraine*, 38th World Conference on Lung Health. 8-12 November, 2007, Cape Town, South Africa, Abstract Book.

denominators are available. Four of these nineteen countries also reported surveillance data, but the XDR-TB case identified was not found during the years for which surveillance data are reported.

A total of 45 countries and 1 SAR have identified at least one case of XDR-TB since 2000. Of the settings conducting routine surveillance, three countries and one oblast of the Russian Federation reported between 25 and 58 cases over a four-year period representing 6.6% (95% CLs, 4.5–9.2) of the MDR-TB burden in Tomsk Oblast (Russian Federation) to 23.7% (95% CLs, 18.5–29.5). The United States reported 17 cases over a six-year period, representing 1.9% (95% CLs, 1.1–3.1) of MDR-TB cases tested for second-line anti-TB drugs during this time. Over a four-year period, Barcelona, Spain reported three cases and the Czech Republic reported five cases; these cases represented 8.1% (95% CLs, 1.7–21.9), and 20.0% (95% CLs, 6.8–40.7) of MDR-TB cases, respectively. Nine countries conducting routine surveillance detected between one and two cases of XDR-TB over a four-year period. During this time, Australia, France, Ireland, the Netherlands, Slovenia and Sweden reported one case; and Israel, Romania, and Canada reported two cases. Aragon, Spain reported one case in 2005. Eight countries (Belgium, Croatia, Denmark, Norway, Poland, Switzerland, Singapore and the United Kingdom) reported no XDR-TB cases over a four-year period. Four settings — China, Macao SAR, Galicia (Spain) and New Zealand — also reported no cases, but the reporting period was only one year. Of the countries conducting surveys, the proportion of XDR-TB among MDR-TB ranged from 0.0% in Rwanda and UR Tanzania to 12.8% (95% CLs, 9.8–16.3) or 55/431 in Baku City, Azerbaijan, and 15.0% (95% CLs, 3.2–37.9), or 3/20 in Donetsk Oblast, Ukraine. Table 4 indicates the country, the source of the data, the number of MDR-TB cases tested, the years in which data were reported and the confidence levels.

Table 4: Countries reporting data on XDR-TB, 2002–2007.

Country	Source	Region	Year	Method	MDR	MDR tested	FLQ	FLQ%	lower CI	upper CI	XDR	XDR%	lower CI	upper CI
Representative survey or surveillance data														
Japan	Global Project, SRL Japan	WPR	2002	sentinel	60	55	21	38,2	-	-	17	30,9	-	-
Estonia	EuroTB	EEUR	2003-2006	surveillance	248	245		0,0	-	-	58	23,7	-	-
Latvia	Global Project	EEUR	2003-2006	surveillance	712	688		0,0	-	-	53	7,7	-	-
Tomsk Oblast, RF	Global Project, SRL Boston, USA	EEUR	2003-2005	surveillance	468	458	33	7,2	-	-	30	6,6	-	-
Lithuania	EuroTB	EEUR	2003-2006	surveillance	656	173		0,0	-	-	25	14,5	-	-
USA	National Tuberculosis Surveillance System	AMR	2000-2006	surveillance	925	601	55	9,2	-	-	18	3,0	-	-
Hong Kong SAR, China	Global Project, SRL Hong Kong, SAR	WPR	2005	surveillance	41	41	12	29,3	-	-	6	14,6	-	-
Czech Republic	EuroTB	EUR	2003-2006	surveillance	38	25		0,0	-	-	5	20,0	-	-
Spain, Barcelona	Global Project, SRL Spain	EUR	2002-2005	surveillance	43	37	4	10,8	-	-	3	8,1	-	-
Romania	EuroTB	EUR	2003-2006	surveillance	50	44		0,0	-	-	2	4,5	-	-
Israel	EuroTB	EUR	2003-2006	surveillance	45	44		0,0	-	-	2	4,5	-	-
Ireland	EuroTB	EUR	2003-2006	surveillance	8	3		0,0	-	-	1	33,3	-	-
Slovenia	EuroTB	EUR	2003-2007	surveillance	3	3		0,0	-	-	1	33,3	-	-
Sweden	EuroTB	EUR	2003-2006	surveillance		18		0,0	-	-	1	5,6	-	-
Netherlands	EuroTB	EUR	2003-2006	surveillance	34	33		0,0	-	-	1	3,0	-	-
France	EuroTB	EUR	2003-2006	surveillance	152	149		0,0	-	-	1	0,7	-	-
Australia	Global Project, SRLs Australia	WPR	2002-2005	surveillance	43	43	4	9,3	-	-	1	2,3	-	-
Canada	Global Project	AMR	2003-2006	surveillance	55	55		0,0	-	-	2	3,6	-	-
UK	EuroTB	EUR	2003-2006	surveillance	174	62		0,0	-	-	0	0,0	-	-
Belgium	EuroTB	EUR	2003-2006	surveillance	31	12		0,0	-	-	0	0,0	-	-
Switzerland	EuroTB	EUR	2003-2006	surveillance	25	22		0,0	-	-	0	0,0	-	-
Poland	EuroTB	EUR	2003-2006	surveillance	17	6		0,0	-	-	0	0,0	-	-
Norway	EuroTB	EUR	2003-2006	surveillance	11	11		0,0	-	-	0	0,0	-	-
Croatia	EuroTB	EUR	2003-2006	surveillance	5	1		0,0	-	-	0	0,0	-	-
Denmark	EuroTB	EUR	2003-2006	surveillance	5	5		0,0	-	-	0	0,0	-	-
Singapore	Global Project	WPR	2002-2005	surveillance	14	14	1	7,1	-	-	0	0,0	-	-
Macao SAR, China	Global Project	WPR	2005	surveillance	9	9	1	11,1	-	-	0	0,0	-	-
New Zealand	Global Project	WPR	2005	surveillance	4	4	2	50,0	-	-	0	0,0	-	-
Spain, Galicia	Global Project	EUR	2006	surveillance	2	2	0	0,0	-	-	0	0,0	-	-
Baku, Azerbaijan	Global Project, SRL Borstel, Germany	EEUR	2007	survey	431	431	125	29,0	24,8	33,5	55	12,8	9,8	16,3
Armenia	Global Project, SRL Borstel, Germany	EEUR	2007	survey	199	199	15	7,5	4,3	12,1	8	4,0	1,8	7,8
Donetsk, Ukraine	Global Project, SRL Gauting, Germany	EEUR	2006	survey	379	20	3	15,0	3,2	37,9	3	15,0	3,2	37,9
Georgia	Global Project, SRL Belgium	EEUR	2006	survey	105	70	3	4,3	0,9	12,0	3	4,3	0,9	12,0
Republic of Moldova	Global Project, SRL Borstel, Germany	EUR	2006	survey	203	47	11	23,4	12,3	38,0	3	6,4	1,3	17,5
Argentina	Global Project, SRL Argentina	AMR	2005	survey	36	36	3	8,3	1,8	22,5	2	5,6	0,7	18,7
Republic of Korea	Global Project	WPR	2004	survey	110	110	13	11,8	0,1	19,3	2	1,8	0,0	6,4
Spain, Aragon	Global Project	EUR	2005	survey	4	4	1	25,0	0,6	80,6	1	25,0	0,6	80,6
Rwanda	Global Project, SRL Belgium	AFR	2005	survey	32	32	3	9,4	2,0	25,0	0	0,0	0,0	8,9
UR Tanzania	Global Project, SRL Belgium	AFR	2007	survey	6	6	0	0,0	0,0	39,3	0	0,0	0,0	39,3

Table 5: Countries reporting data on XDR-TB, non-nationally representative samples 2002–2007.

Country	Source	Region	Year	Method	MDR	MDR tested	FLQ	FLQ%	lower CI	upper CI	XDR	XDR%	lower CI	upper CI
Routine laboratory data (non nationally representative)														
South Africa	National Health Laboratory System	AFR	2004-2007	retrospective review		17615	0	0,0	0,0	0,0	996	5,7	5,3	6,0
Risk groups and MDR-TB treatment programmes														
Philippines	Global Project, GLC program	WPR	2005-2006	Confirmed MDR for Tx		293	149	50,9	45,0	56,7	10	3,4	1,6	6,2
DR Congo, Kinshasa	Global Project, SRL Belgium	AFR	2006-2007	Selection of CatI failures		144	2	1,4	0,0	9,1	0	0,0	0,0	5,0
Burundi	Global Project, SRL Belgium	AFR	2006-2007	Selection of CatII failures		23	0	0,0	0,0	12,2	0	0,0	0,0	12,2
Myanmar	Global Project, SRL Belgium	SEAR	2007	Selection of CatII failures		43	4	9,3	2,6	22,1	0	0,0	0,0	6,7
Bangladesh	Global Project, Damien Foundation, SRL Belgium	SEAR	2003-2006	Retreatment		300	31	10,3	7,1	14,3	3	1,0	0,2	2,9

Table 6: Countries reporting at least one case 2002–2007.

Country	Source	Region
Countries reporting at least one case		
Brazil	(1)	AMR
Chile	(1)	AMR
Ecuador	(1)	AMR
Germany	(1)	EUR
Iran	(2)	EMR
Italy	(3)	EUR
Peru	(1)	AMR
Portugal	(1)	EUR
Vietnam	NTP report	WPR
Mozambique	NTP report	AFR
India	(4)	SEAR
Thailand	NTP report	SEAR
Mexico	(1)	SEAR
UK*	(1)	EUR
Poland*	NTP report	EUR
Norway*	NTP report	EUR
Canada*	NTP report	AMR
Botswana	NTP report	AFR
Nepal	NTP report	SEAR

* one case reported outside of surveillance data reported to EuroTB

1. Emergence of Mycobacterium tuberculosis with Extensive Resistance to Second-Line Drugs – Worldwide, 2000–2004. MMWR 2006;55:301-305
2. Masjedi MR, Farnia P, Sorooch S, et al. Extensively drug-resistant tuberculosis: 2 years of surveillance in Iran. Clin Infect Dis 2006;43(7):841-7.
3. Migliori GB, Ortmann J, Girardi E, et al. Extensively drug-resistant tuberculosis, Italy and Germany. Emerg Infect Dis 2007;13(5):780-2.
4. Thomas A, Ramachandran R, Rehaman F, et al. Management of multi drug resistance tuberculosis in the field: Tuberculosis Research Centre experience. Indian J Tuberc 2007;54(3):117-24.

AFR = WHO African Region; AMR = WHO Region of the Americas; CL = confidence level; EMR = WHO Eastern Mediterranean Region; EUR= WHO European Region; EEUR = Eastern WHO European Region; FLQ = fluoroquinolone; MDR = multidrug resistant; RF = Russian Federation; SEAR = WHO South-East Asia Region; SRL = supranational reference laboratory WPR = WHO Western Pacific Region; XDR = extensively drug resistant.

DATA REPORTED TO THE GLOBAL PROJECT 1994–2007, AND ESTIMATED GLOBAL AND REGIONAL MEANS OF RESISTANCE

Since the start of the global project in 1994, data have been collected from 138 settings in 114 countries and 2 SARs of China worldwide. To estimate the global and regional means of resistance, and to examine the distribution of resistance within a region, this report includes data obtained since the beginning of the project, weighted by the population they represent. Twenty countries reported data before the year 2000.

Data from the 114 countries and 2 SARs of China represent 48% of the world's population and 46% of the total TB burden. Table 7 describes global and regional population coverage. The figures given in Table 7 correspond to the population-weighted means described in Table 8 and shown in Figures 14–17.

Table 7: Population coverage of drug-resistance data reported to WHO, 1994–2007.

	Total population	Total TB cases	Total ss+ TB cases	Total retreatment TB cases	Number of countries
AFR	370.004.932	908.305	349.414	102.657	22
(%)	50%	72%	64%	81%	
AMR	854.140.969	222.731	109.666	21.282	21
(%)	96%	93%	88%	94%	
EMR	227.704.004	62.416	27.737	1.725	9
(%)	42%	24%	25%	15%	
EUR (E)	71.113.271	103.783	33.978	23.387	13
(%)	23%	31%	48%	31%	
EUR (WC)	363.241.951	46.408	12.993	3.693	27
(%)	64%	55%	50%	44%	
SEAR	318.225.607	450.687	163.774	34.463	6
(%)	19%	23%	19%	14%	
WPR	929.919.476	723.940	391.264	58.930	19
(%)	53%	52%	58%	35%	
Global	3.134.350.210	2.518.270	1.088.826	246.137	117
(%)	49%	46%	45%	37%	55%

AFR = WHO African Region; AMR = WHO Region of the Americas; EMR = WHO Eastern Mediterranean Region; EUR= WHO European Region; SEAR = WHO South-East Asia Region; WPR = WHO Western Pacific Region; SS+ = smear-positive sputum

The weighted mean of resistance to individual drugs varied across WHO regions. The proportion of resistance to every drug and of MDR-TB was highest in Eastern Europe, and lowest in Africa and Central and Western Europe. The global weighted mean of MDR-TB was 2.9% (95% CLs, 2.2–3.6) among new cases, 15.3% (95% CLs, 9.6–21.0) among previously treated cases and 5.3%(95% CLs, 3.9–6.7) among all TB cases.

Table 6 shows that the relationship between resistance to specific drugs across regions and by history of previous treatment was similar, with the highest proportions of resistance to isoniazid and streptomycin, followed by rifampicin and ethambutol. This was true for all regions, without regard to treatment history, with the exception of previously treated cases in the Eastern Mediterranean region, where rifampicin resistance was higher than isoniazid resistance. Figures 18–20 shows the distribution of proportions of MDR-TB, any resistance and isoniazid resistance among combined cases within region.

Table 8: Weighted mean of resistance to first-line anti-TB drug by treatment history and by WHO region, 1994–2007.

Global	New	Previous	Combined
Countries	105	94	114
Settings	127	109	138
Any H	10,3 (8.4-12.1)	27,7 (18.7-36.7)	13,3 (10.9-15.8)
Any R	3,7 (2.8-4.5)	17,5 (11.1-23.9)	6,3 (4.7-7.8)
Any S	10,9 (8.0-13.7)	20,1 (12.2-28.0)	12,6 (9.3-16.0)
Any E	2,5 (1.7-3.2)	10,3 (5.0-15.6)	3,9 (2.6-5.2)
Any res.	17,0 (13.6-20.4)	35,0 (24.1-45.8)	20,0 (16.1-23.9)
MDR	2,9 (2.2-3.6)	15,3 (9.6-21.0)	5,3 (3.9-6.6)

AFR	New	Previous	Combined
Countries	21	18	22
Settings	21	18	22
Any H	6,7 (5.2-8.1)	16,9 (8.8-25.0)	8,3 (6.8-9.9)
Any R	1,9 (1.2-2.6)	6,7 (4.4-9.0)	2,7 (1.6-3.8)
Any S	6,9 (2.2-11.6)	9,7 (6.3-13.2)	8,3 (2.6-14.1)
Any E	1,3 (0.6-2.0)	3,5 (1.8-5.1)	2,0 (0.9-3.0)
Any res.	11,4 (6.4-16.5)	21,4 (12.5-30.3)	13,8 (8.0-19.5)
MDR	1,5 (1.0-2.0)	5,8 (3.9-7.7)	2,2 (1.4-3.1)

AMR	New	Previous	Combined
Countries	19	18	21
Settings	19	18	21
Any H	7,9 (5.6-10.3)	20,1 (9.4-30.7)	9,9 (7.0-12.9)
Any R	3,2 (1.0-5.4)	16,4 (4.5-28.2)	5,3 (2.2-8.3)
Any S	9,0 (3.1-14.9)	14,9 (2.8-27.1)	9,6 (3.5-15.6)
Any E	1,5 (0.2-2.8)	5,2 (0.0-10.8)	2,0 (0.2-3.9)
Any res.	14,9 (8.4-21.4)	28,1 (12.4-43.7)	16,7 (9.9-23.4)
MDR	2,2 (0.6-3.8)	13,2 (3.5-22.8)	4,0 (1.7-6.3)

EMR	New	Previous	Combined
Countries	7	7	8
Settings	7	7	8
Any H	6,3 (2.5-10.1)	40,3 (19.8-60.8)	9,9 (3.2-16.7)
Any R	3,3 (0.0-7.3)	41,7 (18.3-65.1)	7,2 (0.0-15.1)
Any S	10,1 (0.8-19.5)	42,2 (21.7-62.8)	13,3 (1.5-25.1)
Any E	1,9 (0.0-4.5)	26,2 (12.0-40.3)	4,2 (0.0-9.2)
Any res.	13,7 (1.3-26.1)	54,4 (26.5-82.3)	17,6 (2.3-33.0)
MDR	2,0 (0.0-4.3)	35,3 (16.4-54.3)	5,4 (0.5-10.4)

EUR (E)	New	Previous	Combined
Countries	13	13	13
Settings	16	15	16
Any H	25,6 (9.5-41.8)	52,2 (30.4-74.0)	38,3 (18.9-57.6)
Any R	11,4 (5.6-17.1)	40,9 (13.8-68.0)	24,7 (10.1-39.2)
Any S	28,8 (8.5-49.0)	52,6 (20.7-84.6)	40,7 (15.7-65.6)
Any E	10,4 (0.9-20.0)	31,2 (6.7-55.8)	19,7 (3.7-35.7)
Any res.	35,8 (15.8-55.7)	62,8 (35.6-90.1)	48,8 (25.3-72.2)
MDR	10,0 (3.8-16.1)	37,7 (12.3-63.0)	22,6 (8.6-36.6)

EUR (WC)	New	Previous	Combined
Countries	27	24	27
Settings	28	25	29
Any H	5,2 (4.0-6.4)	13,9 (11.0-16.8)	6,2 (5.2-7.2)
Any R	1,1 (0.7-1.5)	8,9 (6.8-11.0)	1,9 (1.4-2.3)
Any S	4,0 (1.9-6.0)	9,7 (5.6-13.8)	4,4 (2.1-6.7)
Any E	0,7 (0.3-1.1)	3,9 (2.0-5.8)	1,0 (0.5-1.6)
Any res.	7,9 (5.9-10.0)	17,8 (14.4-21.3)	8,9 (7.2-10.7)
MDR	0,9 (0.5-1.2)	7,7 (5.7-9.8)	1,5 (1.1-2.0)

SEAR	New	Previous	Combined
Countries	6	5	6
Settings	13	6	14
Any H	10,3 (6.9-13.7)	36,8 (26.7-47.0)	15,7 (10.5-20.9)
Any R	3,4 (2.4-4.4)	19,3 (14.1-24.5)	6,9 (4.8-9.0)
Any S	8,9 (5.9-11.8)	21,7 (13.3-30.2)	11,7 (7.5-16.0)
Any E	3,0 (0.7-5.4)	13,8 (0.3-27.3)	4,7 (2.2-7.2)
Any res.	15,8 (11.6-20.0)	42,3 (32.3-52.3)	20,8 (14.2-27.4)
MDR	2,8 (1.9-3.6)	18,8 (13.3-24.3)	6,3 (4.2-8.4)

WPR	New	Previous	Combined
Countries	12	9	17
Settings	23	20	28
Any H	13,3 (10.6-16.0)	34,9 (28.3-41.4)	16,5 (13.3-19.6)
Any R	5,0 (3.4-6.6)	26,6 (20.2-32.9)	8,3 (5.7-11.0)
Any S	14,6 (10.2-19.0)	26,3 (17.2-35.4)	16,2 (11.0-21.2)
Any E	3,0 (2.0-4.0)	13,8 (10.2-17.3)	4,5 (3.3-5.8)
Any res.	22,0 (17.3-26.8)	46,5 (37.7-55.2)	25,3 (19.9-30.7)
MDR	3,9 (2.6-5.2)	21,6 (16.8-26.4)	6,7 (4.6-8.8)

95% confidence levels are given between brackets

AFR = WHO African Region; AMR = WHO Region of the Americas; Any E = any resistance to ethambutol; Any H = any resistance to isoniazid; Any R = any resistance to rifampicin; Any res. = any resistance; Any S = any resistance to streptomycin; EMR = WHO Eastern Mediterranean Region; EUR= WHO European Region; MDR = multidrug resistant; SEAR = WHO South-East Asia Region; WPR = WHO Western Pacific Region.

Figure 14: Weighted mean of resistance to specific drugs among new cases, by WHO region, 1994–2007.

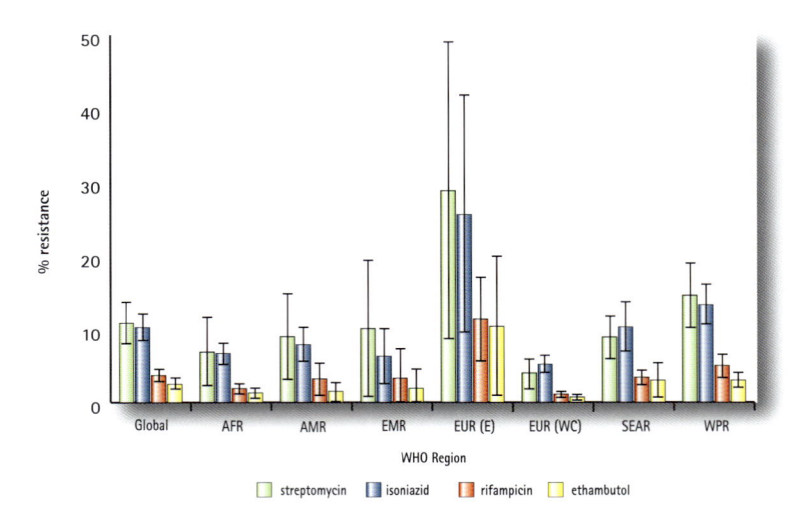

AFR = WHO African Region; AMR = WHO Region of the Americas; EMR = WHO Eastern Mediterranean Region; EUR(E) = WHO European Region (Eastern); EUR(WC) = WHO European Region (Western and Central); SEAR = WHO South-East Asia Region; WPR = WHO Western Pacific Region

Figure 15: Weighted mean of resistance to specific drugs among previously treated cases, by WHO region, 1994–2007.

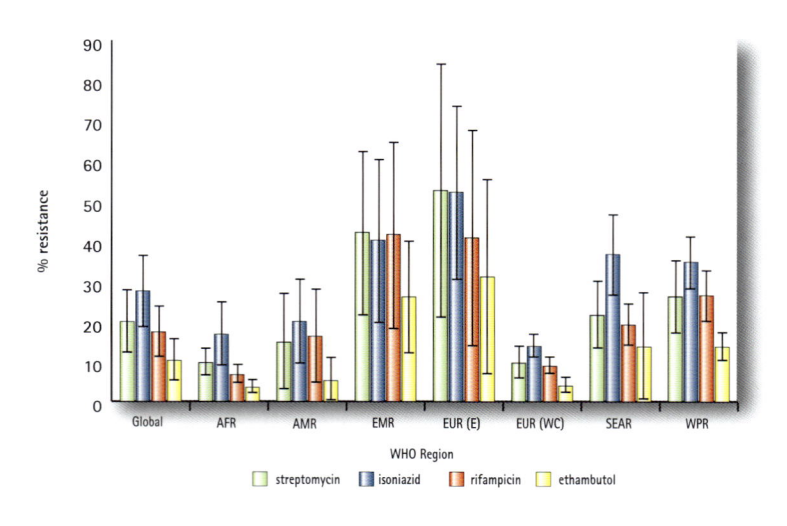

AFR = WHO African Region; AMR = WHO Region of the Americas; EMR = WHO Eastern Mediterranean Region; EUR(E) = WHO European Region (Eastern); EUR(WC) = WHO European Region (Western and Central); SEAR = WHO South-East Asia Region; WPR = WHO Western Pacific Region.

Figure 16: Weighted mean of resistance to specific drugs among all TB cases treated cases, by WHO region, 1994–2007.

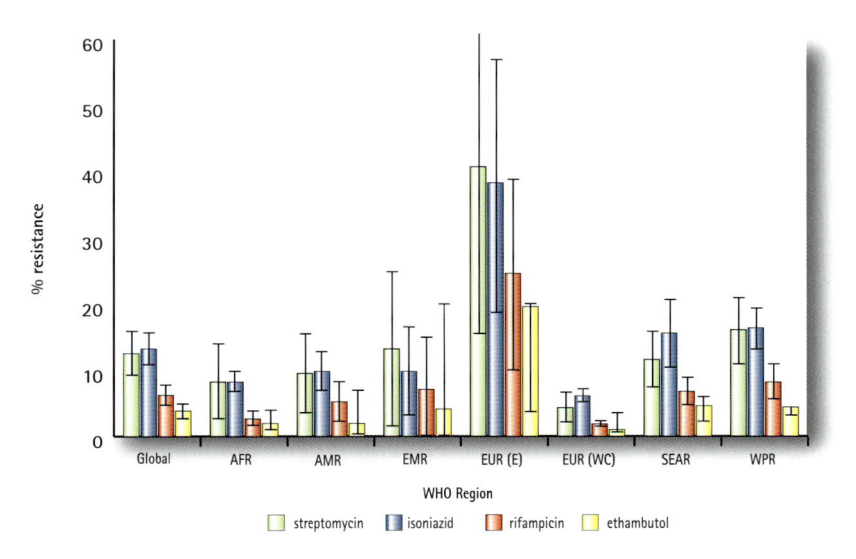

AFR = WHO African Region; AMR = WHO Region of the Americas; EMR = WHO Eastern Mediterranean Region; EUR(E) = WHO European Region (Eastern); EUR(WC) = WHO European Region (Western and Central); SEAR = WHO South-East Asia Region; WPR = WHO Western Pacific Region.

Figure 17: Weighted mean of multidrug-resistant TB among new, previous treated and combined TB cases by WHO region, 1994–2007.

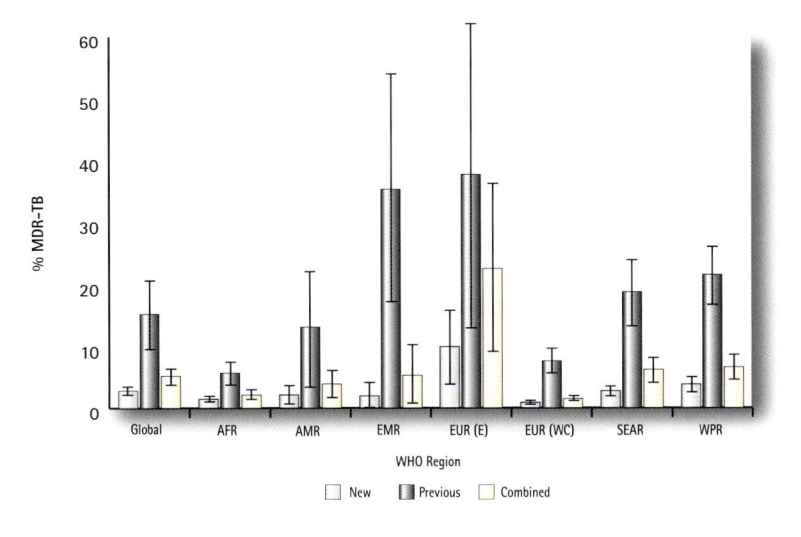

AFR = WHO African Region; AMR = WHO Region of the Americas; EMR = WHO Eastern Mediterranean Region; EUR(E) = WHO European Region (Eastern); EUR(WC) = WHO European Region (Western and Central); SEAR = WHO South-East Asia Region; WPR = WHO Western Pacific Region

A box plot is one way of graphically depicting groups of numerical data through their five-number summaries — that is, the smallest observation, lower quartile (Q1), median, upper quartile (Q3), and largest observation. A box plot also indicates which observations, if any, might be considered outliers. Outliers may present valuable epidemiological clues or information about the validity of data. Box plots are able to visually show different types of populations, without making any assumptions of the underlying statistical distribution. The spacings between the different parts of the box help to indicate variance and skewness, and to identify outliers. Figure 18 shows the distribution of MDR-TB within regions. The widest distribution is in the WHO Eastern European Region, while the narrowest distribution is found in the WHO regions of Central and Western Europe, and Africa. Box plots in Figures 19 and 20 — which show the distribution of any resistance and isoniazid resistance — also show the widest distribution in the WHO Eastern European Region and the narrowest distribution in the WHO regions of Central and Western Europe, and Africa, although these are not as narrow as the distribution of MDR-TB.

Figure 18: Box plot distribution of MDR-TB among combined TB cases by WHO region, 1994–2007.

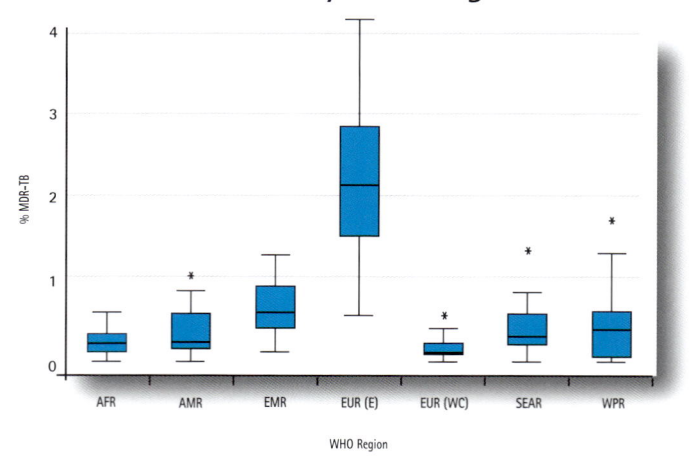

AFR = WHO African Region; AMR = WHO Region of the Americas; EMR = WHO Eastern Mediterranean Region; EUR(E) = WHO European Region (Eastern); EUR(WC) = WHO European Region (Western and Central); SEAR = WHO South-East Asia Region; WPR = WHO Western Pacific Region.

Figure 19: Box plot distribution of any resistance among combined TB cases by WHO region, 1994–2007.

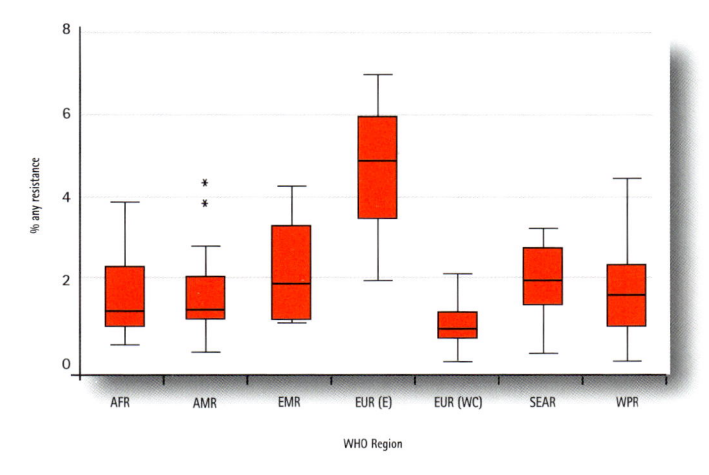

AFR = WHO African Region; AMR = WHO Region of the Americas; EMR = WHO Eastern Mediterranean Region; EUR(E) = WHO European Region (Eastern); EUR(WC) = WHO European Region (Western and Central); SEAR = WHO South-East Asia Region; WPR = WHO Western Pacific Region.

Figure 20: Box plot distribution of any resistance to isoniazid among combined TB cases by WHO region, 1994–2007.

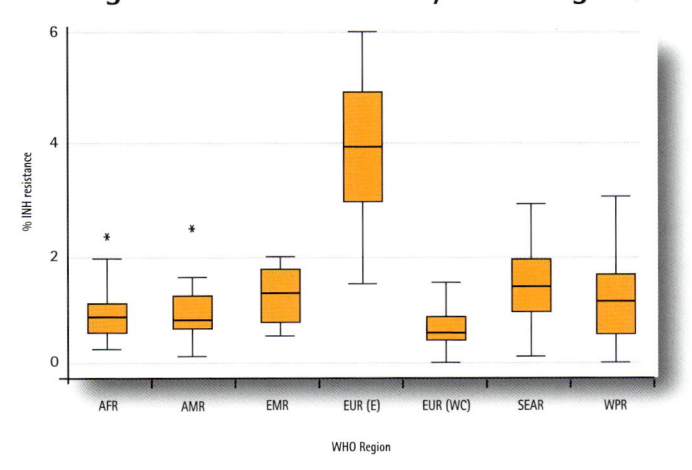

AFR = WHO African Region; AMR = WHO Region of the Americas; EMR = WHO Eastern Mediterranean Region; EUR(E) = WHO European Region (Eastern); EUR(WC) = WHO European Region (Western and Central); SEAR = WHO South-East Asia Region; WPR = WHO Western Pacific Region.

Correlation between multidrug-resistant TB cases in national registers and survey data

The proportion of MDR-TB reported in national registers of cases receiving DST was compared to the proportion of MDR-TB estimated through surveys. The aim was to examine whether routine data can be used to estimate the proportion of MDR-TB in the population. The only region that showed a significant correlation between proportion of MDR-TB reported and the proportion of MDR-TB estimated through surveys was the WHO European Region, suggesting that estimations of MDR-TB are either already based on routine data, or can be in the future. Other regions are not routinely testing for MDR-TB, and surveys will thus continue to play an important role in estimating the MDR-TB burden in these regions.

Figure 21: Correlation of drug resistance survey data with routine notification of multidrug-resistant TB.

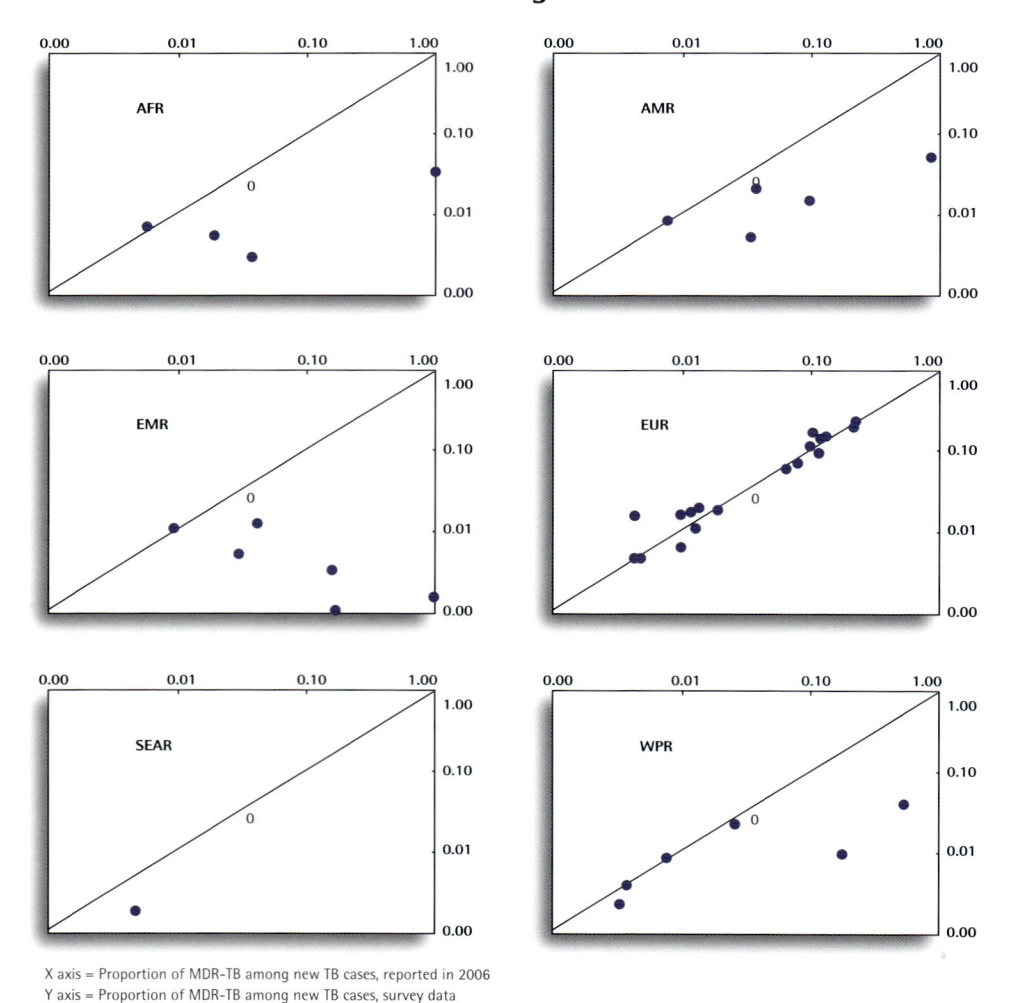

X axis = Proportion of MDR-TB among new TB cases, reported in 2006
Y axis = Proportion of MDR-TB among new TB cases, survey data

AFR = WHO African Region; AMR = WHO Region of the Americas; EMR = WHO Eastern Mediterranean Region; EUR = WHO European Region; SEAR = WHO South-East Asia Region; WPR = WHO Western Pacific Region.

Dynamics of drug resistance over time, 1994–2007

The global project has collected data from 114 countries and 2 SARs of China. The following analysis includes data from all global reports, as well as data provided between the publication of reports. It thus reflects both published and previously unpublished data. This analysis is limited to countries reporting three data points or more (Table 9). Trend information on MDR-TB and resistance to any drug are available for countries reporting more than one year of information in Annexes 6 and 7. A total of 50 countries have reported three or more years of data, 8 countries have reported on two years and 58 countries have reported baseline data only. In countries conducting surveillance on all TB cases, trends are reported on both new and combined cases. In settings conducting surveys, trends are reported on new cases only. Proportions of MDR-TB, isoniazid resistance and any resistance were examined.

Table 9: Data points available for trend analysis by WHO region, 1994–2007.

WHO region	1	2	≥3	Total
Africa	19	2	1	22
Americas	12	3	6	21
Eastern Mediterranean	6	0	2	8
Europe	9	1	30	40
South East Asia	4	0	2	6
Western Pacific	8	2	9	19
Total	**58**	**8**	**50**	**116**

Annexes 6 and 7 provide numbers and proportions of any resistant and MDR-TB for new and combined cases for all settings reporting two data points or more.

Declining trends in resistance

The United States and Hong Kong SAR reported significant decreasing trends in MDR-TB among all TB cases. Hong Kong SAR also showed significant decreases in any resistance among all cases, and isoniazid resistance and MDR-TB among new cases. Both settings report declining TB notifications. Denmark showed significant declines in any drug resistance in both new and combined TB cases. Puerto Rico showed declining trends in any resistance and MDR-TB among combined cases. Singapore showed a significant decrease in prevalence of MDR-TB among all TB cases; however, numbers were small.

Figure 22: Hong Kong SAR, China 1994–2005.

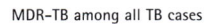

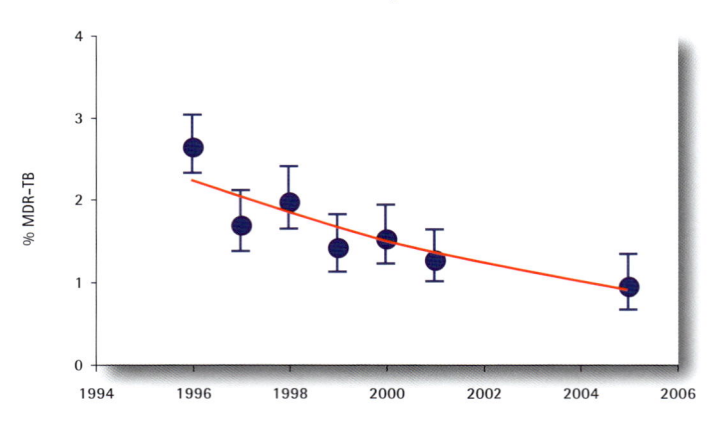

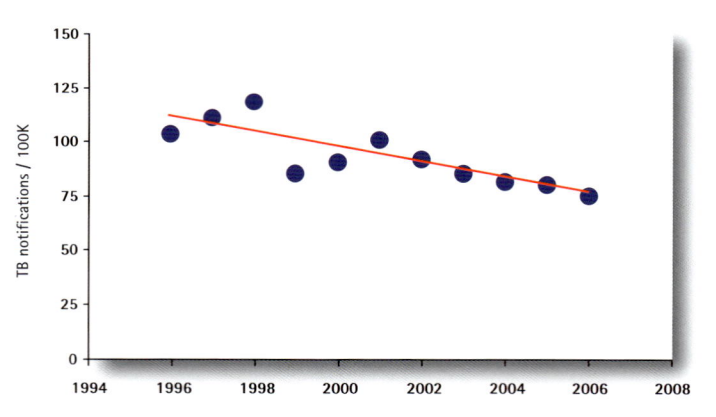

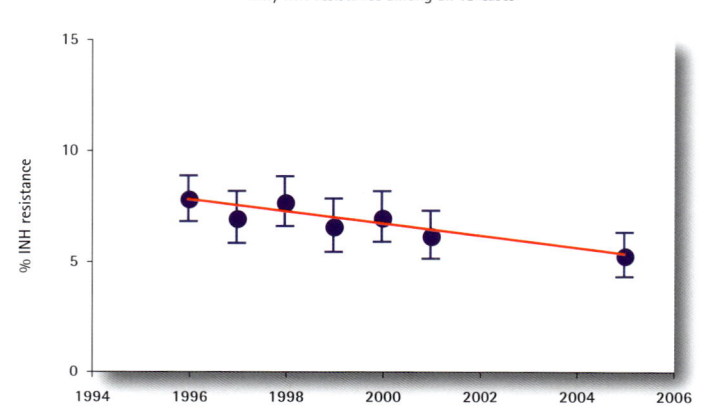

INH = isoniazid; MDR = multidrug resistance; SAR = special administrative region

Figure 23: United States, 1994–2005.

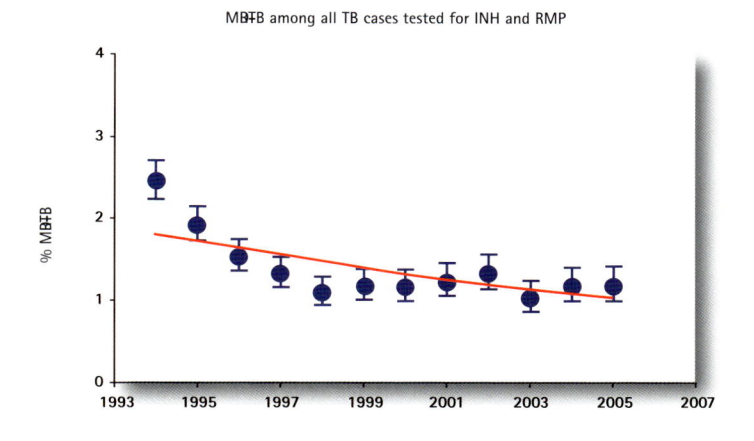

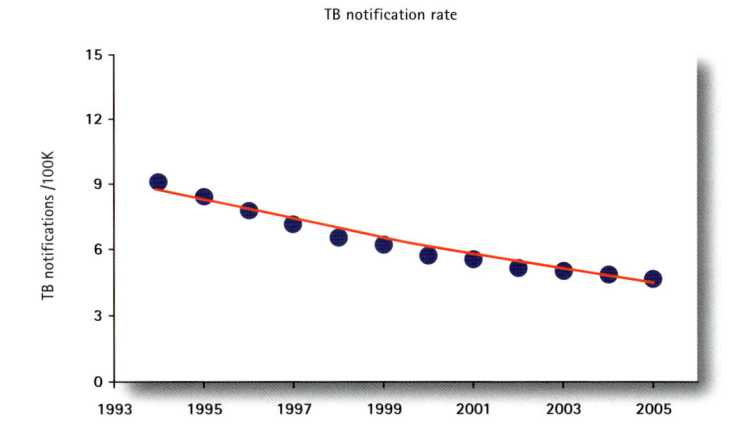

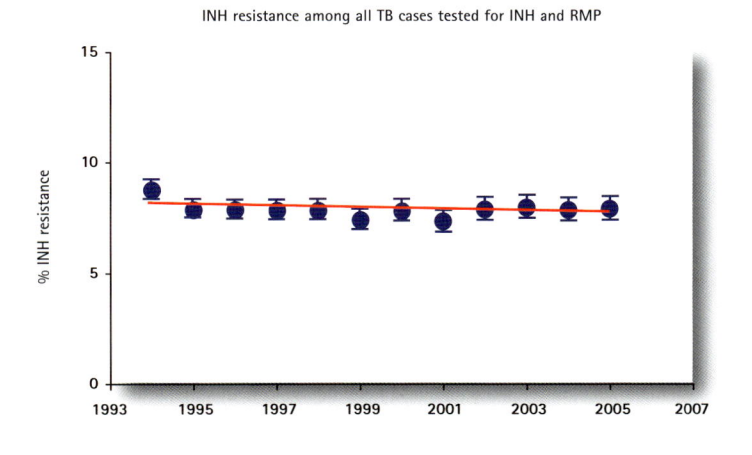

MDR-TB among all TB cases tested for INH and RMP

TB notification rate

INH resistance among all TB cases tested for INH and RMP

INH = isoniazid; MDR = multidrug resistance; RMP = rifampicin; SAR = special administrative region

Stable trends in resistance

Several countries are showing either stable proportion of resistance over time or stable absolute numbers of cases. Many low TB prevalence countries may show fluctuating trends in prevalence of resistance because their overall burden of TB is low; however, most of these countries report small absolute numbers of MDR-TB per year (Figure 24).

Countries of the Baltic region (Estonia, Latvia and Lithuania) are showing relatively stable trends in MDR-TB among new cases, with a slow but significant increase in MDR-TB among new cases in Lithuania. The proportion of resistance remains high in these countries, ranging from 9.8% (CLs, 8.2–11.7) in Lithuania to 13.2% (CLs, 9.7–17.5) in Estonia. These trends in MDR-TB are coupled with declining TB notification rates in all three countries. Estonia has shown the most rapid decline, at about 8% per year, and the TB notification rate declined from 59 per 100 000 in 1998 to 31 per 100 000 in 2006. Latvia has shown a decline of about 6% per year, from 91 TB cases per 100 000 in 1998 to 56 cases in 2006. The notification rate in Lithuania has declined at just under 5.0% per year, from 79 per 100 000 in 1999 to 56 per 100 000 in 2006.

Figure 24: Absolute numbers and proportions of multidrug-resistant TB among low TB prevalence countries, 1994–2007.

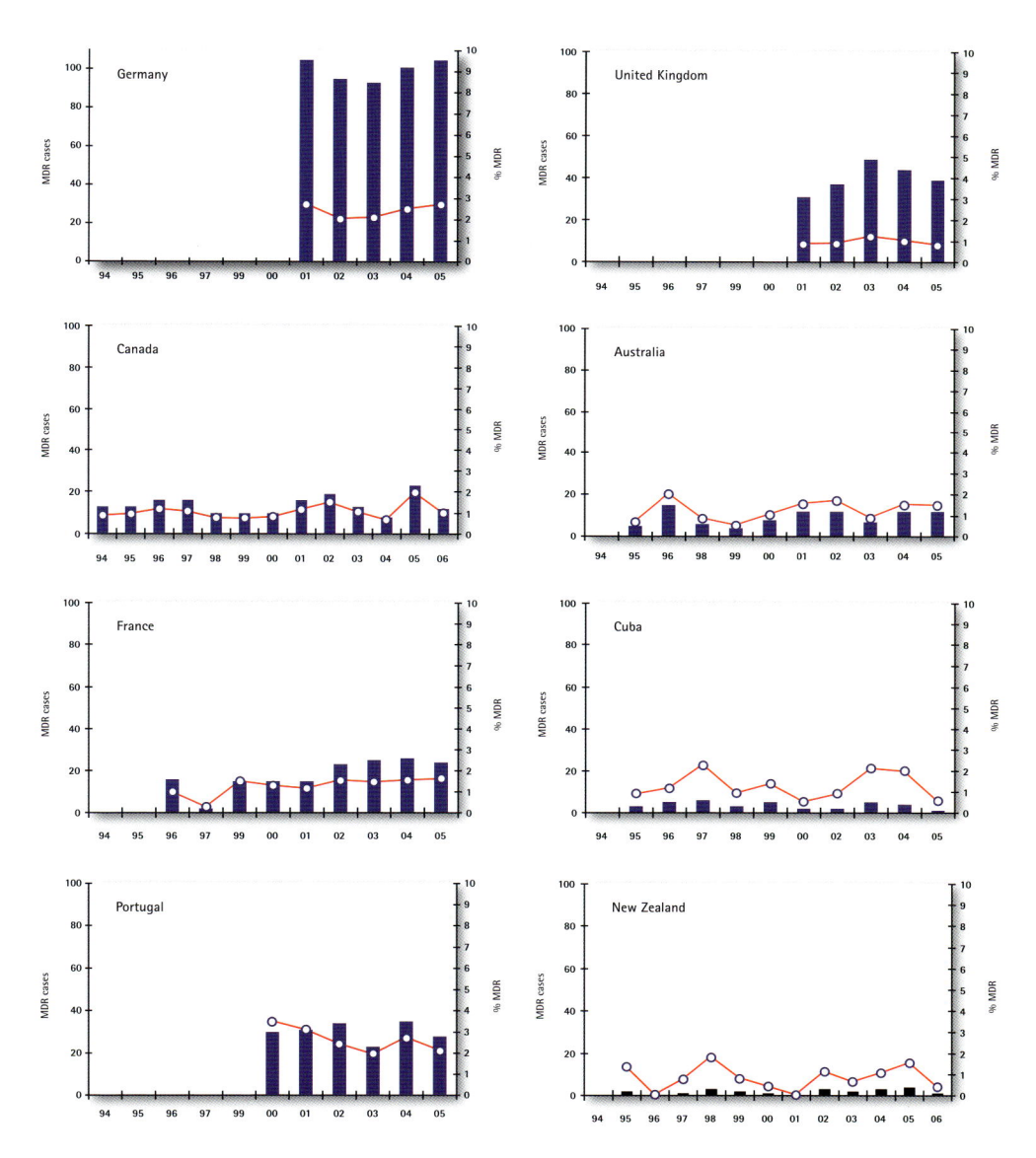

MDR = multidrug resistant

Figure 25: Absolute numbers and proportions of multidrug-resistant TB among new TB cases in the Baltic countries, 1997–2007.

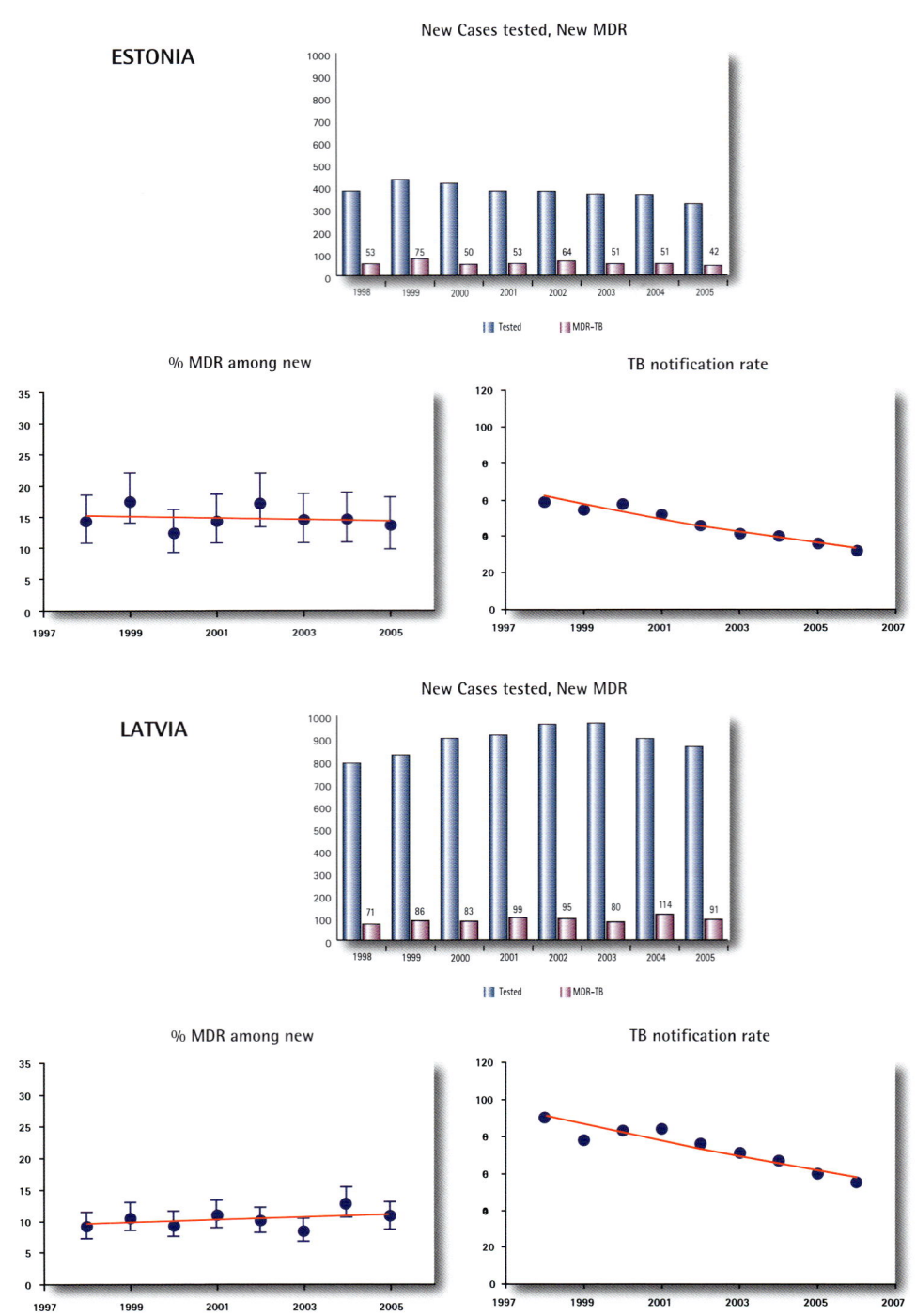

LITHUANIA

New Cases tested, New MDR

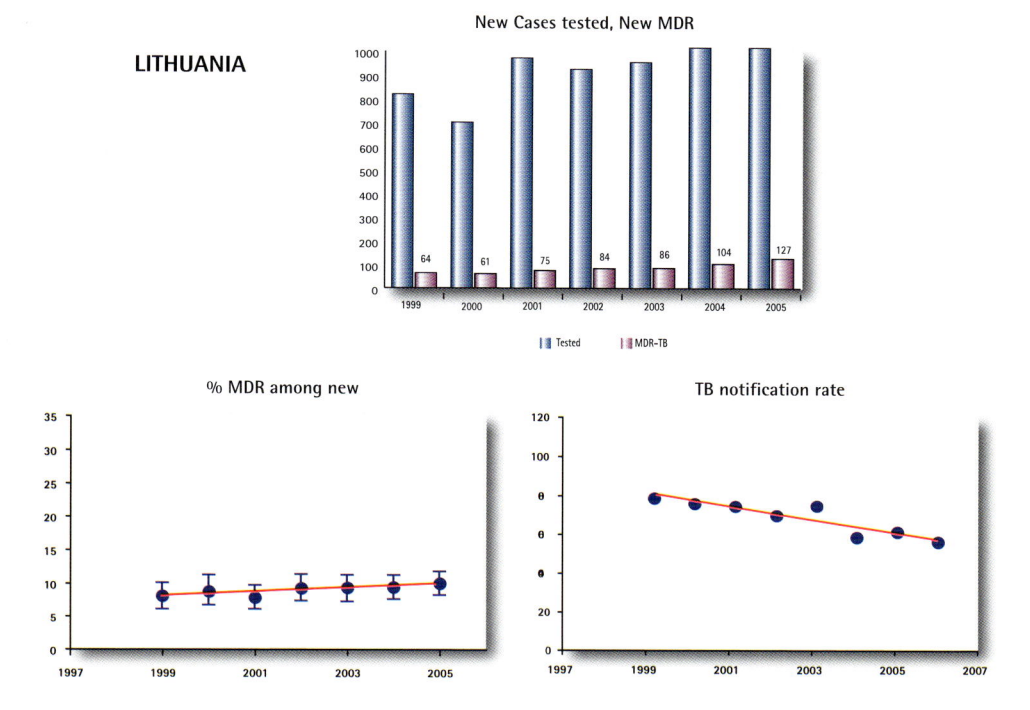

MDR = multidrug resistance

Increasing trends in resistance

In contrast to the stable proportions of MDR-TB reported among new cases in the Baltic countries, data reported to the global project from the Orel and Tomsk oblasts (Russian Federation) indicate statistically significant increases in the proportion of MDR-TB among new TB cases, as well as increases in absolute numbers of cases. Both regions showed increases in isoniazid resistance, though neither were statistically significant. Both regions are showing a slowly declining TB notification rate. In Orel Oblast, the TB notification rate declined from 81 per 100 000 in 2000 to 59 per 100 000 in 2006 — a rate of more than 3% per year. Tomsk Oblast declined by a steady 1.3% per year, from 117 per 100 000 in 2000 to 108 per 100 000 in 2006. During this same period, TB notification rates for the whole of the Russian Federation remained stable.

Figure 26: Absolute numbers and proportions of multidrug-resistant TB among new TB cases in oblasts of the Russian federation, 1997–2007.

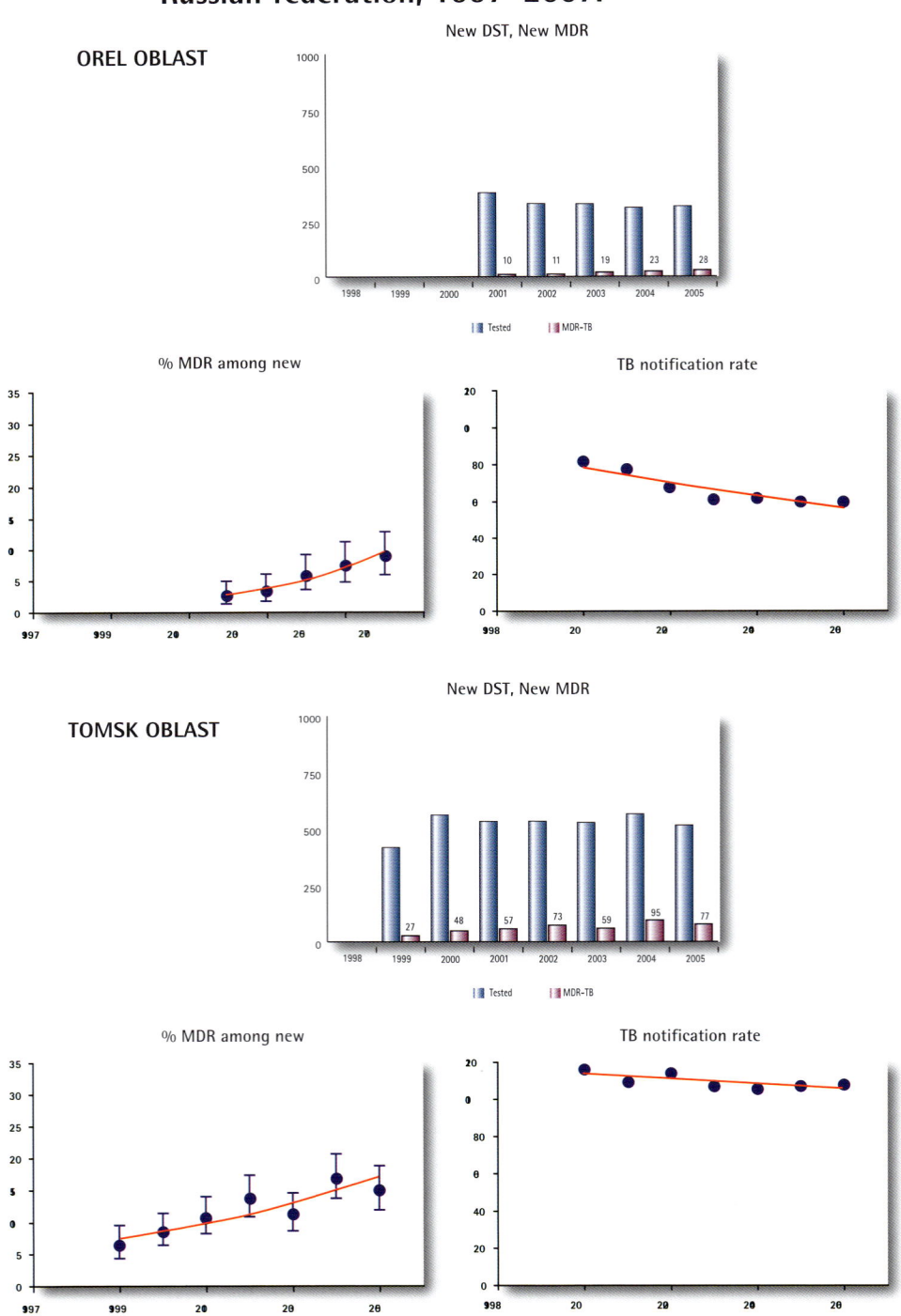

DST = drug susceptibility test; MDR = multidrug resistance

Two countries — the Republic of Korea and Peru — have shown increasing trends in MDR-TB, any resistance and isoniazid resistance among new cases. The data have been reported from three (Peru) and four (Republic of Korea) periodic surveys, and confidence levels are wide; nevertheless, increases in isoniazid and any resistance were statistically significant in both settings[25]. The increase in MDR-TB was statistically significant in the Republic of Korea, which showed a steadily declining TB notification rate from 1994 to 2003. However, from 2004, the TB notification rate has increased slowly, possibly due to expansion of the national surveillance system into the private sector. Similarly, in Peru, the notification rate dropped from 172 per 100 000 in 1996 to 117 per 100 000 in 2003. From 2004 through 2006, the notification rate has stayed around 123–124 per 100 000.

Figure 27: The Republic of Korea, 1996–2005.

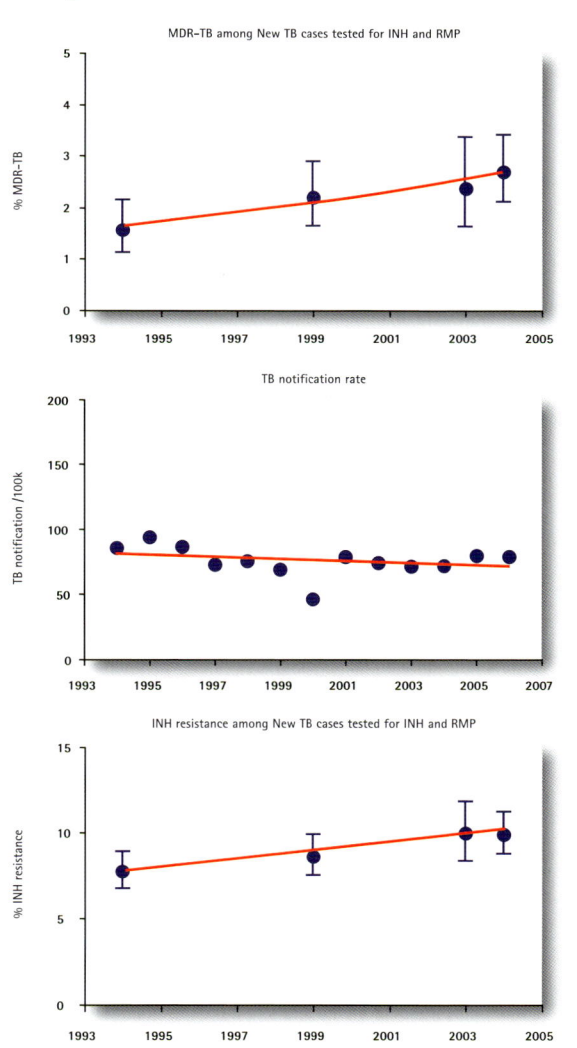

INH = isoniazid; MDR = multidrug resistance

[25] At the time of this report, Peru had not completed rechecking of laboratory results.

Figure 28: Peru, 1996–2005.

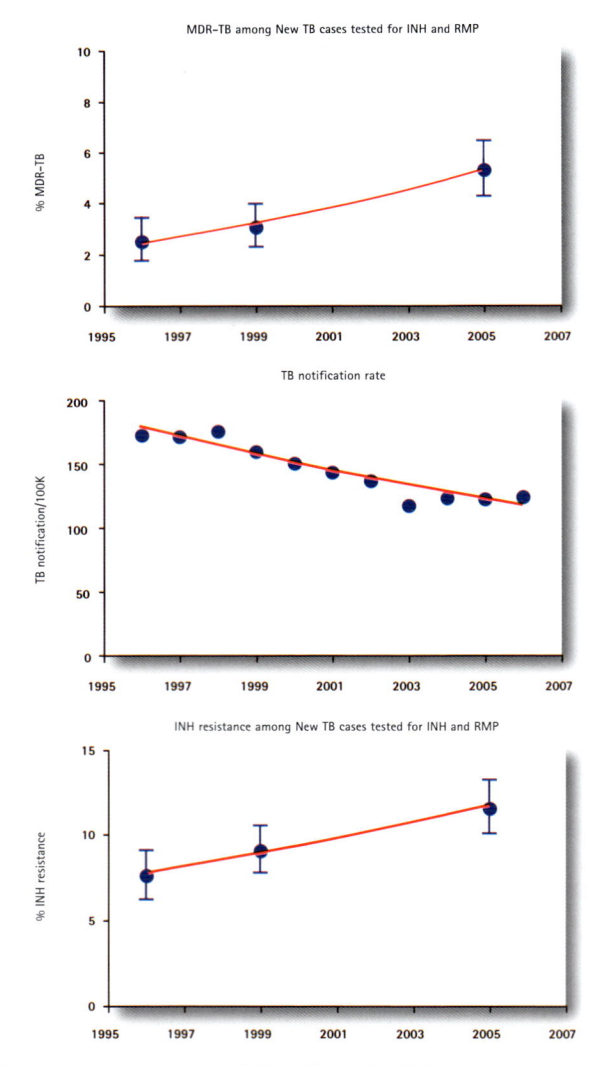

INH = isoniazid; MDR = multidrug resistance; RMP = rifampicin; SAR = special administrative region

GLOBAL ESTIMATES OF MULTIDRUG-RESISTANT TB

Based on drug-resistance data reported from 114 countries and 2 SARs of China, we used a model to:
- estimate the proportion of MDR-TB among new, previously treated and combined TB cases for a further 69 countries
- develop a global estimated burden of incident MDR-TB cases.

New cases

The total number of MDR-TB cases estimated to have occurred in 2006 among newly diagnosed TB cases was 285 718 (95% CLs, 256 072–399 224), or 3.1% (95% CLs, 2.9–4.3) of the total number of new TB cases estimated in 2006 in the 175 countries (9 123 922). The numbers and proportions of MDR-TB among new cases by country are given in Annex 8.

Previously treated cases

The total number of MDR-TB cases among previously treated cases was estimated to be 203 230 (95% CLs, 172 935–242 177) or 19.3% (95% CLs, 18.2–21.3) of the estimated number of previously treated cases in 2006 in the 175 countries (1 052 145). Annex 9 gives the numbers and proportions of MDR-TB among previously treated cases by country.

Total cases

The global estimated number of incident MDR-TB cases in 2006 is 489 139 (95% CLs, 455 093–614 215), which is 4.8% (95% CLs, 4.6–6.0) of the total number of estimated incident TB cases in 2006 in 185 countries (10 229 315)[26]. Two high TB burden countries, China and India, are estimated to have 240 680 cases (95% CLs, 177 608–307 286), which together account for 50% of all estimated incident cases of MDR-TB. The distribution of all MDR-TB cases by country can be found in Annex 10. The numbers and proportions of MDR-TB among new, previously treated and all TB cases by epidemiological region can be found in Annex 11.

Table 10: Estimated numbers and proportions of multidrug-resistant TB among all TB cases by epidemiological region.

Regions	No. of All TB cases	No. of MDR-TB cases	Low 95% CL	High 95% CL	% MDR-TB	Low 95% CL	High 95% CL
Established market economies	105,795	1,317	1,147	1,557	1.2	1.1	1.5
Central Europe	50,502	1,201	623	3,694	2.4	1.3	7.2
Eastern Europe	416,316	80,057	71,893	97,623	19.2	18.0	22.2
Latin America	349,278	12,070	10,523	15,526	3.5	3.0	4.4
Eastern Mediterranean Region	601,225	25,475	15,737	73,132	4.2	2.6	11.9
Africa, low HIV incidence	375,801	8,415	6,889	18,758	2.2	1.9	5.0
Africa, high HIV incidence	2,656,422	58,296	48,718	118,506	2.2	1.9	4.5
South-East Asia	3,464,313	149,615	114,780	217,921	4.3	3.5	6.2
Western Pacific Region	2,173,333	152,694	119,886	188,014	7.0	6.1	8.1
Surveyed countries	7,953,603	408,325	361,264	464,069	5.1	4.7	5.7
Non surveyed countries	2,239,383	80,814	71,684	188,605	3.6	3.2	8.4
All countries (n=185)	10,192,986	489,139	455,093	614,215	4.8	4.6	6.0

CL = confidence level; MDR-TB = multidrug resistant tuberculosis

Supranational Reference Laboratory Network

Performance – as measured by average sensitivity, specificity, efficiency and reproducibility of proficiency testing results – of the SRLN has been at a

---

[26] The number of all estimated TB cases, includes estimated re-treatment cases.

consistently high level over the last five years. On average, specificity, sensitivity, efficiency and reproducibility have stayed between 98–100% for isoniazid, and between 98–100% for rifampicin resistance, with the exception of round 12, where the average specificity was 97%. Performance for ethambutol and streptomycin testing was generally lower. The average sensitivity for ethambutol ranged from 92–96%. Specificity, efficiency and reproducibility were generally between 96% and 98%, except for round 12, where the average reproducibility was 95%. Sensitivity, specificity, efficiency and reproducibility for streptomycin testing were generally between 95% and 98% with the exception of sensitivity in round 12, which was 92%. Network averages are shown in Table 11.

Network averages are important to consider when looking at the overall performance of the network, but disguise variation within the network by round of laboratory proficiency testing. Table 12 shows the variation within the network for the 13th round of proficiency testing; however, in previous rounds, at least one or two laboratories per round showed suboptimal performance. Because results are determined judicially, strains with less than 80% concordance within the network are excluded from standard evaluation; however, these strains have been examined in subsequent studies to determine the reason for borderline results. The number of strains excluded in recent rounds were 9 (rounds 9 and 10), 7 (round 11), 12 (round 12) and 3 (round 13), representing approximately 7% (40/600) of the total strains tested.

Table 11: Average performance of Supranational Reference Laboratory Network laboratories over five rounds of proficiency testing.

Year		No of Laboratories	isoniazid	rifampicin	ethambutol	streptomycin	
	SENSITIVITY						
2002	Round 9	20	99	100	95	96	(%)
2003	Round 10	21	100	99	92	97	(%)
2004	Round 11	23	100	100	96	99	(%)
2005	Round 12	26	98,5	97,8	95	92	(%)
2006	Round 13	26	100	100	93,2	98	(%)
	SPECIFICITY						
2002	Round 9	20	99	99	98	97	(%)
2003	Round 10	21	99	98	99	98	(%)
2004	Round 11	23	100	100	97	99	(%)
2005	Round 12	26	98	97	97	95	(%)
2006	Round 13	26	100	99,6	98,3	97	(%)
	EFFICIENCY						
2002	Round 9	20	99	100	96	96	(%)
2003	Round 10	21	99	99	97	98	(%)
2004	Round 11	23	100	100	97	99	(%)
2005	Round 12	26	98	98	97	94	(%)
2006	Round 13	26	100	100	97	98	(%)
	REPRODUCIBILITY						
2002	Round 9	20	100	100	96	98	(%)
2003	Round 10	21	99	98	99	98	(%)
2004	Round 11	23	99	100	97	100	(%)
2005	Round 12	26	100	98	95	98	(%)
2006	Round 13	26	100	100	96	97	(%)

Table 12: Proficiency testing Round 13 within the Supranational Reference Laboratory Network.

Summary statistics, discordant strains excluded

Round 13

Total participating laboratories: 26

Method used:	No. of labs
1 Proportion method LJ	14
2 Proportion method agar	3
3 Bactec 460	3
4 Resistance ratio	1
5 Absolute concentration	2
6 MGIT	3

Judicial results

ISONIAZID

	\multicolumn{5}{c}{Number of laboratories with results in the range of}	Average score
	100%	95-99%	90-94%	80-89%	<80%	
Sensitivity	26	0	0	0	0	100%
Specificity	26	0	0	0	0	100%
Predictive value resistant	26	0	0	0	0	100%
Predictive value susceptibile	26	0	0	0	0	100%
Efficiency	26	0	0	2	0	100%
Reproductibility	26	1	1	0	0	100%

RIFAMPICIN

	100%	95-99%	90-94%	80-89%	<80%	Average score
Sensitivity	26	0	0	0	0	100%
Specificity	24	0	2	0	0	100%
Predictive value resistant	24	0	2	0	0	99%
Predictive value susceptibile	26	0	0	0	0	100%
Efficiency	24	2	0	1	0	100%
Reproductibility	25	0	1	1	0	100%

STREPTOMYCIN

	100%	95-99%	90-94%	80-89%	<80%	Average score
Sensitivity	21	0	4	1	0	98%
Specificity	20	0	4	0	2	97%
Predictive value resistant	20	0	4	0	2	96%
Predictive value susceptibile	21	0	5	0	2	99%
Efficiency	15	9	0	2	1	98%
Reproductibility	20	0	5	1	1	97%

ETHAMBUTOL

	100%	95-99%	90-94%	80-89%	<80%	Average score
Sensitivity	18	0	0	5	3	93%
Specificity	20	5	0	1	0	98%
Predictive value resistant	20	0	0	5	1	96%
Predictive value susceptibile	18	5	2	1	0	97%
Efficiency	14	6	4	2	0	97%
Reproductibility	17	0	8	0	1	96%

Table 13: Links within the Supranational Reference Laboratory Network.

Country	WHO region	Laboratory	Routine
Algeria	AFR	Laboratoire de la Tuberculose, Institut Pasteur d'Algérie, Alger, Algeria	Benin, Jordan, Syria Mauritania, Morocco
Argentina	AMR	Mycobacteria Laboratory, National Institute of Infectious Diseases ANLIS "Dr Carlos G. Malbran," Buenos Aires, Argentina	Brazil, Cuba, Paraguay Uruguay, Venezuela
Australia	WPR	Mycobacterium Reference Laboratory, Institute of Medical and Veterinary Science, Adelaide, Australia	Indonesia
Australia	WPR	Queensland Mycobacterium Reference Laboratory, Brisbane, Australia	Eritrea, New Zealand, Kenya
Belgium	EUR	Département de Microbiologie, Unité de Mycobactériologie Institut de Médecine Tropicale, Antwerp, Belgium	Bangladesh, Benin, Brazil, Burundi, Cameroon, DR Congo, Mali, Rwanda, Senegal, Slovakia, Sudan, Tanzania, Zimbabwe
Chile	AMR	Instituto de Salud Publica de Chile, Santiago, Chile	Bolivia, Colombia, Dominican Republic, Ecuador, Peru
Czech Republic	EUR	National Institute of Public Health, Prague, Czech Republic	Slovakia
Egypt	EMR	Central Health Laboratory, Ministry opf Health and Population, Cairo, Egypt	Jordan, Libya, Pakistan, Sudan, Syria, Yemen
France	EUR	Institut Pasteur, Centre National de Référencen des Mycobacteries, Paris, France	Côte d'Ivoire, Central African Repoublic, Guinea Lebanon, New Caledonia
Germany	EUR	Kuratorium Tuberkulose in der Welt e.V., IML (Institut für Mikrobiologie und Laboratoriumsdiagnostik) Gauting, Germany	Bhutan, Nepal,Tajikistan, Ukraine (Donetsk), Uzbekistan
Germany	EUR	National Reference Center for Mycobacteria, Borstel, Germany	Austria, Armenia, Azerbaijan, Bosnia and Herzegovina, Croatia, Cyprus, Kazakhstan, Kyrgyzstan, Moldova, Nukus region (UZB and TKM), Serbia, Slovenia Slovakia, South Sudan (MSF)
China, Hong Kong SAR,	WPR	TB Reference Laboratory Department of Health, SAR Hong Kong, China	Provincial surveys China Nationwide survey China
India	SEAR	TB Research Centre (TRC), Indian Council of Medical Research, Chennai, India	Provincial surveys India, DPR Korea, Maldives, Sri Lanka
Italy	EUR	Istituto Superiore di Sanità Dipartimento di Malattie Infettive, Parassitarie e Immunomediate, Rome, Italy and Laboratory of Bacteriology & Medical Mycology and San Raffaele del Monte Tabor Foundation (hSR), Milan, Italy	Albania, Bahrain, Bulgaria, Burkina Faso, Kosovo, Mozambique, Nigeria, Oman, Turkey, TFYR Macedonia, Qatar
Japan	WPR	Research Institute of Tuberculosis Japan Anti-Tuberculosis Association, Tokya, Japan	Cambodia, Mongolia, Philippines Singapore, Yemen
Korea	WPR	Korean Institute of Tuberculosis, Seoul, Korea	Philippines
Mexico	AMR	Departamento de Micobacterias Instituto de Diagnostico y Referencia Epidemiologicos (INDRE), Mexico	Belize, Costa Rica, El Salvador, Guatemala, Nicaragua, Panama
Netherlands	EUR	National Institute of Public Health and the Environment (RIVM), Bilthoven, Netherlands	Ethiopia, Poland, Viet Nam
Portugal	EUR	Centro de Tuberculose e Micobacterias (CTM) Instituto Nacional de Saude, Porto, Portugal	
South Africa	AFR	The Medical Research Council, TB Research Lead Programme Operational and Policy Research, Pretoria, South Africa	Lesotho, Malawi, Namibia, Zambia, Zimbabwe
Spain	EUR	Servicio de Microbiologia, Hospital Universitaris, Vall d'Hebron, Barcelona, Spain	Provincial surveys Spain
Sweden	EUR	Swedish Institute for Infectious Disease Control (SIDC), Solna, Sweden	Belarus, Estonia, Denmark, Finland Iceland, Islamic Republic of Iran Latvia, Lithuania, Norway, Romania Russian Federation
Thailand	SEA	National TB Reference Laboratory Center Tuberculosis Cluster, Bangkok, Thailand	Bangladesh, Indonesia, Myanmar
United Kingdom of Great Britain and Northern Ireland	EUR	Health Protection Agency , National Mycobacterium Reference Unit Department of Infectious Diseases, United Kingdom	Belgium, France, Hungary Ireland, Israel, Malta, Samara Oblast, Russian Federation Switzerland, The Gambia, Seychelles
United States of America	AMR	Centers for Disease Control and Prevention, Mycobacteriology/ Tuberculosis Laboratory, Georgia, USA	Botswana, CAREC, Guyana, Haiti, Orel Oblast, Russian Federation, Mexico, Puerto Rico Surinam
United States of America	AMR	Massachusetts State Laboratory, Massachusetts, USA	Peru, Tomsk Oblast, Russian Federation

AFR = WHO African Region; AMR = WHO Region of the Americas; EMR = WHO Eastern Mediterranean Region; EUR = WHO European Region; SEAR = WHO South-East Asia Region; WPR = WHO Western Pacific Region.

DISCUSSION

OVERVIEW

From 1994 through 2007, the global project has collected data from areas representing almost 50% of the world's TB cases. On the whole, coverage of the project is increasing, with notable expansion in high TB burden countries and in countries with high MDR-TB prevalence; however, coverage varies widely. The number of countries submitting survey protocols through national ethics committees has increased, as has attention to quality assurance of patient classification, laboratory results and data entry.

The areas represented in this project are those with at least the minimum requirements to conduct drug resistance surveys. Laboratory capacity remains the largest obstacle, but other operational components required to conduct surveys also strain the capacity of most NTPs, resulting most importantly in the inability to determine trends in most high-burden countries. HIV testing continues to scale up, but has proven difficult to incorporate where testing and treatment are not already an established component of routine care. DST to second-line anti-TB drugs is not available in most countries. Newly available policy guidance will assist in developing capacity; however, SRLs will continue to play an important role in providing second-line testing of selected isolates.

The primary success of the project has been its ability to collect comparative baseline data on resistance to first-line anti-TB drugs from areas representing half of the world's TB population; the project has also strengthened laboratories through the SRLN. However, the project has generally not achieved its primary objective, which is to measure trends in drug resistance in high-burden countries. As part of the Global Plan to Stop TB, 2006–2015, all countries are committed to scaling up diagnostic networks. Nevertheless, until culture and drug-susceptibility testing are the standard of diagnosis everywhere, surveys will continue to be important for monitoring resistance, as is clearly shown by the poor correlation of survey data to routine reporting of MDR-TB in most regions. However, operational difficulties in the implementation of repeated surveys show that it may be time to re-evaluate the survey methods used, and to coordinate supplementary research to answer the epidemiological questions that routine drug resistance surveillance cannot.

SURVEY METHODS

There are operational, technical and methodological barriers to the implementation and repetition of drug-resistance surveys in most high-burden

countries. The foremost operational barrier is the laboratory capacity. Other operational barriers include:
- the considerable human resources needed to interview and verify patient classification
- the extensive national and international transport networks required to ship sputum specimens, cultures and *M. tuberculosis* isolates within and across national borders.

Some desirable components of surveys – for example, larger sample sizes, better differentiation of subcategories of previously treated cases, HIV testing and DST to second-line drugs – come at great additional expense and workload to the NTP. Therefore, surveys tend to be repeated infrequently.

Current survey methods are based on smear-positive cases for operational reasons; that is, smear-positive cases are more likely to result in a positive culture required for drug-susceptibility testing. Inclusion of smear-negative TB cases may increase survey sample sizes by up to 10 times. Currently, there is no evidence to suggest that smear-negative cases may have different proportions of resistance than smear-positive cases; however, HIV-coinfected TB cases are more frequently smear negative, which means that exclusion of smear-negative cases from surveys may underestimate the proportion of resistance in HIV-coinfected populations.

Current survey methods are based on patients notified in the public sector; they do not attempt to evaluate prevalent cases, chronic populations of patients or patients in the private sector. There are significant operational difficulties in designing such surveys within the context of routine programmes, and the resulting information may not warrant the expense required. Additional research may be useful to explore the prevalence of drug resistance in these three populations.

Another limitation of current methodology has been the ability to determine true acquired resistance. Previous reports have suggested that resistance among previously treated cases may be a useful proxy for acquired resistance. Previously treated cases are a heterogeneous group that may also represent cases that were primarily infected with a resistant strain, failed therapy and acquired further resistance. These cases also may include patients re-infected with resistant isolates [7, 8, 15]. Without the ability to repeat drug-susceptibility testing, and without the use of molecular tools, it is difficult to determine true acquired resistance. Risk factors for acquisition of resistance, particularly in HIV coinfected populations, warrant further research.

If surveillance coverage and determination of trends is to be scaled up in high-burden countries, we need to simplify the process of surveys for NTPs. A study in UR Tanzania is attempting to validate rapid molecular methods against phenotypic methods in the context of drug resistance surveys, and assess feasibility. Because understanding of the mutations causing resistance is incomplete, use of molecular methods alone would limit the amount of information obtained to one or two drugs. However, a substantial advantage would be the reduced laboratory capacity required and the transportation of non-infectious material. Laboratory testing could be carried out within or outside of the country.

When considering the number of drugs tested in routine surveys, it is important to keep in mind that, at present, the ability to adjust regimens for TB treatment is limited in most countries, and generally four primary regimens are all

that is provided:
- category I for smear-positive cases
- category III for smear-negative cases
- category II for re-treatment cases
- category IV for MDR-TB cases.

In terms of programmes, surveillance of rifampicin resistance, isoniazid resistance (MDR-TB) and XDR-TB are the most critical trends to follow.

If rapid rifampicin and isoniazid testing could be used in the context of surveillance (where MDR-TB treatment programmes exist), patients identified with MDR-TB could be rapidly enrolled into a treatment programme, and further culture and drug-susceptibility testing could be undertaken to determine resistance to second-line drugs. Where phenotypic methods are used, another option could be to add a fluroquinolone and one or two second-line injectable agents to the panel of drugs tested, or replace streptomycin and ethambutol with a fluroquinolone and an injectable agent.To enable better assessment of trends in drug resistance over time, one option might be to keep population-based clusters open throughout the year. Patients would be classified by treatment history on a routine basis, and sputum samples or smears could be transported to the NRL for a period of time each year. Alternatively, molecular testing for rifampicin, or rifampicin and isoniazid, could be conducted for a determined number of cases per month. If a point-of-care test were available, this could simplify the process even further. All cases with rifampicin resistance would be further screened for resistance to second-line drugs, and enrolled on treatment. These sites could also develop capacity for programme management, and be used for screening all treatment-failure cases and cases classified as high risk for drug resistance, as outlined in the Global Plan to Stop TB, 2006–2015.

It is important to distinguish between population-based surveys used for epidemiological purposes, surveys used for programme-related reasons and studies designed to answer research questions. Many countries are conducting both epidemiological surveys and surveys designed to answer relevant programme-related questions; for example, they are:
- determining the proportion of category I and category II failure cases that have MDR-TB, to develop a case-finding strategy for MDR-TB cases
- conducting second-line DST on risk groups (e.g. chronic cases, prison populations) and known MDR-TB cases, to:
  - examine the extent of second-line anti-TB drug resistance in these populations
  - inform MDR-TB treatment regimens, where regimens are standardized.

Transmission dynamics and acquisition of resistance are areas that undoubtedly require further research, but are difficult to answer in the context of routine surveillance in most settings. A subgroup on research for MDR-TB has recently been set up with the Stop TB Working Group on MDR-TB; the subgroup may play a key role in protocol development, and in coordinating and implementing global research studies.

There are several possibilities for improving current surveillance mechanisms using new molecular tools as well as modified survey methods. WHO plans to coordinate a meeting in 2008 to evaluate current methods and develop recommendations for revisions of the current surveillance strategies.

MAGNITUDE AND TRENDS

Survey data indicate that proportions of resistance to any TB drug and MDR-TB are lowest in Central and Western Europe, followed by African countries and then the Americas. The Eastern Mediterranean and South-East Asia regions show moderate proportions of resistance, followed by the Western Pacific region. Eastern Europe continues to report the highest proportions of resistance globally and for all first-line drugs. There are important variations within regions, particularly in the Eastern Mediterranean and the Western Pacific regions, and in Europe if Central, Eastern and Western Europe are grouped together (although Central and Western Europe show little variation in resistance across the region). All WHO regions have reported outliers.

Trends are showing a range of scenarios. Rapid decreases in MDR-TB are reported from Hong Kong SAR and the United States. Stable trends in MDR-TB are seen in Thailand, in limited data from Viet Nam, in three Baltic countries and in many low TB prevalence countries. Increases in MDR-TB and a slowing in the decline in the TB notification rates have been seen in the Republic of Korea and in Peru. Supporting data suggest weaknesses in TB control in Peru. In the Republic of Korea, the slowing in the decline of the notification rate has been attributed to an expanding surveillance system that reaches the private sector. Meanwhile, case detection and success rates remain high, and the burden of TB is shifting to the older population, which is inconsistent with the recent increase in MDR-TB among new TB cases. The two oblasts in the Russian Federation are showing increases in the proportion of MDR-TB among new cases at a rapid rate, while the TB notification rate in these regions is falling slowly. Although the global burden of MDR-TB can be estimated, it is not possible to estimate global trends in MDR-TB, because of the few trends available from high-burden countries.

The data reflect TB programmes at various stages of implementation; thus, trends must be interpreted in the context of additional relevant programme indicators. Programme improvement can affect the prevalence of resistance in several ways. A better programme can reduce the overall number of cases, particularly re-treated cases; however, difficult (resistant) cases may persist. Thus, in some instances, an increase in MDR-TB proportion in a population may reflect a stable number of MDR-TB cases but a decrease in the overall re-treatment population. Alternatively, it may be the result of successful treatment of susceptible cases, with insufficient case management of MDR-TB cases. It is also possible that, as diagnostic systems improve, coverage and reporting of culture and DST may result in increases in reported case numbers. Improvement in laboratory proficiency, particularly the sensitivity and specificity of drug-susceptibility testing, may also affect the observed prevalence of resistance. The scenarios outlined above highlight the importance of evaluating trends in prevalence of drug resistance within the context of relevant programme developments.

EXTENSIVELY DRUG-RESISTANT TB

XDR-TB is more expensive and difficult to treat than MDR-TB, and outcomes for patients are much worse[16, 17]. Understanding the magnitude and distribution of XDR-TB is therefore important.

Data included in this report are the first representative information available on XDR-TB, but have limitations. One limitation is the insufficient quality assurance of drug-susceptibility testing for second-line drugs. A number of settings reported results that were tested by an SRL, but this was not the case for most settings. Another limitation is that second-line drug-susceptibility testing is not available in most countries. The cost of shipping of isolates and the cost of second-line testing is significant. Therefore, in most settings, only MDR-TB isolates are tested for resistance to second-line drugs. Even in countries where second-line drug-susceptibility testing is routinely conducted, usually only isolates with MDR-TB or other extensive resistance patterns will receive DST to selected second-line drugs. This situation limits our understanding of the emergence of second-line resistance to all but the highest risk cases; this may be particularly relevant for fluroquinolones, which are widely used and are an important component of second-line anti-TB therapy.

There are problems in using MDR-TB cases tested for second-line drugs as a denominator in survey settings where the number of MDR-TB cases detected in the nationwide survey sample may be small, and may not reflect the true proportion of XDR-TB among all MDR-TB cases. Alternatively, examining cases in MDR-TB treatment programmes may also be biased towards chronic cases and may overestimate the proportion of XDR-TB among all MDR-TB cases.

The current recommendation in the context of surveys is to conduct second-line DST on the sample MDR-TB cases detected in the survey, and to conduct separate surveys relevant to the programme within MDR-TB treatment programmes or within risk groups such as treatment failures.

Despite limitations in the quality assurance of laboratory testing, data from this report indicate that XDR-TB is widespread, with 45 countries having reported at least one case. Most countries that reported were low TB burden countries that reported very few cases, and therefore do not give an indication of global magnitude. Japan and the Republic of Korea (in a previous study) have shown a high proportion of XDR-TB among MDR; however, these countries have a small underlying population of MDR-TB cases. The sentinel system in Japan is hospital based, and previous data reported from the Republic of Korea — based on the national laboratory register that represents 70% of cases in the country — may be biased towards the most ill patients and may be overestimating the proportion of all MDR-TB cases that are XDR-TB. Data from a nationwide survey in the Republic of Korea, examining 110 MDR-TB patients, showed a significantly lower prevalence of XDR-TB among MDR-TB cases.

Data on second-line drug resistance are currently unavailable from China, although there are plans to conduct second-line DST on MDR-TB cases detected in an ongoing nationwide survey. Second line-DST from the nationwide survey in the Philippines was not completed at the time of this publication; however, the level of resistance to fluoroquinolones in the MDR-TB patients under treatment (50%) suggests that further investigation is required.

Although the numbers are small, most of the data available from African countries reveal a low proportion of XDR-TB among MDR-TB cases. South Africa is the outlier in the region. Although a moderate proportion of XDR-TB was reported, and there are known biases related to the selection of cases for testing[27], this constitutes a large burden of cases, most of whom are HIV positive.

No countries from the WHO Eastern Mediterranean Region have yet reported representative data on second-line drug resistance, although studies are planned, and Morocco is having all MDR-TB isolates from the nationwide survey further tested.

India has conducted second-line DST in surveys in both Gujarat and Maharasthra, but data are not yet available. Myanmar is surveying risk populations, but is currently showing low proportions of second-line drug resistance. Quinolones are widely available in this region; therefore, determining the extent of resistance to this class of drug is a priority, as is establishing cross-resistance between early and later generations of quinolones.

The high proportion of XDR-TB among MDR-TB (ranging from 4.0% to >20%), and the large underlying burden of MDR-TB, suggests a significant problem within the countries of the former Soviet Union, where drug resistance is widespread. Second-line drugs are locally available in most of the countries of the former Soviet Union and have been widely used for a long time.

These data highlight the need to strengthen global capacity for both diagnosis and surveillance of resistance to second-line drugs if the true magnitude and distribution of XDR-TB are to be understood.

DRUG RESISTANCE AND HIV

There is a well-documented association between TB and HIV. However, although outbreaks of drug-resistant TB among HIV-positive patients have been widely documented in nosocomial and other congregate settings[18, 19], little information is available about the association of HIV and drug-resistant TB on a population level.[20-22] The primary reason for the lack of information is that HIV and anti-TB drug-susceptibility testing have not been sufficiently accessible for joint surveys under routine conditions. The scale up of HIV testing has opened up possibilities for joint surveys; however, in this report only seven countries were able to provide information on drug-susceptibility testing disaggregated by HIV status. In most settings with a high TB burden, either drug-resistant TB or HIV (or both) are rare; thus, routine surveys may not capture a sufficiently large number of either drug-resistant TB patients or HIV-positive patients to examine an association with sufficient statistical power[3]. To examine the association on a population level, it may be necessary to sample HIV-positive and HIV-negative TB patients separately.

There are two main reasons why drug resistant-TB may be associated with HIV. The first is the documented acquisition of rifamycin resistance among TB patients living with HIV and under treatment for TB, although this may also be due to intermittent therapy. Anti-TB drug malabsorption has also been documented in

---

[27] Data from a retrospective review of the National Health Laboratory Service of South Africa were presented at the 38th World Conference on Lung Health. 8-12 November 2007. Cape Town, South Africa.

patient cohorts in settings of high HIV prevalence, which suggests that HIV-positive TB patients may be at greater risk of acquiring resistance. The second reason relates to exposure. HIV-positive patients and drug-resistant TB patients may have similar risk factors, such as history of hospitalization, which may mean that HIV-positive TB patients are at a higher risk of exposure to resistant forms of disease. It is also possible that HIV-positive patients may be more susceptible to TB infection once exposed, although there are no data to show this.

The epidemiological impact of HIV on the epidemic of drug-resistant TB is not known, and may depend on several factors. HIV-positive TB cases are more likely to be smear negative; also, delayed diagnosis of drug resistance and unavailability of treatment have led to high death rates in people living with HIV. Both of these factors, smear negativity and shorter duration of disease due to mortality, may suggest a lower rate of general transmission. However, HIV-positive cases progress rapidly to disease, and in settings where MDR-TB is prevalent — either in the general population, or in the local population such as a hospital or a district — this may lead to rapid development of a pool of drug-resistant TB patients, or an outbreak.

The data reported from the majority of countries were not strong enough to examine an association between HIV and drug resistance. However, the data available from Donetsk Oblast, Ukraine and from Latvia indicated a significant association between HIV and MDR-TB. Additional information on risk factors, including history of hospitalization or imprisonment, was not available for this analysis, so the specific reasons for the association are not known. Both countries have a high underlying prevalence of MDR-TB, as well as an emerging HIV epidemic, which initially was concentrated among risk groups, but has now become more generalized. Despite some of the weakness in these data and in subsequent analysis, the association between HIV and MDR-TB is concerning, particularly given the implications for the clinical management of these patients. As both countries have well-developed diagnostic infrastructure, continued monitoring of the epidemic will be crucial, to gain a better understanding of how HIV may affect the epidemiology of drug resistance in the region.

Rapid progression to death in HIV-positive MDR-TB patients in both outbreaks and treatment cohorts has been widely documented[18, 23]. Anti-retroviral treatment for HIV does appear to benefit coinfected MDR-TB patients; however, co-management of treatment for both diseases is complicated. Currently, most TB control programmes in high-burden countries have neither the diagnostic infrastructure to detect an outbreak nor the programme capacity to manage one. Given the impact on mortality, outbreaks should be avoided at all cost. Development of infection control measures in congregate settings and diagnostic screening tools for rapid identification of drug-resistant TB is a priority for all countries, but particularly for those with high prevalence of HIV or MDR-TB.

From a global perspective, routine diagnosis of both HIV and drug-resistant TB should be scaled up for patient benefit. Better surveillance data may help in developing an understanding of the relationship between these epidemics; however, additional studies should be undertaken in several settings to answer the questions that surveys cannot.

GLOBAL ESTIMATES

It is estimated that 489 139 (95% CLs, 455 093–614 215) cases emerged in 2006, and the global proportion of resistance among all incident TB cases was 4.8% (95% CLs, 4.6–6.0). China and India are estimated to carry 50% of the global burden, with the Russian Federation carrying a further 7%. The difference between the estimated number of cases, and between the proportions published in 2004 and those published in this report, can be accounted for by revisions in underlying estimations of TB incidence and by more recent survey and surveillance data. In this report, as in previous publications, we have estimated the incidence rather than the prevalence of MDR-TB. Prevalence can be estimated by multiplying incidence by the average duration of the disease. The duration of MDR-TB is not known, and is likely to vary, depending on diagnostics, treatment available and HIV coinfection; however, it is expected to be longer than 1.75 years, the current estimated duration of an episode of drug-susceptible TB. In general, duration is expected to be longer because most patients will receive some treatment that will contribute to prolongation of disease rather than curing it. A modelling exercise estimated MDR-TB prevalence to be three times the annual MDR-TB incidence[24]. If we assume that the duration of the disease is 2–3 years, the global prevalence of MDR-TB would range from 1 000 000 to 1 500 000 cases.

SUPRANATIONAL REFERENCE LABORATORY NETWORK

The SRLN, which currently comprises 26 laboratories in six regions, provides a wide range of support to more than 150 laboratories worldwide. The network has completed 13 rounds of proficiency testing since 1994; and cumulative results indicate an overall high performance. Although overall performance of the network is good, annually, one or two laboratories within the network will show suboptimal performance. This indicates the difficulty of executing high-quality drug-susceptibility testing year after year, and also highlights the importance of internal quality assurance.

Results are determined judicially, and through the course of 13 rounds of proficiency testing, "borderline" strains have been encountered, where up to half the network has found these strains to be susceptible and the other laboratories have found them to be resistant. Since round 9, thorough pretesting has been used to exclude such strains from panels, but has not always been successful. Therefore, strains with less than 80% concordance within the network have been excluded from overall performance measures, so that judicial results are not distorted. Over a five-year period, 40 of 600 strains, or approximately 7% of strains included in annual panels, have been excluded. Although the network acknowledges that these strains are present in routine care of TB patients, it was decided to examine them outside of annual proficiency, partly to determine the reasons for the results, but also to ensure reliable evaluation of national and other reference laboratories that subsequently receive these panels. The study on borderline strains has been useful in confirming that the most important factor explaining the variation of the results of panel testing is strain selection. Results of the borderline study are not yet published. Currently, there is no established gold standard to replace the judicial system. One possible solution would be a definition of "intermediary" resistant results; however, this would require testing at two concentrations. Many high-income countries will test drugs (at least isoniazid) at two concentrations. However, this is not the case in most low-income countries.

The use of DST for first-line anti-TB drugs has been thoroughly studied and consensus has been reached on appropriate methodologies. However, surveys on current practices for second-line DST in the SRLN and in some multicentre studies, have indicated a range of methods, critical concentrations of drugs and critical proportions of resistance used in drug-susceptibility testing. To date, no study has systematically evaluated all available methods for testing, established critical concentrations for all available second-line drugs, or evaluated a large number of clinical isolates for microbiological and clinical end-points. Despite the absence of this critical information, there is a clear and urgent need to provide guidance to countries engaging in MDR-TB treatment programmes, and to develop mechanisms for external quality assurance of DST for second-line drugs.

In July 2007, guidance was developed for the selection of and testing for second-line drugs [13]. Based on evidence or expert consensus (where no evidence was available), a hierarchy was developed recommending drug-susceptibility testing based on both clinical relevance and reliability of the test available. Rifampicin and isoniazid were prioritized, followed by ethambutol, streptomycin and pyrazinamide, and then the second-line injectables (amikacin, kanamycin and capreomycin) and fluroquinolones. The policy guidance is available, and full technical guidelines for the drug-susceptibility testing of second-line drugs became available in 2008. At the same time, the SRLN began to include isolates with second-line drug resistance into the 14th round of proficiency testing for the SRLN and selected NRLs. Results of this first exercise will be available in mid-2008.

Newer, rapid methods for phenotypic and genotypic DST hold considerable promise for the rapid diagnosis of MDR-TB, as well as opportunities for scaling up surveillance of resistance, discussed previously. While several of these tests are in a validation stage, many countries are already using some these methods to identify MDR-TB patients. Tests for rapid identification of second-line drug resistance are not yet available.

The SRLN continues to play a critical role in capacity strengthening of laboratories worldwide, and provides the backbone for surveillance activities. The network is still largely supported by host governments; however, an increasing number of countries are obtaining funding for services provided by the SRLN through Global Fund grants. Inadequate laboratory capacity now presents one of the greatest obstacles to achieving the targets set out in the Global Plan to Stop TB, 2006–2015. The Subgroup on Laboratory Capacity Strengthening has become a more substantive movement, and has been renamed the Global Laboratory Initiative, with a secretariat based at WHO; the initiative has a wider base of technical partners and is seeking the interest and engagement of donor agencies. Since 2007, the SRLN has been fully integrated into this initiative. The main priority for the SRLN is expansion within regions, to fulfil the demand for reference laboratories and obtain sustainable financing, so that services can continue to be delivered to countries requiring assistance. All WHO regions are committed to expansion, and most have identified laboratories to be evaluated for integration into the SRLN.

WHO REGIONS

WHO African Region

In the WHO African Region, six countries have reported data since 2002 – Côte d'Ivoire, Ethiopia, Madagascar, Rwanda, Senegal and UR Tanzania. Data from UR Tanzania and Madagascar are considered preliminary. Rwanda was the outlier, reporting 3.9% (95% CLs, 2.5–5.8) MDR-TB among new cases. Senegal reported 2.1% (95% CLs, 0.7–4.9) among new cases, but all other countries reported less than 2.0% MDR-TB. Since 1994, 22 of 46 African countries have reported drug-resistance data from areas representing 72% of all TB cases in the region. The population-weighted mean of MDR-TB based on countries reporting in the region is 1.5% (95% CLs, 1.0–2.0) among new cases, 5.8% among previously treated cases (95% CLs, 3.9–7.7) and 2.2% (95% CLs, 1.4–3.1) among combined cases. The variation in resistance among countries within the region is relatively narrow; however, roughly half of the data points used to look at the distribution are at least five years old. It is possible that current survey methodology, which is based on smear-positive cases, may underrepresent HIV coinfected TB cases, who are more likely to be smear negative. In addition, transmission dynamics of drug-resistant TB in a heavily HIV-infected population are not well understood. These and other factors, described in detail in the HIV and MDR-TB section of this report (above), make estimation of the true burden of MDR-TB difficult in high HIV prevalence settings. With the exception of Botswana, Mozambique and South Africa, HIV testing has not been a component of drug-resistance surveys. However, as routine HIV testing rapidly scales up in the region (from 11% of TB cases tested in 2005 to 22% in 2006), HIV information will become a more routine component of anti-TB drug-resistance surveys. It is estimated that there were 66 711 (95% CLs, 55 606–137 263) incident MDR-TB cases in the region in 2006, with almost 90% of these cases emerging in high HIV prevalence settings.

The WHO African Region has the fewest settings for which trends can be identified. Only Botswana, Côte d'Ivoire, Sierra Leone and Mpumalanga Province, South Africa, have carried out repeat surveys. In the surveys reported previously, Botswana showed a significant increase in drug resistance among new cases, and an increase, though not significant, in the proportion of MDR-TB cases. A fourth survey is under way in Botswana, the results of which will be important in understanding the trends in drug resistance in this country, and other countries where HIV is prevalent. Côte d'Ivoire showed a decrease in the proportion of MDR-TB cases between surveys, but an increase in resistance to streptomycin and ethambutol, and an increase in isoniazid monoresistance[28]. Survey methods remained the same between the surveys, and most of the MDR-TB cases captured in the first survey had an identical resistance pattern, suggesting that a cluster of cases may be have been included. Further surveys are required to interpret trends in Côte d'Ivoire.

The low median proportions of drug resistance and limited trend data may underestimate the importance of drug-resistant TB in high HIV prevalence settings. A large outbreak of XDR-TB in an HIV-positive population in the province

---

[28] Mono resistance is defined as resistance to a single drug

of KwaZulu-Natal, South Africa, was associated with extremely high mortality[25] and highlighted the vulnerability of TB patients coinfected with HIV. Detection of this outbreak was only possible because of the extensive laboratory infrastructure available in the country. It is likely that similar outbreaks of drug resistance with associated high mortality are taking place in other countries, but are not being detected due to insufficient laboratory capacity.

Botswana, Mauritania and Mozambique have nationwide surveys under way, and Angola, Burundi, Lesotho, Malawi, Namibia, South Africa, Uganda and Zambia have plans to initiate nationwide surveys over the next year. Nigeria and the Congo plan to begin a survey covering selected districts in their respective countries in 2008. All protocols stipulate second-line drug-susceptibility testing for MDR-TB isolates, and most surveys are being financed through Global Fund grants. Currently, Botswana and Swaziland are surveying high-risk populations to examine the extent of first and second-line drug resistance; results should be available in early 2008. The Congo, Burundi and Rwanda[26–28], with the assistance of an SRL, are routinely examining second-line resistance among treatment failure cases; so far they have detected limited second-line resistance; however, samples are relatively small. Malawi, Mozambique, Zambia and Zimbabwe all have plans to conduct similar studies. South Africa has recently conducted a review of the country's laboratory database and found that 996 (5.6%) of 17 615 MDR-TB isolates collected over a four-year period were XDR-TB. Proportions varied across provinces, with KwaZulu-Natal reporting 656 (14%) of 4701 MDR-TB cases as XDR-TB. Selection and testing practices varied across the country and with time; however, all isolates correspond to individual cases[29]. UR Tanzania, with the support of an SRL, is evaluating the use of rapid rifampicin testing for the purposes of surveillance. Data from this project will be available in early 2008 and, if shown to be comparable with phenotypic testing, may be a useful tool in the expansion of survey coverage in the region as well as in trend analysis.

The most critical factor in addressing drug resistance in African countries is the lack of laboratory infrastructure and transport networks that can provide rapid diagnosis. The Global Plan to Stop TB, 2006–2015 stipulates expansion of culture and DST to all re-treatment cases and to 90% of new cases that are at high risk of MDR-TB (i.e. contacts and treatment failures at 3 months). Most countries in the region are far from reaching this target. In 2006, it was reported that 9% of re-treatment cases received DST in the WHO African Region. Most countries have, at most, one laboratory able to conduct culture and drug-susceptibility testing in the public sector, let alone DST for second-line drugs. There are two SRLs in the region, one in Algeria and one in South Africa; however, the National Health Laboratory service of South Africa and laboratories outside the region are playing an important role in providing quality assurance, as well as DST for second-line drugs. There are plans to upgrade national laboratory networks in most countries; also, the identification and upgrade of at least three SRLs are planned for the region over the nxt two years. Reviews of existing laboratories have already begun. Pilot projects led by the Foundation for Innovative New Diagnostics (FIND) and other partners are paving the way for the integration of new and more rapid diagnostics

---

[29] Data from a retrospective review of the National Health Laboratory Service of South Africa were presented at the 38th World Conference on Lung Health. 8–12 November 2007. Cape Town, South Africa.

in the region, and funding from the United States President's Plan for Emergency AIDS Relief (PEPFAR) and the Global Fund are filling critical gaps. However, if laboratories are to scale up rapidly, coordination of funding and technical agencies will be critical, as will concerted efforts to address the widespread constraints in human-resource capacity in the region.

Currently, Burkina Faso, the Congo, Guinea, Kenya, Lesotho, Malawi, Rwanda and Uganda have approved GLC projects. Mozambique has submitted an application, which is under review. Benin, Ethiopia, Mali, Namibia, UR Tanzania and Zambia have Global Fund approved grants for the management of MDR-TB, and have plans to apply to the GLC in 2008.

WHO Region of the Americas

In the WHO Region of the Americas, 11 countries have reported data since 2002, including never previously reported data from Costa Rica, Guatemala (final data), Honduras and Paraguay. Since 1994, 21 countries have reported drug-resistance data from areas representing 93% of all TB cases in the region, but covering 48% of the countries. The population-weighted mean of MDR-TB based on all countries that have reported in the Americas is 2.2% (95% CLs, 0.6–3.8) among new cases, 13.2% (95% CLs, 3.5–22.8) among previously treated cases and 4.0% (95% CLs, 1.7–6.3) among combined cases.

To a great extent, as found in previous reports, the prevalence of MDR-TB is low in the region as a whole; however, there are important outliers. In this report, Guatemala reported 3.0% (95% CLs, 1.8–4.6), and Peru showed 5.3% (95% CLs, 4.2–6.4) among new TB cases. In the last report — though in the same reporting period (2002) — Ecuador showed 4.9% (95% CLs, 3.5–6.7) MDR-TB among new cases.

In North America, Canada has shown low proportions of resistance and relatively steady trends in resistance among both new and previously treated cases. TB case notification has decreased since 1997 and, in 2006, 12 MDR-TB cases were identified. The United States has shown decreases in overall TB notifications, as well as overall numbers of MDR-TB cases since 1995. The United States reported significant decreases in MDR-TB among all TB cases. A total of 124 MDR-TB cases were recorded in 2005.

Argentina showed a slight, but not statistically significant, increase in MDR-TB among new cases from 1.8% (95% CLs, 0.9–3.0) in 1999 to 2.2 (95% CLs, 1.2–3.6) in 2005, and the TB notification rate has steadily decreased over the past decade. Uruguay showed a decrease in resistance to any drug, but this was not significant. The prevalence of any resistance remains low in this country at 2.1% (95% CLs, 0.8–4.3) among new TB cases. Cuba continues to show low prevalence of resistance in the population, with MDR-TB never reaching much above 2.0% among all TB patients. Cuba was one of the few countries able to report on DST results disaggregated both by HIV status, subcategory of re-treatment and prison status[29]. Peru reported increases in any resistance, isoniazid resistance and MDR-TB among new cases, though only the increase in any resistance and isoniazid resistance were significant. MDR-TB increased from 2.4% (95% CLs, 1.7–3.4) in 1996 to 5.3% (95% CLs, 4.2–6.4) in 2006. Peru showed a yearly reduction in the TB notification rate between 1994 and 2002 of approximately 4–6%; however, since 2003, the notification rate has slightly increased, at 123–124 per 100 000.

The recent rise in the notification rate and the increase in drug resistance may be due to weakness in management of TB cases (both new and MDR-TB) in previous years, and to weakness in the entire health system, particularly in the years 2003 and 2004. The GLC-approved project has operated primarily in Lima, until expanded nationally in 2006.

A nationwide drug resistance survey, by state, is currently under way in Brazil, and includes HIV testing. A repeat survey in the Dominican Republic is also ongoing and will help better establish the prevalence of MDR-TB, which was shown to be 6.6% among new TB cases in the first survey more than a decade ago. Mexico has started a nationwide survey that will include HIV testing. Panama also has plans for a nationwide survey. All surveys have plans to test MDR-TB isolates for second-line drug resistance at an SRL.

At present, there are five SRLs in the WHO Region of the Americas, with plans to expand the network to one or two additional laboratories over the next two years. This network provides annual proficiency testing panels to almost all NRLs in the region. Many countries plan to upgrade laboratory networks because there is increased demand for development of second-line testing capacity.

In 2006, there were an estimated 12 070 (95% CLs, 10 523–15 526) incident MDR-TB cases in Latin America, 3972 (95% CLs, 2842–5192) in Peru, 1483 (95% CLs, 1034–1998) in Ecuador and 1464 (95% CLs, 945–2077) in Brazil. The WHO Region of the Americas has the largest number of GLC-approved projects, with programmes in Belize, Bolivia, Costa Rica, Dominican Republic, Ecuador, Guatemala, Haiti, Honduras, Mexico, Nicaragua, Paraguay, Peru (nationwide), El Salvador and Uruguay. Though not GLC approved, MDR-TB management is fully integrated in Brazil, and the country has an extensive laboratory network able to conduct culture and drug-susceptibility testing. Treatment success of MDR-TB patients reported from Brazil was 60% for the 2003 cohort.

WHO Eastern Mediterranean Region

The WHO Eastern Mediterranean Region has made strong progress in survey coverage since 2002, reporting data from six countries, including never previously reported data from Lebanon, Jordan, Morocco (nationwide survey data) and Yemen. Since 1994, eight countries have reported drug-resistance data from areas representing 22% of all TB cases in the region, but covering 36% of the countries in the region. The population-weighted mean of MDR-TB based on all countries that have reported in the WHO Eastern Mediterranean Region is 2.0% (95% CLs, 0.0–4.3) among new cases, 35.3% (95% CLs, 16.4–54.3) among previously treated cases and 5.4% (95% CLs, 0.5–10.4) among combined cases. There were an estimated 25 475 (95% CLs, 15 737–73 132) incident MDR-TB cases in the region in 2006, with almost 60% of these cases estimated to be in Pakistan.

Lebanon, Morocco and Oman reported low proportions of MDR-TB among new cases, with levels ranging from 0.5% (95% CLs, 0.2–1.1) in Morocco to 1.3% (95% CLs, 0.2–4.7) in Oman. Yemen reported a higher proportion of resistance (2.9%; 95% CLs, 1.6–4.9) and Jordan reported 5.4% (95% CLs, 2.0–11.4) MDR-TB among new cases. Jordan, Lebanon and Oman reported high proportions of resistance among re-treated cases, though sample sizes were small and confidence levels were wide. The high proportions of resistance found in Jordan are similar to those reported from the Islamic Republic of Iran in 1998. Jordan reports high success rates and low proportions of re-treatment cases, suggesting that further evaluation is needed to confirm the high proportion of MDR-TB found among new cases.

Trends are available only for the Gulf States of Oman and Qatar, both with small numbers of total cases and low-to-moderate levels of resistance, much of which is imported. Trends are difficult to interpret because of the small numbers of cases, though drug resistance does not appear to be a problem in either of these countries. The extent of second-line drug resistance is not known in the region. The only available data have been reported from the Islamic Republic of Iran, which showed the existence of XDR-TB, but denominators were not available. Morocco plans to have MDR-TB isolates collected from its nationwide survey tested for second-line drug resistance.

The primary limiting factor to expanding survey coverage in the region is the high number of countries currently addressing conflict situations. In many of these countries, basic health services must be prioritized over expansion of surveillance. Another limiting factor is the poor laboratory infrastructure in many countries. Currently, there is only one SRL in the region, but one candidate SRL has been nominated and is undergoing evaluation, and there are plans to identify another candidate in the region in the next year.

Pakistan has expanded external quality assurance of microscopy laboratories and is in the process of identifying an NRL, which is a prerequisite for a nationwide survey, and is also desirable for the successful implementation of a MDR-TB treatment programme under the NTP. The Islamic Republic of Iran has been planning a second nationwide survey for several years; however, to date the survey has not taken place. The Libyan Arab Jamahiriya, Saudi Arabia and Somalia will start preparation for drug-resistance surveys in 2008. Sudan has recently begun a survey.

Currently, Egypt, Jordan, Lebanon, the Syrian Arab Republic and Tunisia, have GLC-approved projects. Djibouti, Egypt, Iraq, Morocco and Sudan have Global Fund approved grants for MDR-TB management, which will result in GLC applications shortly.

WHO European Region

In the WHO European Region, 38 countries have reported data since 2002, including never previously reported data from Armenia, Baku City (Azerbaijan), Donetsk Oblast within Ukraine, Georgia, the Republic of Moldova, Tashkent, Uzbekistan and three oblasts in the Russian Federation. Since 1994, 40 countries have reported drug-resistance data from areas representing 35% of all TB cases in the region (31% of the cases in Eastern European countries, and 55% of the cases in Central and Western European countries). The population-weighted mean of MDR-TB based on all countries that have reported in Central and Western Europe is 9% (95% CLs, 0.5–1.2) among new cases, 7.7% (95% CLs, 5.7–9.8) among previously treated cases and 1.5% (95% CLs, 1.1–2.0) among combined cases. The proportion of MDR-TB was significantly higher in the Eastern European and Central Asian countries, with the following population-weighted means: 10.0% MDR-TB (95% CLs, 3.8–16.1) among new cases, 37.7% (95% CLs, 12.3–63.0) among previously treated cases and 22.6% (95% CLs, 8.6–36.6) among combined cases.

Based on important differences in epidemiology, Central and Western

Europe are discussed separately from Eastern Europe and Central Asia. Most Central and Western European countries are reporting routine surveillance data. Both proportions and absolute numbers of drug-resistant cases remain low in most of Central and Western Europe. Germany reports the highest number of MDR-TB cases, recording approximately 100 cases per year. Most of the drug-resistant cases recorded are imported cases. Israel is an outlier, presenting the highest levels of resistance to all drugs. However, the situation of this country is unique, because of the high levels of immigration from areas of the former Soviet Union. Between 80% and 85% of TB patients in Israel are foreign born, mainly from Ethiopia and countries of the former Soviet Union. Therefore, most MDR-TB cases in the country were likely to have been infected abroad before immigrating to Israel[30]. A 1994 survey in Romania showed 2.4% MDR-TB among new cases, and 5.4% among all TB cases, and the absolute number of incident cases estimated in 2006 was 1546 (95% CLs, 1047–2138). Turkey has never carried out a nationwide survey, although there are plans to do so. The number of cases estimated to have emerged in 2006 is 889 (95% CLs, 284–3320). Importantly, almost all countries in Central and Western Europe are now linked to an SRL and are participating in annual external quality assurance for drug-susceptibility testing.

Eastern Europe

Since the beginning of this project, countries of Eastern Europe and Central Asia have reported the highest proportions of resistance to anti-TB drugs. It has been speculated that one of the most important factors in the resurgence of TB in the region, and the emergence of the drug-resistance epidemic, was the disintegration of the Union of Soviet Socialist Republics in 1991 and the economic crisis that followed. This crisis resulted in interruptions in drug supply and overall deterioration of the health sector, which also had an impact on transmission of infection and susceptibility to disease. The lack of standardized treatment regimens in many countries is also likely to have contributed to the development of drug resistance, and there is extensive documentation of spread of drug resistance throughout the prison sector. In this report, data reported from Georgia show the lowest proportion of resistance in the region at 6.8% (95% CLs, 5.1–8.8) among new cases. Georgia has continued to use the systems developed for the survey to improve its routine surveillance system. Data from Baku City, Azerbaijan, as well as data from the Republic of Moldova, showed proportions of MDR-TB of 20.0% and higher among new cases. Data from several of the countries surveyed showed that between 4.0% (Armenia) and 23.7% (Estonia) of MDR-TB cases were XDR-TB. Donetsk Oblast, Ukraine conducted a joint drug-resistance and HIV survey among TB patients, which showed a significant association between drug resistance and HIV. Currently, it is estimated that 80 057 (95% CLs, 71 893–97 623) MDR-TB cases emerged in Eastern Europe and Central Asia in 2006.

Though most countries in the region conduct routine culture and drug-susceptibility testing on all, or at least most TB cases notified, practices do not follow the criteria required for inclusion in this report. These countries are not

---

[30] Chemtob D. Multi and extensive drug-resistant tuberculosis burden in Israel, a country with immigration from high endemic areas. 4th Congress of the IUATLD, European Region, Riga, Latvia, June 2007, pp. 19.

participating in annual quality assurance of laboratory results, patients may not be classified according to treatment history, and culture and DST coverage may not be sufficiently high. Nevertheless, data on notification of MDR-TB cases collected through annual reporting to WHO correlate well with survey data collected from the region, which indicates that relying on routine data collection for surveillance of drug resistance will be possible in the future. In the meantime, surveys are important to estimate the burden of MDR-TB in these countries.

Currently, robust trend information is available only from the Baltic countries and two oblasts in the Russian Federation. Trends in MDR-TB among new cases in the Baltic countries appear to be relatively stable, at 9.8% in Lithuania and 13.2% in Estonia, with a slow decrease indicated in Estonia and slow but significant increase in MDR-TB in Lithuania. The TB notification rate is falling by 5.0% (Lithuania) to 8.0% (Estonia) per year. Treatment success of new smear-positive cases over the same period has been relatively stable at around 70–74%, but fell slightly in Lithuania (from 74 to 70%) over the last four years. DOTS was initiated in 1996 (Latvia), 1998 (Lithuania) and 2000 (Estonia), and DOTS-Plus was initiated in 1998 (Latvia), 2002 (Estonia) and 2005 (Lithuania). Success rates for patients with MDR-TB in 2003 were highest in Latvia, at 69%, but quite low in Lithuania, at around 36%.

The TB scenario in the Baltics, especially in Latvia and Estonia, probably reflects improved TB control over the past 10 years, including better management of MDR-TB, with more rapid diagnosis and infection control (particularly in hospitals). Economic growth and investment in health has also probably contributed to the decline in TB over this period. Absolute numbers of chronic cases and defaulters have steadily declined in the years 2003 through 2006[30, 31].

All three countries struggle with social issues among TB patients, such as alcohol, drug abuse and homelessness. Social issues have been identified as a limiting factor in reduction of default and failure rates. Social support must continue to be a key aspect in reducing poor treatment outcomes. Reduction in the proportion of MDR, if sustained in the Baltic countries, particularly in Latvia and Estonia, may provide an important model for other countries in the region that struggle with MDR-TB epidemics.

The scenario in the Russian Federation differs from the picture indicated in the Baltic countries. TB notification rates for the whole of the Russian Federation have been relatively stable from 1997 (81/100 000) through 2006 (87/100 000), and data from selected oblasts where TB control has been well implemented are showing declines in TB. In Orel Oblast, the TB notification rate has declined by more than 3% per year for the last six years. Tomsk Oblast showed a steady decline in TB notification rate, by 1.3% over the same period.

Trend data are currently available from the Tomsk and Orel oblasts. The data from these regions are considered reliable because culture and drug-susceptibility testing has been provided to 85–100% of the new TB cases over this period, new and previously treated cases are reliably differentiated, and there is evidence of good laboratory performance over the period of data collection.

In addition, an exercise was undertaken to examine quarterly data from 10 oblasts with the aim of using routine data as a basis for surveillance of drug resistance. Based on a validation exercise to determine the population coverage of culture, DST and other quality indicators, and combined with external quality assurance results from the laboratory, data on new cases in the civilian sector from Mary El Oblast were also included in this report. Data are representative only for the populations covered and cannot be extrapolated to the whole of the country. The exercise showed that the national reporting system and laboratory registers correlate well for new cases; therefore, as quality-assured diagnostic coverage of the population expands, routine data from additional regions in Russian Federation could be included in future reports[31].

While overall notifications of TB in Orel and Tomsk oblasts are declining, trends in the proportion of drug resistance are showing important increases, ranging from an average 13.0% per year increase in Tomsk to 32.0% increase per year in Orel. Absolute numbers of new TB cases with MDR-TB are also increasing. Both regions have strong and improving TB control programs, as well as GLC-approved MDR-TB management programmes. It is possible that, while susceptible cases are being successfully treated, MDR-TB cases have not been successfully reduced, leaving drug-resistant cases as an increasing reservoir of TB transmission. Data reported do not allow disaggregation of cases by place of origin, or by previous history of hospitalization or imprisonment, both of which may have an impact on trends in resistance in these oblasts. Supporting the trend data reported from these oblasts is a report jointly published in 2006 by the Russian Ministry of Health and WHO. The report indicated an increase in MDR-TB both in proportion and absolute numbers of cases, and highlighted the variation in proportions of resistance across oblasts, indicating that up to 20% of new TB cases in Samara Oblast[32–34] may have MDR-TB. According to this report, approximately 40% of TB patients in the Russian Federation were categorized as chronic cases in the national register. Although some of the increase in numbers of MDR-TB cases in the national system may be due to better laboratory detection, this probably does not explain the size of the increase. The enormous pool of chronic cases constitutes an important reservoir of transmission of MDR-TB.

Over recent years, the Russian Federation has made important progress in addressing TB, including implementation of World Bank and Global Fund projects. The revised TB control strategy is being implemented in 85 of 88 regions, and new TB treatment standards and forms have been introduced. Currently, 14 of 89 regions have GLC-approved applications (and many more are in the pipeline). The Russian Federation forecasts that 3200 MDR-TB cases will be enrolled on MDR-TB treatment by 2008, with designation of five federal centres of excellence for the treatment of MDR-TB in the civilian sector, and eight in the penal system. The strengthening and upgrading of laboratory services have been prioritized, and 120 laboratories have been enrolled in external quality-assurance programmes. Despite the current momentum, the epidemiological picture available from the Russian Federation suggests extraordinary measures will be necessary to accelerate and strengthen the implementation of the Stop TB strategy, if MDR-TB is to be reduced in the population.

Commitment to TB control varies across the region but, in general, progress has been made. A regional laboratory task force has been developed to improve

---

[31] According to official statistics, the prevalence of MDR-TB among new cases in the Russian Federation is 9.4%. These data do not currently conform to global project methodology and therefore have not been included in this report.

laboratory networks through:
- development of new accreditation procedures
- development of guidance on laboratory biosafety and infection control
- identification of additional SRLs specifically to serve this region
- expansion of quality-assurance practices and integration of new tools.

Currently, all countries in this subregion are linked to an SRL, with the exception of Bulgaria and Turkmenistan. Despite progress, further efforts are needed to accelerate the roll out of GLC-approved programmes to treat the large burden of MDR-TB cases. Also needed are better supply and management of good-quality second-line anti-TB drugs, improved infection control and continued improvement in rapid detection of resistant cases.

Belarus, Bulgaria, Tajikistan and Turkmenistan are priority countries for drug-resistance surveys. Kazakhstan is repeating a nationwide survey, Kyrgyzstan is starting with a survey of Bishkek, and Uzbekistan is planning a nationwide survey following the survey in Tashkent. MDR-TB treatment through the GLC mechanism is expanding, with 13 countries (including 14 regions in Russia) currently approved by the GLC. Partners are willing and are coordinated to improve community involvement and links to prisons, but additional investment will be needed to scale up and meet the targets outlines in the Global Plan to Stop TB, 2006–2015.

WHO South-East Asia Region

In the WHO South-East Asia Region, six countries reported data since 2002 – India, Indonesia, Myanmar, Nepal, Sri Lanka and Thailand. India reported data from three districts and one state, and Indonesia reported data from one district. Of the countries reporting, Mayhurbhanj district in Orissa State[35], India, Sri Lanka, and Thailand reported less than 2.0% MDR-TB among new cases. Ernakulam district in Kerala State[36], Hoogli district in West Bengal State[35], and Gujarat State, India as well as Mimika district, of Papua province in Indonesia and Nepal reported between 2.0–3.0% MDR-TB among new cases. Myanmar was the outlier, reporting 3.9% (95% CLs, 2.6–5.7) MDR-TB among new cases. Since 1994, 6 of 11 countries have reported drug-resistance data, from areas representing 23% of all TB cases in the region, but covering 55% of the countries in the region. The population-weighted mean of MDR-TB based on all countries that have reported in the WHO South-East Asia Region is 2.8% (95% CLs, 1.9–3.6) among new cases, 18.8% (95% CLs, 13.3–24.3) among previously treated cases and 6.3% (95% CLs, 4.2–8.4) among combined cases. There were an estimated 149 615 (95% CLs, 114 780–217 921) incident MDR-TB cases in the region in 2006, with 74% of these cases estimated to be in India.

Based on results from a nationwide survey in Myanmar[37] showing 3.9% (95% CLs, 2.6–5.7) MDR-TB among new cases and 15.5% (95% CLs, 9.5–23.4) among re-treatment cases, it is estimated that there were 4251 (95% CLs, 2648–6187) incident MDR-TB cases in Myanmar in 2006. Myanmar has made good progress in TB control, with case detection reaching 61% and treatment success reaching 86%; and the proportion of re-treatment cases comprises approximately 5% of the notified cases. Despite resource constraints, Myanmar is moving quickly towards implementing management of MDR-TB under the NTP. Currently, there are only two laboratories in the public sector providing culture, and only one of these conducts DST; however, plans are under way to extend DST capacity to the second laboratory. A second drug-resistance survey is ongoing, as well as a survey of category II failure cases and chronics, to determine the extent of second-line drug resistance in this population and to inform the development of a treatment regimen. A GLC application has been approved.

The results from the recent survey in Gujarat State in India show low-to-moderate levels of MDR-TB among new TB cases 2.4% (95% CLs, 1.7–3.2) and 17.2% (95% CLs, 14.8–19.9) among re-treatment cases. However, India reports that re-treatment cases comprise 13.7% of notified cases in the country, suggesting a considerable burden of MDR-TB in this population. It is widely thought, though little documented, that a large number of registered re-treatment cases are reporting from the private sector.

In general, the TB control programme is performing well. The Revised National TB Control Programme has achieved population coverage of DOTS in all districts in the country in 2006, case detection is about 61% and treatment success is 86%. However, plans for scaling up 24 inter-regional laboratories capable of culture and DST, attached to 24 MDR-TB management sites capable of managing some 5000 cases per year, are behind schedule. Currently, most MDR-TB is managed in an unregulated private sector that has access to second-line drugs that are manufactured locally and are of variable quality. XDR-TB has been reported in the country[38], and results of second-line testing from the state-wide survey in Gujarat and a nearly completed survey in Maharashtra will provide further evidence as to the extent of second-line resistance in the country.

A GLC application has been approved for two sites in the states of Andhra Pradesh and Haryana. Laboratory capacity is seen as the biggest bottleneck in the country's ability to respond to MDR-TB. There is consensus that the private sector, including private laboratories and medical colleges, must be more involved, but accreditation under the public system as well as formal linkages may take time. The concern is that, unless MDR-TB management develops rapidly in the public sector, an increasing number of MDR-TB cases will be managed by the unregulated private sector.

The data available from Mimika district of Papua province in Indonesia[39] show moderate levels of resistance; however, the sample for this survey was small and represented a small proportion of the population. Soon-to-be-available data from a drug-resistance survey in central Java should provide a better estimate of drug resistance in Indonesia. A survey of treatment-failure cases is also under way to determine the extent of second-line resistance in this population. Case detection is just under the target of 70%, and cure rates in the country are high. Indonesia, like Myanmar and India, is struggling with the upgrade, expansion and quality assurance of its laboratory network. A GLC application has been approved, but patients have not yet been enrolled.

The new survey data available from Sri Lanka are showing exceptionally low proportions of resistance. While these data have not yet been fully quality assured, other indicators from the program support this estimate. All treatment failure cases receive culture and DST, and identified MDR-TB cases are managed by the public sector. Sri Lanka is the only country in the region routinely reporting MDR-TB cases. The success rate among MDR-TB cases is not known, but the country has plans to submit an application to the GLC.

Nepal and Thailand are the only two countries reporting trend data in this report. The proportion of MDR-TB among new cases in Nepal has fluctuated from a little over 1.0% to 3.0% in the four surveys that have been conducted since 1996, making trends difficult to interpret. The current estimate is 2.9% (95% CLs, 1.8–4.3) among new cases and 11.7% (95% CLs, 7.2–17.7) among re-treatment cases. Nepal has had a well-functioning TB control programme for more than a decade, and both case detection and treatment success remain high. Nepal has proven to be the leader in MDR-TB control in the region, establishing the first MDR-TB control programme in the public sector and expanding its coverage to 100% of the country by the end of 2006. Currently, there is one MDR-TB treatment centre and at least three to four subcentres in all the five regions of the country. Cure rates among registered MDR-TB cases for whom treatment outcomes are available are 75%. Like other countries in the region, the ability to expand MDR-TB services has been limited by laboratory capacity; however, there are plans to expand the culture network.

Thailand has also reported data from three surveys showing stable trends in resistance, with MDR-TB just under 2.0% among new TB cases. Data from a separate surveillance network with roughly the same population coverage are showing similar proportions of resistance in the population; however, data from border regions with Myanmar are showing higher proportions of resistance[32]. Unlike the other countries in the region, Thailand has an extensive and well-developed laboratory network. Due the decentralized nature of laboratory services and an abundance of private sector laboratories, maintaining a high level of performance is one of the major challenges of the NTP. The Thai NRL currently serves as an SRL for the region and is one of only a few laboratories in the region able to perform second-line DST. Currently, MDR-TB patients are managed in the public sector, but practices do not conform to international guidelines.

Although survey data are not included in this report for Bangladesh, the Damien Foundation has been monitoring drug resistance in a rural population of the country for the past 10 years, and levels of drug resistance appear to be low[40]. An NRL has recently been recognized and upgraded, and there are plans to conduct a nationwide survey in the coming year. A GLC application has been approved. The Republic of Korea has developed plans to improve the capacity of the NRL in order to conduct culture and drug-susceptibility testing. The primary obstacle to achieving this goal is the lack of sustainable funding for the development and operation of the laboratory. The Republic of Korea reports that re-treatment cases comprise 18% of notified cases in the country, suggesting a considerable burden of MDR-TB in this population, and indicating that drug resistance may be higher than in other countries in the region. A total of 3472 (95% CLs, 1136–11 248) MDR-TB cases were estimated to have emerged in 2006 in The Republic of Korea or 6.8% of all cases (95% CLs, 2.3–21.7). Additional assistance will be required to upgrade the NRL and to measure the burden of resistance in this country.

The WHO South-East Asia Region is home to four high-burden countries. Though resistance in the region is moderate, the overall burden of MDR-TB is

---

[32] Personal communication with Somsak and Dhanida Reinthong of the National Reference Laboratory, Bangkok, Thailand.

considerable. Important progress has been made throughout the region in initiating plans for MDR-TB treatment, and almost all countries in the region have GLC applications approved or in the pipeline. However, with the exception of Thailand, all countries have identified laboratory capacity as the primary bottleneck to scaling up diagnosis and treatment to reach the targets outlines in the Global Plan to Stop TB, 2006-2015. In addition, many countries in the region have growing private sectors that are currently managing most of the MDR-TB cases in the region, and second-line drugs are widely available through the private sector. Coordinated efforts on behalf of NTPs as well as partners will be required to solve the laboratory capacity shortage in the region.

WHO Western Pacific region

In the WHO Western Pacific Region, 14 countries and 2 SARs reported data since 2002, including data from one province, one SAR, and two municipalities in China, the Philippines and Viet Nam. Of the countries reporting, Fiji, Guam, New Caledonia, New Zealand, the Northern Mariana Islands, Singapore, Solomon Islands and Vanuatu reported the fewest cases, with between 0 and 3 cases of MDR-TB per year. Australia reported 12 cases in 2005 and Macao SAR, China reported 9 cases of MDR-TB. Hong Kong SAR reported 41 MDR-TB cases in 2005 among all cases or 1.2% (95% CLs, 0.9-1.6) and Japan, through its sentinel survey, reported that 1.9% (95% CLs, 1.5-2.5) of all notified cases were MDR-TB. China, the Philippines and Viet Nam reported higher proportions of resistance.

Since 1994, 19 countries have reported drug-resistance data from areas representing 52% of all TB cases in the region, but covering 53% of the countries in the region. The population-weighted mean of MDR-TB based on all countries that have reported in the WHO Western Pacific Region is 3.9% (95% CLs, 2.6-5.2) among new cases, 21.6% (95% CLs, 16.8-26.4) among previously treated cases and 6.7% (95% CLs, 4.6-8.8) among combined cases. There were and estimated 152 694 (95% CLs, 119 886-188 014) incident MDR-TB cases in the region in 2006, with almost 85% of these cases estimated to be in China.

Viet Nam reported 2.7% (95% CLs, 2.0-3.6) MDR-TB among new cases in the country's 2006 survey, and 2.3% (95% CLs, 1.3-3.9) in a survey carried out a decade ago, which suggests that MDR-TB has not significantly increased among new cases over this time. Any resistance was shown to have decreased, though not significantly. There were no results for re-treatment cases in the first survey, and the 2006 survey shows a considerable proportion of MDR-TB among previously treated cases, at 19.3% (95% CLs, 14.2-25.4). A survey in southern Viet Nam in 2001 also showed that any drug resistance had actually decreased since 1996, and there had been no increase in MDR-TB[41].

The Philippines conducted its first nationwide survey in 2004, which showed 4.0% (95% CLs, 2.9-5.5) MDR-TB among new cases and 20.9% (95% CLs, 14.3-29.0) among previously treated cases. MDR-TB isolates from this survey are being further tested to second-line drugs at the SRL. Given the underlying high TB burden, it is estimated that there were 11 848 (95% CLs, 7428-17 106) incident MDR-TB in 2006. TB notifications in the country are stable and treatment success is high. Importantly, the Philippines have had a long-running GLC-approved programme for the management of MDR-TB patients, and this programme is now expanding. Treatment success in the programme is high, at 73% in the 2003 cohort. Based on data from the GLC programme[33], 50.0% of the MDR-TB patients enrolled in the GLC programme were resistant to a fluoroquinolone, and 3.4% (95% CLs, 1.6–6.1) were XDR-TB. The high proportion of resistance to quinolones among MDR-TB cases is concerning and should be monitored in subsequent surveys.

Since 1994, China has reported data on 8of 31 provinces, 2 major municipalities, and 2 SARs. Several other provincial surveys are under way, as well as a nationwide drug-resistance survey that is due to be completed in 2008.

Data from surveys in Heilongjiang Province, Inner Mongolia Autonomous Region, and Beijing and Shanghai municipalities are included in this report. These data support findings from previous surveys in other provinces. Heilongjiang Province showed 7.2% (95% CLs, 5.9–8.6) MDR-TB among new cases and Inner Mongolia Autonomous Region showed 7.3% (95% CLs, 5.6–9.4). These proportions are similar to those reported from Liaoning province, also in North Eastern China. Lower proportions of resistance were reported from Beijing (2.3%; 95% CLs, 1.5–3.4) and Shanghai (3.9%; 95% CLs, 2.6–5.6). This is one of the first reports of lower proportions of drug resistance in urban settings. A nationwide survey, based on a random selection of 70 clusters representing counties or districts, is scheduled to complete in 2008. Surveys in Chongqing, Hunan and Xinjiang provinces will be finalized shortly. Despite reaching the global targets for case detection and cure, China has proportions of resistance that are among the highest in the world, only second to rates found in countries of the former Soviet Union. The plan for expansion of MDR-TB treatment under the NTP includes the launch of pilot projects in 31 prefectures in six provinces, with plans to enrol 5000 MDR-TB patients by 2009, and scale up to 50 prefectures in 10 additional provinces, treating 10 000 MDR-TB patients by 2011. China, is not on target to meet this goal, even though MDR-TB management guidelines, in line with international standards, have been published and a GLC application has been approved.

The extent of resistance to second-line drugs is currently unknown; however, the NRL is developing capacity to conduct second-line testing, and MDR-TB isolates from the nationwide survey will be evaluated. China has spent considerable time expanding quality assurance for smear microscopy in the country and now has plans to upgrade culture and DST laboratories, as well as quality assurance for drug-susceptibility testing.

Trends are available from Hong Kong SAR and the Republic of Korea. Trends in resistance to any drug, isoniazid and MDR-TB continue to decline in Hong Kong SAR[42] at a faster rate than TB. The TB notification rate decreased from 103 per 100 000 in 1996 to 81 per 100 000 in 2005. The Republic of Korea has conducted four nationwide surveys. The surveys have shown a gradual but significant increase in MDR-TB[43], any resistance and isoniazid resistance among new cases. The TB notification rate has declined since 1994, but has been relatively stable for the past three years. The slowing in the decline in the overall TB notification rate probably reflects the expansion of the routine registration of TB patients from the private sector. The TB notification rate in the public sector alone continued to show a

---

[33] Drug susceptibility testing data were reported from a local laboratory currently conducting external quality assurance for first-line drugs, but second-line results have not been rechecked by an SRL.

decline for those same years. The last two drug-resistance surveys were carried out one year apart, so future surveys will be needed to better understand if this is a true increase in population prevalence. The Korean Institute of Tuberculosis, which is an NRL as well as an SRL, conducts nearly 70% of culture and DST in the country, for both the public and private sectors. Data reported in the Centers for Disease Control and Prevention (CDC) Morbidity and Mortality Weekly Report[44] showing results of a global survey of SRLs showed that 15.4% of MDR-TB cases in Korea were XDR-TB. Because these data were biased towards hospitalized patients in the private sector, it is likely that it overestimated the proportion of MDR-TB among total isolates tested, and of MDR-TB cases that are XDR-TB. Data from the nationwide survey showed that only 1.8% of MDR-TB cases detected in the survey had XDR-TB. Therefore, if culture and DST coverage are not complete, routine laboratory investigations may be biased towards chronic cases and treatment failure.

Currently, information on resistance to second-line drugs is limited. Australia, Hong Kong and Macao SARs, Japan and the Republic of Korea are able to report data on second-line drug resistance routinely. The Philippines has been able to report data on a GLC cohort, and Viet Nam has identified one case. Thus far, the data are difficult to interpret. The proportion of XDR-TB among MDR-TB was highest in Japan, at 30.9% (95% CLs, 19.1–44.9), and in Hong Kong SAR, at 14.6 (95% CLs, 13.7–16.1). Where absolute numbers of MDR-TB are low, XDR-TB may not represent a significant obstacle for TB control. However, in high-burden countries where second-line drugs are widely available, such as China and the Philippines, further assessment of resistance to second-line drugs will be a critical component of designing the strategy for the management of MDR-TB.

Currently, Cambodia, China, the Federated States of Micronesia, Mongolia, the Philippines, Samoa and Viet Nam have GLC-approved programmes.

Like the WHO South-East Asia Region, the Western Pacific is also faced with limited capacity for culture and drug-susceptibility testing. China, Viet Nam and the Republic of Korea have extensive culture networks in the public sector, but only China has a significant number of laboratories able to conduct drug-susceptibility testing. Quality assurance of DST and links with the private sector may also prove critical in this region for building the capacity necessary for the scale up outlined in the Global Plan to Stop TB, 2006–2015. The Western Pacific region currently has five very active SRLs and has plans to add one more over the next year.

REFERENCES

1. World Health Organization, *Global tuberculosis control: surveillance, planning, financing. WHO Report 2008*. World Health Organization Document, 2008. **WHO/HTM/ TB/2008.393**.

2. World Health Organization, *The Global MDR-TB & XDR-TB response Plan 2007-2008*. World Health Organization Document, 2007. **WHO/HTM/TB/2007.387**.

3. Wells, C. et al., *HIV infection and multidrug-resistant tuberculosis: the perfect storm*. J Infect Dis, 2007. **196**(Suppl 1): p. S86–107.

5. World Health Organization, *Guidelines for the surveillance of drug resistance in tuberculosis*. World Health Organization Document, 2003. **WHO/TB/2003.320**: p. 1–21.

6. World Health Organization., *Interim Recommendations for the Surveillance of Drug Resistance in Tuberculosis*. World Health Organization Document, 2007. **WHO/HTM/TB/2007.385**.

7. Van Deun, A. et al., *Evaluation of tuberculosis control by periodic or routine susceptibility testing in previously treated cases*. Int.J.Tuberc.Lung Dis., 2001. **5**: p. 329–338.

8. van Rie, A. et al., *Classification of drug-resistant tuberculosis in an epidemic area*. Lancet, 2000. **356**: p. 22–25.

9. World Health Organization, *Laboratory services in tuberculosis control. Part III: Culture*. 1 ed, ed. W.H. Organization. 1998, Geneva: World Health Organization. 1–95.

10. Vestal, A. and G. Kubica, *Differential identification of mycobacteria. 3. Use of thiacetazone, thiophen-2-carboxylic acid hydrazide, and triphenyltetrazolium chloride*. Scand J Respir Dis, 1967. **48**(2): p. 142–8.

11. Canetti, G. et al., *Mycobacteria: laboratory methods for testing drug sensitivity and resistance*. 1963. **29**: p. 565–578.

12. Canetti, G. et al., *Advances in techniques of testing mycobacterial drug sensitivity, and the use of sensitivity tests in tuberculosis control programmes.* 1969. **41**: p. 21–43.

13. World Health Organization, *Interim Policy Guidance on Drug Susceptibility Testing (DST) of Second-line Anti-Tuberculosis Drugs.* World Health Organization Document, 2008. **WHO/HTM/ TB/2008.392**.

14. Zignol, M. et al., *Global incidence of multidrug-resistant tuberculosis.* 2006. **194**: p. 479–485.

15. Li, X. et al., *Transmission of drug-resistant tuberculosis among treated patients in Shanghai, China.* J Infect Dis, 2007. **195**(6): p. 864–9.

16. Jeon, C. et al., *Extensively drug-resistant tuberculosis in South Korea: risk factors and treatment outcomes among patients at a tertiary referral hospital.* Clin Infect Dis, 2008. **46**(1): p. 42–9.

17. Cox, H. et al., *Multidrug-Resistant Tuberculosis Treatment Outcomes in Karakalpakstan, Uzbekistan: Treatment Complexity and XDR-TB among Treatment Failures.* PLoS ONE, 2007. **2**(11): p. e1126.

18. Edlin, B.R. et al., *An outbreak of multidrug-resistant tuberculosis among hospitalized patients with the acquired immunodeficiency syndrome.* 1992. **326**: p. 1514–1521.

19. Moro, M.L. et al., *An outbreak of multidrug-resistant tuberculosis involving HIV-infected patients of two hospitals in Milan, Italy.* AIDS, 1998. **12**: p. 1095–1102.

20. Kenyon, T.A. et al., *Low levels of drug resistance amidst rapidly increasing tuberculosis and human immunodeficiency virus co-epidemics in Botswana.* Int.J.Tuberc.Lung Dis., 1999. **3**: p. 4–11.

21. Chum, H.J. et al., *An epidemiological study of tuberculosis and HIV infection in Tanzania, 1991–1993.* AIDS, 1996. **10**: p. 299–309.

22. Mac-Arthur, A., Jr. et al., *Characteristics of drug resistance and HIV among tuberculosis patients in Mozambique.* Int.J.Tuberc.Lung Dis., 2001. **5**: p. 894–902.

23. Gandhi, N.R. et al., *Extensively drug-resistant tuberculosis as a cause of death in patients coinfected with tuberculosis in a rural area of South Africa.* Lancet, 2006. **368**: p. 1575–1580.

24. Blower, S.M. and T. Chou, *Modeling the emergence of the "hot zones'" tuberculosis and the amplification dynamics of drug resistance.* Nat Med, 2004. **10**(10): p. 1111–6.

25. Gandhi, N.R. et al., *Extensively drug-resistant tuberculosis as a cause of death in patients coinfected with tuberculosis and HIV in a rural area of South Africa.* Lancet, 2006. **368**(9547): p. 1575–80.

26. Umubyeyi, A. et al., *Low levels of second-line drug resistance among multidrug-resistant Mycobacterium tuberculosis isolates from Rwanda.* Int J Infect Dis, 2007.

27. Umubyeyi, A.N. et al., *Limited fluoroquinolone resistance among Mycobacterium tuberculosis isolates from Rwanda: results of a national survey.* J Antimicrob Chemother, 2007. **59**(5): p. 1031–3.

28. Umubyeyi, A.N. et al., *Results of a national survey on drug resistance among pulmonary tuberculosis patients in Rwanda.* Int J Tuberc Lung Dis, 2007. **11**(2): p. 189–94.

29. Montoro, E. et al., *Drug-resistant tuberculosis in Cuba. Results of the three global projects.* Tuberculosis (Edinb), 2006. **86**(3–4): p. 319–23.

30. Blöndal, K., *Barriers to reaching the targets for tuberculosis control: multidrug-resistant tuberculosis.* Bull World Health Organ, 2007. **85**(5): p. 387–90.

31. Leimane, V. and J. Leimans, *Tuberculosis control in Latvia: itnegrated DOTS and DOTS-Plus programmes.* Eurosurveillance, 2006. **11**: p. 29–33.

32. Balabanova Ia, M. et al., *[Analysis of risk factors of the occurrence of drug resistance in patients with tuberculosis from civil and penitentiary sectors in the Samara Region].* Probl Tuberk Bolezn Legk, 2005(5): p. 25–31.

33. Drobniewski, F. et al., *Drug-resistant tuberculosis, clinical virulence, and the dominance of the Beijing strain family in Russia.* JAMA, 2005. **293**: p. 2726–2731.

34. Drobniewski, F.A. et al., *Tuberculosis, HIV seroprevalence and intravenous drug abuse in prisoners.* 2005. **26**: p. 298–304.

35. Mahadev, B. et al., *Surveillance of drug resistance to anti-tuberculosis drugs in districts of Hoogli in West Bengal and Mayurbhanj in Orissa.* Indian J Tuberc., 2004. **52**: p. 5–10.

36. Joseph, M. et al., *Surveillance of anti-tuberculosis drug resistance in Ernakulam District, Kerala State, South India.* Int J Tuberc Lung Dis, 2007. **11**(4): p. 443–9.

37. Ti, T. et al., *National anti-tuberculosis drug resistance survey, 2002, in Myanmar.* Int J Tuberc Lung Dis, 2006. **10**(10): p. 1111–6.

38. Thomas, A. et al., *Management of multi drug resistance tuberculosis in the field: Tuberculosis Research Centre experience.* Indian J Tuberc, 2007. **54**(3): p. 117–24.

39. Kelly, P.M. et al., *A community-based TB drug susceptibility study in Mimika District, Papua Province, Indonesia.* Int J Tuberc Lung Dis, 2006. **10**(2): p. 167–71.

40. Van Deun, A. et al., *Drug resistance monitoring: combined rates may be the best indicator of programme performance.* Int.J.Tuberc.Lung Dis., 2004. **8**: p. 23–30.

41. Huong, N.T. et al., *Antituberculosis drug resistance in the south of Vietnam: prevalence and trends.* J Infect Dis, 2006. **194**(9): p. 1226–32.

42. Kam, K.M. and C.W. Yip, *Surveillance of Mycobacterium tuberculosis drug resistance in Hong Kong, 1986–1999, after the implementation of directly observed treatment.* Int.J.Tuberc.Lung Dis., 2001. **5**: p. 815–823.

43. Bai, G.H. et al., *Trend of anti-tuberculosis drug resistance in Korea, 1994–2004.* Int J Tuberc Lung Dis, 2007. **11**(5): p. 571–6.

44. *Emergence of Mycobacterium tuberculosis with extensive resistance to second-line drugs--worldwide, 2000–2004.* MMWR Morb Mortal Wkly Rep, 2006. **55**(11): p. 301–5.

ANNEXES

Annex 1: Notified prevalence of resistance to specific drugs among new TB cases tested for resistance to at least INH and RIF (1) 1994–2007

Country	Sub-National	Year	Method	Patients Tested	Susceptible	%	Any Res.	%	Any H	%	Any R	%	Any E	%	Any S	%	Mono	%	Mono H	%	Mono R	%
AFRICA																						
Algeria	Countrywide	2001	Survey	518	486	93,8	32	6,2	16	3,1	6	1,2	0	0,0	27	5,2	21	4,1	5	1,0	0	0,0
Benin	Countrywide	1997	Survey	333	305	91,6	28	8,4	18	5,4	1	0,3	2	0,6	16	4,8	20	6,0	11	3,3	0	0,0
Botswana	Countrywide	2002	Survey	1182	1.059	89,6	123	10,4	53	4,5	24	2,0	15	1,3	82	6,9	86	7,3	22	1,9	10	0,8
Central African Republic	Bangui	1998	Survey	464	388	83,6	76	16,4	44	9,5	6	1,3	11	2,4	51	11,0	50	10,8	19	4,1	1	0,2
Côte d'Ivoire	Countrywide	2006	Survey	320	244	76,3	76	23,8	39	12,2	10	3,1	22	6,9	32	10,0	53	16,6	23	7,2	0	0,0
DR Congo	Kinshasa	1999	comb. only																			
Ethiopia	Countrywide	2005	Survey	804	588	73,1	216	26,9	62	7,7	22	2,7	19	2,4	187	23,3	165	20,5	16	2,0	8	1,0
Gambia	Countrywide	2000	Survey	210	201	95,7	9	4,3	5	2,4	2	1,0	0	0,0	3	1,4	8	3,8	4	1,9	1	0,5
Guinea	Sentinel sites	1998	Survey	539	460	85,3	79	14,7	50	9,3	4	0,7	3	0,6	51	9,5	53	9,8	24	4,5	1	0,2
Kenya	Nearly Countrywide	1995	Survey	445	417	93,7	28	6,3	28	6,3	0	0,0	0	0,0	4	0,9	24	5,4	24	5,4	0	0,0
Lesotho	Countrywide	1995	Survey	330	301	91,2	29	8,8	26	7,9	3	0,9	0	0,0	10	3,0	20	6,1	17	5,2	0	0,0
Madagascar (2)	Countrywide	2007	Survey	810	759	93,7	51	6,3	37	4,6	4	0,5	4	0,5	26	3,2	42	5,2	28	3,5	0	0,0
Mozambique	Countrywide	1999	Survey	1028	814	79,2	214	20,8	170	16,5	54	5,3	5	0,5	108	10,5	125	12,2	81	7,9	18	1,8
Rwanda	Countrywide	2005	Survey	616	552	89,6	64	10,4	38	6,2	24	3,9	32	5,2	46	7,5	33	5,4	7	1,1	0	0,0
Senegal	Countrywide	2006	Survey	237	212	89,5	25	10,5	10	4,2	5	2,1	8	3,4	18	7,6	18	7,6	3	1,3	0	0,0
Sierra Leone	Nearly Countrywide	1997	Survey	117	88	75,2	29	24,8	12	10,3	1	0,9	0	0,0	25	21,4	21	17,9	4	3,4	0	0,0
South Africa	Countrywide	2002	Survey	4243	3.906	92,1	337	7,9	249	5,9	91	2,1	38	0,9	178	4,2	197	4,6	109	2,6	14	0,3
Swaziland	Countrywide	1995	Survey	334	295	88,3	39	11,7	30	9,0	3	0,9	3	0,9	24	7,2	22	6,6	13	3,9	0	0,0
Uganda	3 GLRA Zones *	1997	Survey	374	300	80,2	74	19,8	25	6,7	3	0,8	23	6,1	50	13,4	48	12,8	12	3,2	1	0,3
UR Tanzania (2)	Countrywide	2007	Survey	369	346	93,8	23	6,2	16	4,3	4	1,1	3	0,8	13	3,5	15	4,1	8	2,2	0	0,0
Zambia	Countrywide	2000	Survey	445	394	88,5	51	11,5	28	6,3	8	1,8	9	2,0	24	5,4	38	8,5	15	3,4	0	0,0
Zimbabwe	Nearly Countrywide	1995	Survey	676	654	96,7	22	3,3	22	3,3	13	1,9	4	0,6	5	0,7	9	1,3	9	1,3	0	0,0
AMERICAS																						
Argentina	Countrywide	2005	Survey	683	615	90,0	68	10,0	39	5,7	16	2,3	4	0,6	44	6,4	43	6,3	14	2,1	1	0,
Bolivia	Countrywide	1996	Survey	498	371	74,5	127	25,5	51	10,2	30	6,0	25	5,0	49	9,8	100	20,1	34	6,8	14	2,8
Brazil	Nearly Countrywide	1996	Survey	2095	1.915	91,4	180	8,6	124	5,9	23	1,1	3	0,1	76	3,6	135	6,4	79	3,8	4	0,
Canada	Countrywide	2006	Surveillance	1058	977	92,3	81	7,7	67	6,3	12	1,1	10	0,9	25	2,4	59	5,6	45	4,3	4	0,
Chile	Countrywide	2001	Survey	867	776	89,5	91	10,5	39	4,5	7	0,8	2	0,2	78	9,0	64	7,4	12	1,4	1	0,
Colombia	Countrywide	2000	Survey	1087	918	84,5	169	15,5	103	9,5	18	1,7	9	0,8	125	11,5	102	9,4	37	3,4	1	0,
Costa Rica	Countrywide	2006	Survey	263	244	92,8	19	7,2	9	3,4	5	1,9	13	4,9	0	0,0	7	2,7	5	1,9	1	0,
Cuba	Countrywide	2005	Sentinel	169	157	92,9	12	7,1	1	0,6	1	0,6	0	0,0	11	6,5	11	6,5	0	0,0	1	0,
Dominican Republic	Countrywide	1995	Survey	303	180	59,4	123	40,6	60	19,8	49	16,2	11	3,6	64	21,1	78	25,7	26	8,6	21	6,
Ecuador	Countrywide	2002	Survey	812	649	79,9	163	20,1	89	11,0	59	7,3	10	1,2	92	11,3	99	12,2	29	3,6	15	1,
El Salvador	Countrywide	2001	Survey	611	576	94,3	35	5,7	8	1,3	7	1,1	2	0,3	23	3,8	30	4,9	3	0,5	5	0,
Guatemala	Countrywide	2002	Survey	668	435	65,1	233	34,9	72	10,8	28	4,2	52	7,8	193	28,9	156	23,4	8	1,2	5	0
Honduras	Countrywide	2004	Survey	457	402	88,0	55	12,0	27	5,9	10	2,2	8	1,8	38	8,3	39	8,5	11	2,4	2	0,
Mexico	Baja California, Sinaloa, Oaxaca	1997	Survey	334	287	85,9	47	14,1	24	7,2	12	3,6	10	3,0	24	7,2	35	10,5	14	4,2	2	0
Nicaragua	Countrywide	2006	Survey	320	278	86,9	42	13,1	21	6,6	3	0,9	4	1,3	25	7,8	33	10,3	13	4,1	1	0,
Paraguay	Countrywide	2001	Survey	235	209	88,9	26	11,1	15	6,4	8	3,4	6	2,6	12	5,1	16	6,8	7	3,0	3	1,
Peru	Countrywide	2006	Survey	1809	1.389	76,8	420	23,2	209	11,6	105	5,8	36	2,0	342	18,9	254	14,0	45	2,5	9	0
Puerto Rico	Countrywide	2005	Surveillance	comb. only																		
Uruguay	Countrywide	2005	Survey	335	328	97,9	7	2,1	4	1,2	1	0,3	1	0,3	1	0,3	7	2,1	4	1,2	1	0
USA	Countrywide	2005	Surveillance	comb. only																		
Venezuela	Countrywide	1999	Survey	769	711	92,5	58	7,5	30	3,9	8	1,0	8	1,0	36	4,7	38	4,9	13	1,7	3	0
EASTERN MEDITERRANEAN																						
Egypt	Countrywide	2002	Survey	632	439	69,5	193	30,5	62	9,8	44	7,0	18	2,8	149	23,6	137	21,7	17	2,7	22	3
Iran	Countrywide	1998	Survey	666	560	84,1	106	15,9	65	9,8	41	6,2	31	4,7	65	9,8	54	8,1	18	2,7	6	0
Jordan	Countrywide	2004	Survey	111	75	67,6	36	32,4	10	9,0	13	11,7	11	9,9	25	22,5	23	20,7	1	0,9	4	3
Lebanon	Countrywide	2003	Survey	190	153	80,5	37	19,5	23	12,1	5	2,6	7	3,7	23	12,1	19	10,0	7	3,7	2	1
Morocco	Countrywide	2006	Survey	1049	976	93,0	73	7,0	43	4,1	8	0,8	2	0,2	56	5,3	43	4,1	14	1,3	2	0
Oman	Countrywide	2006	Surveillance	150	140	93,3	10	6,7	7	4,7	2	1,3	1	0,7	5	3,3	7	4,7	4	2,7	0	0
Qatar	Countrywide	2006	Surveillance	comb. only																		
Yemen	Countrywide	2004	Survey	510	461	90,4	49	9,6	20	3,9	15	2,9	15	2,9	40	7,8	33	6,5	4	0,8	0	0
EUROPE																						
Andorra	Countrywide	2005	Surveillance	9	8	88,9	1	11,1	1	11,1	0	0,0	0	0,0	1	11,1	0	0,0	0	0,0	0	0
Armenia	Countrywide	2007	Survey	552	345	62,5	207	37,5	150	27,2	60	10,9	24	4,3	160	29,0	90	16,3	34	6,2	7	1
Austria	Countrywide	2005	Surveillance	570	501	87,9	69	12,1	54	9,5	14	2,5	9	1,6	39	6,8	40	7,0	27	4,7	2	0
Azerbaijan	Baku City	2007	Survey	551	241	43,7	310	56,3	225	40,8	125	22,7	68	12,3	281	51,0	109	19,8	25	4,5	1	0
Belgium	Countrywide	2005	Surveillance	588	554	94,2	34	5,8	29	4,9	9	1,5	8	1,4	0	0,0	24	4,1	19	3,2	2	0
Bosnia & Herzegovina	Countrywide	2005	Surveillance	1035	1.020	98,6	15	1,4	8	0,8	7	0,7	3	0,3	4	0,4	10	1,0	3	0,3	3	0
Croatia	Countrywide	2005	Surveillance	586	569	97,1	17	2,9	12	2,1	6	1,0	3	0,5	8	1,4	10	1,7	8	1,4	0	0
Czech Republic	Countrywide	2005	Surveillance	562	519	92,3	43	7,7	21	3,7	8	1,4	4	0,7	34	6,1	29	5,2	8	1,4	0	0
Denmark	Countrywide	2005	Surveillance	307	290	94,5	17	5,5	15	4,9	5	1,6	6	2,0	0	0,0	12	3,9	10	3,3	0	0
Estonia	Countrywide	2005	Surveillance	316	225	71,2	91	28,8	65	20,6	42	13,3	42	13,3	83	26,3	34	10,8	8	2,5	0	
Finland	Countrywide	2005	Surveillance	198	190	96,0	8	4,0	7	3,5	2	1,0	2	1,0	1	0,5	6	3,0	5	2,5	0	0
France	Countrywide	2005	Sentinel	1291	1.179	91,3	112	8,7	71	5,5	15	1,2	9	0,7	60	4,6	80	6,2	39	3,0	1	
Georgia	Countrywide	2006	Survey	799	406	50,8	393	49,2	187	23,4	61	7,6	33	4,1	330	41,3	249	31,2	49	6,1	4	
Germany	Countrywide	2005	Surveillance	3094	2.755	89,0	339	11,0	225	7,3	68	2,2	55	1,8	229	7,4	195	6,3	85	2,7	8	

Mono E	%	Mono S	%	Mdr	%	Hr	%	Hre	%	Hrs	%	Hres	%	Poly	%	He	%	Hs	%	Hes	%	Re	%	Rs	%	Res	%	Es	%
0	0,0	16	3,1	6	1,2	0	0,0	0	0,0	6	1,2	0	0,0	5	1,0	0	0,0	5	1,0	0	0,0	0	0,0	0	0,0	0	0,0	0	0,0
0	0,0	9	2,7	1	0,3	0	0,0	1	0,3	0	0,0	0	0,0	7	2,1	0	0,0	6	1,8	0	0,0	0	0,0	0	0,0	0	0,0	1	0,3
2	0,2	52	4,4	10	0,8	3	0,3	2	0,2	3	0,3	2	0,2	27	2,3	2	0,2	15	1,3	4	0,3	0	0,0	3	0,3	1	0,1	2	0,2
0	0,0	30	6,5	5	1,1	2	0,4	2	0,4	0	0,0	1	0,2	21	4,5	1	0,2	13	2,8	6	1,3	0	0,0	0	0,0	0	0,0	1	0,2
13	4,1	17	5,3	8	2,5	4	1,3	1	0,3	3	0,9	0	0,0	15	4,7	3	0,9	5	1,6	0	0,0	0	0,0	2	0,6	0	0,0	5	1,6
1	0,1	140	17,4	13	1,6	3	0,4	0	0,0	1	0,1	9	1,1	38	4,7	1	0,1	28	3,5	4	0,5	0	0,0	1	0,1	0	0,0	4	0,5
0	0,0	3	1,4	1	0,5	1	0,5	0	0,0	0	0,0	0	0,0	0	0,0	0	0,0	0	0,0	0	0,0	0	0,0	0	0,0	0	0,0	0	0,0
0	0,0	28	5,2	3	0,6	1	0,2	0	0,0	2	0,4	0	0,0	23	4,3	2	0,4	20	3,7	1	0,2	0	0,0	0	0,0	0	0,0	0	0,0
0	0,0	0	0,0	0	0,0	0	0,0	0	0,0	0	0,0	0	0,0	4	0,9	0	0,0	4	0,9	0	0,0	0	0,0	0	0,0	0	0,0	0	0,0
0	0,0	3	0,9	3	0,9	2	0,6	0	0,0	1	0,3	0	0,0	6	1,8	0	0,0	6	1,8	0	0,0	0	0,0	0	0,0	0	0,0	0	0,0
0	0,0	20	2,5	4	0,5	1	0,1	1	0,1	0	0,0	2	0,2	5	0,6	1	0,1	4	0,5	0	0,0	0	0,0	0	0,0	0	0,0	0	0,0
0	0,0	26	2,5	36	3,5	7	0,7	0	0,0	24	2,3	5	0,5	53	5,2	0	0,0	53	5,2	0	0,0	0	0,0	0	0,0	0	0,0	0	0,0
10	1,6	16	2,6	24	3,9	1	0,2	0	0,0	2	0,3	21	3,4	7	1,1	0	0,0	6	1,0	1	0,2	0	0,0	0	0,0	0	0,0	0	0,0
3	1,3	12	5,1	5	2,1	0	0,0	1	0,4	1	0,4	3	1,3	2	0,8	0	0,0	1	0,4	1	0,4	0	0,0	0	0,0	0	0,0	0	0,0
0	0,0	17	14,5	1	0,9	0	0,0	0	0,0	1	0,9	0	0,0	7	6,0	0	0,0	7	6,0	0	0,0	0	0,0	0	0,0	0	0,0	0	0,0
0	0,0	74	1,7	77	1,8	21	0,5	10	0,2	26	0,6	20	0,5	63	1,5	5	0,1	55	1,3	3	0,1	0	0,0	0	0,0	0	0,0	0	0,0
1	0,3	8	2,4	3	0,9	0	0,0	1	0,3	2	0,6	0	0,0	14	4,2	0	0,0	13	3,9	1	0,3	0	0,0	0	0,0	0	0,0	0	0,0
9	2,4	26	7,0	2	0,5	1	0,3	1	0,3	0	0,0	0	0,0	24	6,4	0	0,0	11	2,9	0	0,0	0	0,0	0	0,0	0	0,0	13	3,5
0	0,0	7	1,9	4	1,1	0	0,0	1	0,3	2	0,5	1	0,3	4	1,1	1	0,3	3	0,8	0	0,0	0	0,0	0	0,0	0	0,0	0	0,0
3	0,7	20	4,5	8	1,8	4	0,9	3	0,7	0	0,0	1	0,2	5	1,1	2	0,4	3	0,7	0	0,0	0	0,0	0	0,0	0	0,0	0	0,0
0	0,0	0	0,0	13	1,9	8	1,2	0	0,0	1	0,1	4	0,6	0	0,0	0	0,0	0	0,0	0	0,0	0	0,0	0	0,0	0	0,0	0	0,0
1	0,1	27	4,0	15	2,2	7	1,0	1	0,1	5	0,7	2	0,3	10	1,5	0	0,0	10	1,5	0	0,0	0	0,0	0	0,0	0	0,0	0	0,0
18	3,6	34	6,8	6	1,2	5	1,0	0	0,0	1	0,2	0	0,0	21	4,2	2	0,4	9	1,8	0	0,0	5	1,0	5	1,0	0	0,0	0	0,0
2	0,1	50	2,4	19	0,9	18	0,9	0	0,0	1	0,1	0	0,0	26	1,2	1	0,1	25	1,2	0	0,0	0	0,0	0	0,0	0	0,0	0	0,0
3	0,3	7	0,7	8	0,8	3	0,3	0	0,0	3	0,3	2	0,2	14	1,3	1	0,1	9	0,9	4	0,4	0	0,0	0	0,0	0	0,0	0	0,0
0	0,0	51	5,9	6	0,7	0	0,0	0	0,0	4	0,5	2	0,2	21	2,4	0	0,0	21	2,4	0	0,0	0	0,0	0	0,0	0	0,0	0	0,0
0	0,3	61	5,6	16	1,5	1	0,1	2	0,2	11	1,0	2	0,2	51	4,7	0	0,0	48	4,4	2	0,2	0	0,0	1	0,1	0	0,0	0	0,0
9	3,4	0	0,0	4	1,5	0	0,0	4	1,5	0	0,0	0	0,0	8	3,0	0	0,0	0	0,0	0	0,0	0	0,0	0	0,0	0	0,0	0	0,0
0	0,0	10	5,9	0	0,0	0	0,0	0	0,0	0	0,0	0	0,0	1	0,6	0	0,0	1	0,6	0	0,0	0	0,0	0	0,0	0	0,0	0	0,0
1	0,3	30	9,9	20	6,6	9	3,0	1	0,3	6	2,0	4	1,3	25	8,3	0	0,0	13	4,3	1	0,3	1	0,3	7	2,3	0	0,0	3	1,0
2	0,2	53	6,5	40	4,9	20	2,5	4	0,5	14	1,7	2	0,2	24	3,0	0	0,0	20	2,5	0	0,0	1	0,1	2	0,2	1	0,1	0	0,0
2	0,3	20	3,3	2	0,3	2	0,3	0	0,0	0	0,0	0	0,0	3	0,5	0	0,0	3	0,5	0	0,0	0	0,0	0	0,0	0	0,0	0	0,0
23	3,4	120	18,0	20	3,0	2	0,3	1	0,1	7	1,1	10	1,5	57	8,5	1	0,1	37	5,5	6	0,9	0	0,0	2	0,3	1	0,1	10	1,5
0	0,0	26	5,7	8	1,8	1	0,2	2	0,4	0	0,0	5	1,1	8	1,8	1	0,2	7	1,5	0	0,0	0	0,0	0	0,0	0	0,0	0	0,0
1	0,3	18	5,4	8	2,4	1	0,3	1	0,3	2	0,6	4	1,2	4	1,2	2	0,6	0	0,0	0	0,0	2	0,6	0	0,0	0	0,0	0	0,0
1	0,3	18	5,6	2	0,6	0	0,0	2	0,6	0	0,0	0	0,0	7	2,2	0	0,0	6	1,9	0	0,0	0	0,0	0	0,0	0	0,0	1	0,3
0	0,0	6	2,6	5	2,1	1	0,4	2	0,9	1	0,4	1	0,4	5	2,1	1	0,4	2	0,9	0	0,0	0	0,0	0	0,0	0	0,0	2	0,9
0	0,0	200	11,1	95	5,3	17	0,9	6	0,3	45	2,5	27	1,5	71	3,9	1	0,1	67	3,7	1	0,1	0	0,0	1	0,1	0	0,0	1	0,1
1	0,3	1	0,3	0	0,0	0	0,0	0	0,0	0	0,0	0	0,0	0	0,0	0	0,0	0	0,0	0	0,0	0	0,0	0	0,0	0	0,0	0	0,0
1	0,1	21	2,7	4	0,5	2	0,3	0	0,0	1	0,1	1	0,1	16	2,1	2	0,3	10	1,3	1	0,1	1	0,1	0	0,0	0	0,0	2	0,3
3	0,5	95	15,0	14	2,2	0	0,0	0	0,0	5	0,8	9	1,4	42	6,6	2	0,3	28	4,4	1	0,2	0	0,0	8	1,3	0	0,0	3	0,5
2	0,3	28	4,2	33	5,0	8	1,2	1	0,2	6	0,9	18	2,7	19	2,9	5	0,8	8	1,2	1	0,2	1	0,2	1	0,2	0	0,0	3	0,5
2	1,8	16	14,4	6	5,4	1	0,9	1	0,9	1	0,9	3	2,7	7	6,3	1	0,9	1	0,9	1	0,9	1	0,9	1	0,9	1	0,9	1	0,9
3	1,6	7	3,7	2	1,1	0	0,0	1	0,5	0	0,0	1	0,5	16	8,4	0	0,0	14	7,4	0	0,0	1	0,5	0	0,0	0	0,0	1	0,5
0	0,0	27	2,6	5	0,5	1	0,1	0	0,0	3	0,3	1	0,1	25	2,4	0	0,0	23	2,2	1	0,1	0	0,0	1	0,1	0	0,0	0	0,0
0	0,0	3	2,0	2	1,3	1	0,7	0	0,0	0	0,0	1	0,7	1	0,7	0	0,0	1	0,7	0	0,0	0	0,0	0	0,0	0	0,0	0	0,0
2	0,4	27	5,3	15	2,9	1	0,2	1	0,2	2	0,4	11	2,2	1	0,2	1	0,2	0	0,0	0	0,0	0	0,0	0	0,0	0	0,0	0	0,0
0	0,0	0	0,0	0	0,0	0	0,0	0	0,0	0	0,0	0	0,0	1	11,1	0	0,0	1	11,1	0	0,0	0	0,0	0	0,0	0	0,0	0	0,0
1	0,2	48	8,7	52	9,4	4	0,7	0	0,0	37	6,7	11	2,0	65	11,8	1	0,2	52	9,4	11	2,0	0	0,0	1	0,2	0	0,0	0	0,0
0	0,0	11	1,9	11	1,9	0	0,0	1	0,2	4	0,7	6	1,1	18	3,2	0	0,0	15	2,6	2	0,4	0	0,0	1	0,2	0	0,0	0	0,0
0	0,0	83	15,1	123	22,3	2	0,4	1	0,2	63	11,4	57	10,3	78	14,2	0	0,0	67	12,2	10	1,8	0	0,0	1	0,2	0	0,0	0	0,0
3	0,5	0	0,0	7	1,2	5	0,9	2	0,3	0	0,0	0	0,0	3	0,5	3	0,5	0	0,0	0	0,0	0	0,0	0	0,0	0	0,0	0	0,0
0	0,1	9	0,3	4	0,3	3	0,3	0	0,0	0	0,0	0	0,0	1	0,1	1	0,1	0	0,0	0	0,0	0	0,0	0	0,0	0	0,0	0	0,0
0	0,0	2	0,3	3	0,5	0	0,0	1	0,2	2	0,3	0	0,0	4	0,7	0	0,0	1	0,2	0	0,0	0	0,0	0	0,0	2	0,3	0	0,0
1	0,2	20	3,6	7	1,2	0	0,0	0	0,0	4	0,7	3	0,5	7	1,2	0	0,0	6	1,1	0	0,0	0	0,0	0	0,0	0	0,0	0	0,0
2	0,7	0	0,0	5	1,6	1	0,3	4	1,3	0	0,0	0	0,0	0	0,0	0	0,0	0	0,0	0	0,0	0	0,0	0	0,0	0	0,0	0	0,0
0	0,0	26	8,2	42	13,3	0	0,0	0	0,0	3	0,9	39	12,3	15	4,7	0	0,0	12	3,8	3	0,9	0	0,0	0	0,0	0	0,0	0	0,0
1	0,5	0	0,0	2	1,0	1	0,5	0	0,0	0	0,0	1	0,5	0	0,0	0	0,0	0	0,0	0	0,0	0	0,0	0	0,0	0	0,0	0	0,0
3	0,7	37	2,9	14	1,1	6	0,5	2	0,2	4	0,3	2	0,2	18	1,4	1	0,1	16	1,2	0	0,0	2	0,1	0	0,0	0	0,0	0	0,0
3	0,4	193	24,2	54	6,8	6	0,8	0	0,0	27	3,4	21	2,6	90	11,3	1	0,1	78	9,8	5	0,6	0	0,0	3	0,4	0	0,0	3	0,4
6	0,2	96	3,1	57	1,8	6	0,2	2	0,1	20	0,6	29	0,9	87	2,8	1	0,0	68	2,2	14	0,5	2	0,1	0	0,0	0	0,0	1	0,0

Annex 1

Country	Sub-National	Year	Method	Patients Tested	Susceptible	%	Any Res.	%	Any H	%	Any R	%	Any E	%	Any S	%	Mono H	%	Mono R	%	Mono R	%
Iceland	Countrywide	2005	Surveillance	7	7	100	0	0,0	0	0,0	0	0,0	0	0,0	0	0,0	0	0,0	0	0,0	0	0,0
Ireland	Countrywide	2005	Surveillance	200	194	97,0	6	3,0	6	3,0	1	0,5	1	0,5	1	0,5	5	2,5	5	2,5	0	0,0
Israel	Countrywide	2005	Surveillance	211	165	78,2	46	21,8	32	15,2	12	5,7	13	6,2	41	19,4	15	7,1	2	0,9	0	0,0
Italy	Half of the country	2005	Surveillance	485	438	90,3	47	9,7	30	6,2	11	2,3	4	0,8	29	6,0	30	6,2	15	3,1	1	0,2
Kazakhstan	Countrywide	2001	Survey	359	154	42,9	205	57,1	153	42,6	56	15,6	89	24,8	185	51,5	50	13,9	11	3,1	1	0,3
Latvia	Countrywide	2005	Surveillance	873	560	64,1	313	35,9	270	30,9	94	10,8	92	10,5	273	31,3	80	9,2	37	4,2	0	0,0
Lithuania	Countrywide	2005	Surveillance	1293	980	75,8	313	24,2	262	20,3	128	9,9	234	18,1	62	4,8	109	8,4	60	4,6	0	0,0
Luxembourg	Countrywide	2005	Surveillance	36	32	88,9	4	11,1	3	8,3	0	0,0	0	0,0	2	5,6	3	8,3	2	5,6	0	0,0
Malta	Countrywide	2005	Surveillance	11	9	81,8	2	18,2	0	0,0	0	0,0	0	0,0	2	18,2	2	18,2	0	0,0	0	0,0
Netherlands	Countrywide	2005	Surveillance	709	650	91,7	59	8,3	46	6,5	10	1,4	3	0,4	26	3,7	39	5,5	26	3,7	5	0,7
Norway	Countrywide	2005	Surveillance	193	150	77,7	43	22,3	20	10,4	3	1,6	4	2,1	31	16,1	32	16,6	9	4,7	0	0,0
Poland	Countrywide	2004	Surveillance	2716	2.564	94,4	152	5,6	91	3,4	15	0,6	4	0,1	76	2,8	125	4,6	65	2,4	6	0,2
Portugal	Countrywide	2005	Surveillance	1407	1.204	85,6	203	14,4	91	6,5	14	1,0	18	1,3	145	10,3	151	10,7	42	3,0	1	0,1
Republic of Moldova	Countrywide	2006	Surveillance	825	471	57,1	354	42,9	257	31,2	171	20,7	107	13,0	280	33,9	118	14,3	30	3,6	6	0,7
Romania	Countrywide	2004	Surveillance	849	727	85,6	122	14,4	71	8,4	41	4,8	19	2,2	64	7,5	76	9,0	31	3,7	13	1,5
Russian Federation	Ivanovo Oblast	2002	Surveillance	350	197	56,3	153	43,7	109	31,1	47	13,4	41	11,7	144	41,1	41	11,7	5	1,4	1	0,3
Russian Federation	Orel Oblast	2006	Surveillance	317	230	72,6	87	27,4	64	20,2	30	9,5	14	4,4	76	24,0	27	8,5	5	1,6	1	0,3
Russian Federation	Mary El oblast	2006	Surveillance	304	213	70,1	91	29,9	79	26,0	38	12,5	39	12,8	78	25,7	18	5,9				
Russian Federation	Tomsk Oblast	2005	Surveillance	515	333	64,7	182	35,3	136	26,4	86	16,7	33	6,4	167	32,4	50	9,7	12	2,3	1	0,2
Serbia	Countrywide	2005	Surveillance	1112	1.079	97,0	33	3,0	9	0,8	9	0,8	7	0,6	22	2,0	23	2,1	3	0,3	3	0,3
Slovakia	Countrywide	2005	Surveillance	248	230	92,7	18	7,3	13	5,2	7	2,8	0	0,0	9	3,6	9	3,6	6	2,4	1	0,4
Slovenia	Countrywide	2005	Surveillance	217	207	95,4	10	4,6	7	3,2	0	0,0	0	0,0	4	1,8	9	4,1	6	2,8	0	0,0
Spain	Galicia	2005	Surveillance	566	529	93,5	37	6,5	20	3,5	1	0,2	0	0,0	22	3,9	31	5,5	14	2,5	0	0,0
Spain	Aragon	2005	Surveillance	200	187	93,5	13	6,5	11	5,5	1	0,5	1	0,5	2	1,0	11	5,5	9	4,5	1	0,5
Spain	Barcelona	2005	Surveillance	combined only																		
Sweden	Countrywide	2005	Surveillance	425	373	87,8	52	12,2	42	9,9	3	0,7	2	0,5	9	2,1	50	11,8	40	9,4	1	0,2
Switzerland	Countrywide	2005	Surveillance	326	311	95,4	15	4,6	14	4,3	3	0,9	0	0,0	0	0,0	13	4,0	12	3,7	1	0,3
Turkmenistan	Dashoguz Velayat (Aral Sea Region)	2002	Survey	105	73	69,5	32	30,5	16	15,2	4	3,8	2	1,9	26	24,8	22	21,0	6	5,7	0	0,0
Ukraine	Donetsk	2006	Survey	1003	604	60,2	399	39,8	311	31,0	180	17,9	30	3,0	284	28,3	148	14,8	69	6,9	12	1,1
United Kingdom	Countrywide	2005	Surveillance	3428	3.183	92,9	245	7,1	230	6,7	34	1,0	13	0,4	3	0,1	217	6,3	202	5,9	11	0,3
Uzbekistan	Tashkent	2005	Survey	203	99	48,8	104	51,2	86	42,4	32	15,8	25	12,3	88	43,3	31	15,3	14	6,9	1	0,5
SOUTH-EAST ASIA																						
India	Mayhurbhanj District, Orissa State	2001	Survey	282	267	94,7	15	5,3	7	2,5	2	0,7	1	0,4	11	3,9	11	3,9	3	1,1	0	0,0
India	Wardha District, Maharashtra State	2001	Survey	197	158	80,2	39	19,8	30	15,2	1	0,5	2	1,0	15	7,6	30	15,2	21	10,7	0	0,0
India	Delhi State	1995	Survey	combined only																		
India	Raichur District, Karnataka State	1999	Survey	278	217	78,1	61	21,9	52	18,7	7	2,5	9	3,2	20	7,2	43	15,5	34	12,2	0	0,0
India	North Arcot District, Tamil Nadu State	1999	Survey	282	204	72,3	78	27,7	66	23,4	8	2,8	13	4,6	35	12,4	47	16,7	36	12,8	0	0,0
India	Ernakulam district, Kerala State	2004	Survey	305	220	72,1	85	27,9	27	8,9	11	3,6	8	2,6	72	23,6	64	21,0	8	2,6	3	1,0
India	Gujarat State	2006	Survey	1571	1.236	78,7	335	21,3	173	11,0	40	2,5	30	1,9	228	14,5	246	15,7	84	5,3	3	0,2
India	Tamil Nadu State	1997	Survey	384	312	81,3	72	18,8	59	15,4	17	4,4	27	7,0	26	6,8	40	10,4	29	7,6	2	0,5
India	Hoogli district, West Bengal State	2001	Survey	263	219	83,3	44	16,7	27	10,3	8	3,0	5	1,9	36	13,7	23	8,7	6	2,3	0	0,0
Indonesia	Mimika district, Papua Province	2004	Survey	101	87	86,1	14	13,9	13	12,9	2	2,0	2	2,0	9	8,9	4	4,0	3	3,0	0	0,0
Myanmar	Countrywide	2003	Survey	733	660	90,0	73	10,0	48	6,5	34	4,6	9	1,2	50	6,8	27	3,7	7	1,0	0	0,0
Nepal	Countrywide	2007	Survey	766	653	85,2	113	14,8	64	8,4	22	2,9	29	3,8	82	10,7	70	9,1	21	2,7	0	0,0
Sri Lanka	Countrywide	2006	Survey	561	553	98,6	8	1,4	4	0,7	3	0,5	1	0,2	4	0,7	6	1,1	2	0,4	2	0,4
Thailand	Countrywide	2006	Survey	1150	970	84,3	180	15,7	111	9,7	30	2,6	20	1,7	91	7,9	132	11,5	65	5,7	10	0,9
WESTERN PACIFIC																						
Australia	Countrywide	2005	Surveillance	combined only																		
Cambodia	Countrywide	2001	Survey	638	572	89,7	66	10,3	41	6,4	4	0,6	1	0,2	32	5,0	54	8,5	30	4,7	3	0,5
China	Guandong Province	1999	Survey	461	401	87,0	60	13,0	43	9,3	16	3,5	11	2,4	28	6,1	37	8,0	22	4,8	2	0,4
China	Beijing Municipality	2004	Survey	1043	856	82,1	187	17,9	91	8,7	44	4,2	43	4,1	95	9,1	113	10,8	35	3,4	11	1,1
China	Shandong Province	1997	Survey	1009	831	82,4	178	17,6	114	11,3	38	3,8	17	1,7	123	12,2	99	9,8	38	3,8	6	0,6
China	Henan Province	2001	Survey	1222	858	70,2	364	29,8	208	17,0	117	9,6	53	4,3	271	22,2	190	15,5	40	3,3	17	1,4
China (3)	Liaoning Province	1999	Survey	818	474	57,9	344	42,1	207	25,3	93	11,4	31	3,8	279	34,1	177	21,6	44	5,4	4	0,5
China	Heilongjiang Province	2005	Survey	1574	1.005	63,9	569	36,1	268	17,0	167	10,6	93	5,9	383	24,3	340	21,6	61	3,9	34	2,2
China	Hubei Province	1999	Survey	859	709	82,5	150	17,5	83	9,7	33	3,8	5	0,6	98	11,4	94	10,9	32	3,7	10	1,2
China	Zhejiang Province	1999	Survey	802	683	85,2	119	14,8	71	8,9	52	6,5	12	1,5	72	9,0	67	8,4	22	2,7	13	1,6
China	Shanghai Municipality	2005	Survey	764	646	84,6	118	15,4	85	11,1	37	4,8	23	3,0	62	8,1	57	7,5	25	3,3	6	0,8
China	Inner Mongolia Autonomous region	2002	Survey	806	524	65,0	282	35,0	164	20,3	79	9,8	72	8,9	172	21,3	148	18,4	40	5,0	13	1,6
China, Hong Kong SAR	Hong Kong	2005	Surveillance	3271	2.909	88,9	362	11,1	164	5,0	36	1,1	27	0,8	274	8,4	262	8,0	66	2,0	7	0,2
China, Macao SAR	Macao	2005	Surveillance	265	223	84,2	42	15,8	28	10,6	7	2,6	4	1,5	27	10,2	28	10,6	14	5,3	1	0,4
Fiji	Countrywide	2006	Surveillance	combined only																		
Guam	Countrywide	2002	Survey	combined only																		
Japan	Countrywide	2002	Surveillance	2705	2.472	91,4	233	8,6	77	2,8	28	1,0	23	0,9	188	7,0	184	6,8	33	1,2	5	0,2
Malaysia	Peninsular Malaysia	1997	Survey	1001	953	95,2	48	4,8	16	1,6	5	0,5	5	0,5	30	3,0	42	4,2	10	1,0	4	0,4
Mongolia	Countrywide	1999	Survey	405	286	70,6	119	29,4	62	15,3	5	1,2	7	1,7	98	24,2	74	18,3	18	4,4	1	0,2
New Caledonia	Countrywide	2005	Survey	combined only																		

Mono E	%	Mono S	%	Mdr	%	Hr	%	Hre	%	Hrs	%	Hres	%	Poly	%	He	%	Hs	%	Hes	%	Re	%	Rs	%	Res	%	Es	%
0	0,0	0	0,0	0	0,0	0	0,0	0	0,0	0	0,0	0	0,0	0	0,0	0	0,0	0	0,0	0	0,0	0	0,0	0	0,0	0	0,0	0	0,0
0	0,0	0	0,0	1	0,5	0	0,0	0	0,0	0	0,0	1	0,5	0	0,0	0	0,0	0	0,0	0	0,0	0	0,0	0	0,0	0	0,0	0	0,0
1	0,5	12	5,7	12	5,7	1	0,5	1	0,5	2	0,9	8	3,8	19	9,0	0	0,0	16	7,6	2	0,9	0	0,0	0	0,0	0	0,0	1	0,5
0	0,0	14	2,9	8	1,6	2	0,4	0	0,0	3	0,6	3	0,6	9	1,9	0	0,0	6	1,2	1	0,2	0	0,0	2	0,4	0	0,0	0	0,0
3	0,8	35	9,7	51	14,2	2	0,6	0	0,0	17	4,7	32	8,9	104	29,0	2	0,6	50	13,9	39	10,9	1	0,3	0	0,0	3	0,8	9	2,5
1	0,1	42	4,8	94	10,8	1	0,1	1	0,1	10	1,1	82	9,4	139	15,9	0	0,0	131	15,0	8	0,9	0	0,0	0	0,0	0	0,0	0	0,0
49	3,8	0	0,0	127	9,8	14	1,1	60	4,6	2	0,2	51	3,9	77	6,0	68	5,3	3	0,2	4	0,3	0	0,0	0	0,0	1	0,1	1	0,1
0	0,0	1	2,8	0	0,0	0	0,0	0	0,0	0	0,0	0	0,0	1	2,8	0	0,0	1	2,8	0	0,0	0	0,0	0	0,0	0	0,0	0	0,0
0	0,0	2	18,2	0	0,0	0	0,0	0	0,0	0	0,0	0	0,0	0	0,0	0	0,0	0	0,0	0	0,0	0	0,0	0	0,0	0	0,0	0	0,0
0	0,0	8	1,1	5	0,7	1	0,1	0	0,1	1	0,1	2	0,3	15	2,1	0	0,0	15	2,1	0	0,0	0	0,0	0	0,0	0	0,0	0	0,0
3	1,6	20	10,4	3	1,6	0	0,0	0	0,0	3	1,6	0	0,0	8	4,1	0	0,0	7	3,6	1	0,5	0	0,0	0	0,0	0	0,0	0	0,0
2	0,1	52	1,9	8	0,3	3	0,1	0	0,0	3	0,1	2	0,1	19	0,7	0	0,0	18	0,7	0	0,0	0	0,0	1	0,0	0	0,0	0	0,0
9	0,6	99	7,0	12	0,9	3	0,2	2	0,1	4	0,3	3	0,2	40	2,8	1	0,1	35	2,5	1	0,1	0	0,0	1	0,1	0	0,0	2	0,1
13	1,6	69	8,4	160	19,4	14	1,7	75	9,1	2	0,2	69	8,4	76	9,2	9	1,1	48	5,8	10	1,2	0	0,0	5	0,6	0	0,0	4	0,5
2	0,2	30	3,5	24	2,8	9	1,1	2	0,2	4	0,5	9	1,1	22	2,6	1	0,1	13	1,5	2	0,2	0	0,0	3	0,4	1	0,1	2	0,2
0	0,0	35	10,0	43	12,3	0	0,0	1	0,3	15	4,3	27	7,7	69	19,7	2	0,6	54	15,4	7	2,0	0	0,0	2	0,6	1	0,3	3	0,9
0	0,0	21	6,6	28	8,8	3	0,9	1	0,3	14	4,4	10	3,2	32	10,1	1	0,3	28	8,8	2	0,6	0	0,0	1	0,3	0	0,0	0	0,0
				38	12,5									35	11,5														
0	0,0	37	7,2	77	15,0	2	0,4	0	0,0	45	8,7	30	5,8	55	10,7	0	0,0	45	8,7	2	0,4	0	0,0	7	1,4	1	0,2	0	0,0
0	0,0	17	1,5	4	0,4	2	0,2	1	0,1	0	0,0	1	0,1	6	0,5	2	0,2	0	0,0	0	0,0	0	0,0	1	0,1	1	0,1	2	0,2
0	0,0	2	0,8	4	1,6	2	0,8	0	0,0	2	0,8	0	0,0	5	2,0	0	0,0	3	1,2	0	0,0	0	0,0	2	0,8	0	0,0	0	0,0
0	0,0	3	1,4	0	0,0	0	0,0	0	0,0	0	0,0	0	0,0	1	0,5	0	0,0	1	0,5	0	0,0	0	0,0	0	0,0	0	0,0	0	0,0
0	0,0	17	3,0	1	0,2	1	0,2	0	0,0	0	0,0	0	0,0	5	0,9	0	0,0	5	0,9	0	0,0	0	0,0	0	0,0	0	0,0	0	0,0
0	0,0	1	0,5	0	0,0	0	0,0	0	0,0	0	0,0	0	0,0	2	1,0	1	0,5	1	0,5	0	0,0	0	0,0	0	0,0	0	0,0	0	0,0
1	0,2	8	1,9	2	0,5	1	0,2	0	0,0	0	0,0	1	0,2	0	0,0	0	0,0	0	0,0	0	0,0	0	0,0	0	0,0	0	0,0	0	0,0
0	0,0	0	0,0	2	0,6	2	0,6	0	0,0	0	0,0	0	0,0	0	0,0	0	0,0	0	0,0	0	0,0	0	0,0	0	0,0	0	0,0	0	0,0
0	0,0	16	15,2	4	3,8	0	0,0	0	0,0	3	2,9	1	1,0	6	5,7	0	0,0	5	4,8	1	1,0	0	0,0	0	0,0	0	0,0	0	0,0
1	0,1	66	6,6	160	16,0	24	2,4	6	0,6	115	11,5	15	1,5	91	9,1	3	0,3	75	7,5	4	0,4	0	0,0	8	0,8	0	0,0	1	0,1
3	0,1	1	0,0	23	0,7	16	0,5	7	0,2	0	0,0	0	0,0	5	0,1	3	0,1	2	0,1	0	0,0	0	0,0	0	0,0	0	0,0	0	0,0
0	0,0	16	7,9	30	14,8	1	0,5	0	0,0	10	4,9	19	9,4	43	21,2	0	0,0	36	17,7	6	3,0	0	0,0	1	0,5	0	0,0	0	0,0
0	0,0	8	2,8	2	0,7	1	0,4	0	0,0	0	0,0	1	0,4	2	0,7	0	0,0	2	0,7	0	0,0	0	0,0	0	0,0	0	0,0	0	0,0
0	0,0	9	4,6	1	0,5	1	0,5	0	0,0	0	0,0	0	0,0	8	4,1	2	1,0	6	3,1	0	0,0	0	0,0	0	0,0	0	0,0	0	0,0
0	0,0	9	3,2	7	2,5	2	0,7	2	0,7	1	0,4	2	0,7	11	4,0	3	1,1	6	2,2	2	0,7	0	0,0	0	0,0	0	0,0	0	0,0
1	0,4	10	3,5	8	2,8	0	0,0	2	0,7	4	1,4	2	0,7	23	8,2	4	1,4	15	5,3	3	1,1	0	0,0	0	0,0	0	0,0	1	0,4
0	0,0	53	17,4	6	2,0	0	0,0	2	0,7	1	0,3	3	1,0	15	4,9	0	0,0	10	3,3	3	1,0	0	0,0	2	0,7	0	0,0	0	0,0
3	0,2	156	9,9	37	2,4	7	0,4	7	0,4	10	0,6	13	0,8	52	3,3	3	0,2	45	2,9	4	0,3	0	0,0	0	0,0	0	0,0	0	0,0
2	0,5	7	1,8	13	3,4	2	0,5	4	1,0	0	0,0	7	1,8	19	4,9	7	1,8	5	1,3	5	1,3	0	0,0	0	0,0	2	0,5	0	0,0
0	0,0	17	6,5	8	3,0	1	0,4	0	0,0	4	1,5	3	1,1	13	4,9	1	0,4	11	4,2	1	0,4	0	0,0	0	0,0	0	0,0	0	0,0
0	0,0	1	1,0	2	2,0	0	0,0	2	2,0	0	0,0	0	0,0	8	7,9	0	0,0	8	7,9	0	0,0	0	0,0	0	0,0	0	0,0	0	0,0
0	0,0	20	2,7	29	4,0	11	1,5	3	0,4	11	1,5	4	0,5	17	2,3	1	0,1	11	1,5	0	0,0	1	0,1	4	0,5	0	0,0	0	0,0
4	0,5	45	5,9	22	2,9	1	0,1	3	0,4	4	0,5	14	1,8	21	2,7	2	0,3	13	1,7	6	0,8	0	0,0	0	0,0	0	0,0	0	0,0
0	0,0	2	0,4	1	0,2	0	0,0	0	0,0	0	0,0	1	0,2	1	0,2	0	0,0	1	0,2	0	0,0	0	0,0	0	0,0	0	0,0	0	0,0
5	0,4	52	4,5	19	1,7	3	0,3	3	0,3	6	0,5	7	0,6	29	2,5	3	0,3	23	2,0	1	0,1	0	0,0	1	0,1	0	0,0	1	0,1
0	0,0	21	3,3	0	0,0	0	0,0	0	0,0	0	0,0	0	0,0	12	1,9	1	0,2	10	1,6	0	0,0	0	0,0	1	0,2	0	0,0	0	0,0
0	0,0	13	2,8	13	2,8	4	0,9	2	0,4	2	0,4	5	1,1	10	2,2	1	0,2	6	1,3	1	0,2	1	0,2	0	0,0	0	0,0	1	0,2
14	1,3	53	5,1	24	2,3	15	1,4	1	0,1	5	0,5	3	0,3	50	4,8	11	1,1	21	2,0	0	0,0	5	0,5	4	0,4	0	0,0	9	0,9
1	0,1	54	5,4	29	2,9	4	0,4	2	0,2	14	1,4	9	0,9	50	5,0	3	0,3	43	4,3	1	0,1	1	0,1	2	0,2	0	0,0	0	0,0
10	0,8	123	10,1	95	7,8	18	1,5	5	0,4	47	3,8	25	2,1	79	6,5	2	0,2	62	5,1	9	0,7	1	0,1	4	0,3	0	0,0	1	0,1
2	0,2	127	15,5	85	10,4	10	1,2	2	0,2	54	6,6	19	2,3	82	10,0	2	0,2	71	8,7	5	0,6	1	0,1	3	0,4	0	0,0	0	0,0
3	0,2	242	15,4	113	7,2	24	1,5	63	4,0	4	0,3	22	1,4	116	7,4	0	0,0	93	5,9	1	0,1	1	0,1	18	1,1	1	0,1	2	0,1
1	0,1	51	5,9	18	2,1	6	0,7	2	0,2	9	1,1	1	0,1	38	4,4	1	0,1	32	3,7	0	0,0	0	0,0	5	0,6	0	0,0	0	0,0
2	0,2	30	3,7	36	4,5	10	1,2	0	0,0	17	2,1	9	1,1	16	2,0	0	0,0	12	1,5	1	0,1	0	0,0	3	0,4	0	0,0	0	0,0
0	0,0	26	3,4	30	3,9	7	0,9	17	2,2	1	0,1	5	0,7	31	4,1	1	0,1	29	3,8	0	0,0	0	0,0	1	0,1	0	0,0	0	0,0
5	0,6	90	11,2	59	7,3	13	1,6	29	3,6	4	0,5	13	1,6	75	9,3	9	1,1	44	5,5	12	1,5	1	0,1	6	0,7	0	0,0	3	0,4
1	0,0	188	5,7	28	0,9	5	0,2	3	0,1	9	0,3	11	0,3	72	2,2	5	0,2	60	1,8	5	0,2	1	0,0	0	0,0	0	0,0	1	0,0
0	0,0	13	4,9	6	2,3	0	0,0	0	0,0	3	1,1	3	1,1	8	3,0	0	0,0	7	2,6	1	0,4	0	0,0	0	0,0	0	0,0	0	0,0
2	0,1	144	5,3	19	0,7	2	0,1	3	0,1	3	0,1	11	0,4	30	1,1	0	0,0	21	0,8	4	0,1	0	0,0	2	0,1	2	0,1	1	0,0
4	0,4	24	2,4	1	0,1	0	0,0	0	0,0	0	0,0	1	0,1	5	0,5	0	0,0	5	0,5	0	0,0	0	0,0	0	0,0	0	0,0	0	0,0
0	0,0	55	13,6	4	1,0	1	0,2	0	0,0	1	0,2	2	0,5	41	10,1	1	0,2	36	8,9	3	0,7	0	0,0	0	0,0	0	0,0	1	0,2

Annex 1

Country	Sub-National	Year	Method	Patients Tested	Susceptible	%	Any Res.	%	Any H	%	Any R	%	Any E	%	Any S	%	Mono H	%	Mono H	%	Mono R	%
New Zealand	Countrywide	2006	Surveillance	250	224	89,6	26	10,4	17	6,8	1	0,4	1	0,4	18	7,2	17	6,8	8	3,2	0	0,0
Northern Mariana Is	Countrywide	2006	Surveillance	18	4	22,2	4	22,2	3	16,7	2	11,1	0	0,0	2	11,1	1	5,6	0	0,0	0	0,0
Philippines	Countrywide	2004	Survey	965	767	79,5	198	20,5	130	13,5	44	4,6	41	4,2	115	11,9	122	12,6	57	5,9	4	0,4
Rep. Korea	Countrywide	2004	Survey	2636	2.315	87,8	321	12,2	261	9,9	98	3,7	70	2,7	70	2,7	203	7,7	145	5,5	25	0,9
Singapore	Countrywide	2005	Surveillance	895	837	93,5	58	6,5	30	3,4	5	0,6	7	0,8	35	3,9	44	4,9	16	1,8	3	0,
Solomon Islands	Countrywide	2004	Survey	combined only																		
Vanuatu	Countrywide	2006	Surveillance	29	28	96,6	1	3,4	1	3,4	0	0,0	0	0,0	0	0,0	1	3,4	1	3,4	0	0,0
Viet Nam	Countrywide	2006	Survey	1619	1.122	69,3	497	30,7	310	19,1	53	3,3	42	2,6	375	23,2	291	18,0	114	7,0	5	0,

(1) Several countries conducting routine diagnostic surveillance do not routinely test for streptomycin. Where this is the case the proportion tested is indicated in a footnote.
(2) Data from UR Tanzania and Madagascar are preliminary
(3) Based on patient re-interviews it is expected that between 20-30% of resistant cases may have been classified as new when in fact they had been treated previously. Therefore, M among new cases could be reduced from 10% to 8%. The reduction would be

Mono E	%	Mono S	%	Mdr	%	Hr	%	Hre	%	Hrs	%	Hres	%	Poly	%	He	%	Hs	%	Hes	%	Re	%	Rs	%	Res	%	Es	%
0	0,0	9	3,6	1	0,4	0	0,0	0	0,0	0	0,0	1	0,4	8	3,2	0	0,0	8	3,2	0	0,0	0	0,0	0	0,0	0	0,0	0	0,0
0	0,0	1	5,6	2	11,1	2	11,1	0	0,0	0	0,0	0	0,0	1	5,6	0	0,0	1	5,6	0	0,0	0	0,0	0	0,0	0	0,0	2	0,2
1	0,1	60	6,2	39	4,0	10	1,0	5	0,5	5	0,5	19	2,0	37	3,8	5	0,5	21	2,2	8	0,8	1	0,1	0	0,0	0	0,0	2	0,2
7	0,3	26	1,0	71	2,7	24	0,9	33	1,3	4	0,2	10	0,4	47	1,8	16	0,6	26	1,0	3	0,1	1	0,0	1	0,0	0	0,0	0	0,0
2	0,2	23	2,6	2	0,2	0	0,0	0	0,0	0	0,0	2	0,2	12	1,3	2	0,2	9	1,0	1	0,1	0	0,0	0	0,0	0	0,0	0	0,0
.	.	.	.	.	.	.	.	.	.	.	.	.	.	.	.	.	.	.	.	.	.	.	.	.	.	.	.	.	.
0	0,0	0	0,0	0	0,0	0	0,0	0	0,0	0	0,0	0	0,0	0	0,0	0	0,0	0	0,0	0	0,0	0	0,0	0	0,0	0	0,0	0	0,0
3	0,2	169	10,4	44	2,7	0	0,0	0	0,0	20	1,2	24	1,5	162	10,0	0	0,0	143	8,8	9	0,6	0	0,0	4	0,2	0	0,0	6	0,4

Annex 2: Notified prevalence of resistance to specific drugs among previously treated TB cases tested for resistance to at least INH and RIF (1) 1994-2007

Country	Sub-National	Year	Method	Patients Tested	Susceptible	%	Any Res.	%	Any H	%	Any R	%	Any E	%	Any S	%	Mono	%	Mono H	%	Mono R	%
AFRICA																						
Algeria	Countrywide	2001	Survey	new only																		
Benin	Countrywide	1997	Survey	new only																		
Botswana	Countrywide	2002	Survey	106	82	77,4	24	22,6	15	14,2	13	12,3	9	8,5	17	16,0	7	6,6	0	0,0	0	0
Central African Republic	Bangui	1998	Survey	33	21	63,6	12	36,4	10	30,3	7	21,2	6	18,2	4	12,1	4	12,1	3	9,1	0	0
Côte d'Ivoire	Countrywide	2006	Survey	new only																		
DR Congo	Kinshasa	1999	Survey	combined only																		
Ethiopia	Countrywide	2005	Survey	76	39	51,3	37	48,7	19	25,0	11	14,5	11	14,5	29	38,2	21	27,6	4	5,3	1	1
Gambia	Countrywide	2000	Survey	15	15	100,0	0	0,0	0	0,0	0	0,0	0	0,0	0	0,0	0	0,0	0	0,0	0	0
Guinea	Sentinel sites	1998	Survey	32	16	50,0	16	50,0	16	50,0	9	28,1	6	18,8	11	34,4	3	9,4	3	9,4	0	0
Kenya	Nearly Countrywide	1995	Survey	46	29	63,0	17	37,0	17	37,0	0	0,0	0	0,0	3	6,5	14	30,4	14	30,4	0	0
Lesotho	Countrywide	1995	Survey	53	35	66,0	18	34,0	16	30,2	3	5,7	2	3,8	9	17,0	11	20,8	9	17,0	0	0
Madagascar (2)	Countrywide	2007	Survey	51	45	88,2	6	11,8	5	9,8	3	5,9	0	0,0	2	3,9	2	3,9	2	3,9	0	0
Mozambique	Countrywide	1999	Survey	122	67	54,9	55	45,1	50	41,0	5	4,1	1	0,8	30	24,6	27	22,1	22	18,0	1	0
Rwanda	Countrywide	2005	Survey	85	66	77,6	19	22,4	9	10,6	9	10,6	10	11,8	16	18,8	10	11,8	0	0,0	1	1
Senegal	Countrywide	2006	Survey	42	29	69,0	13	31,0	10	23,8	7	16,7	7	16,7	12	28,6	4	9,5	1	2,4	0	0
Sierra Leone	Nearly Countrywide	1997	Survey	13	5	38,5	8	61,5	8	61,5	3	23,1	1	7,7	3	23,1	4	30,8	4	30,8	0	0
South Africa	Countrywide	2002	Survey	1465	1.235	84,3	230	15,7	173	11,8	116	7,9	41	2,8	120	8,2	97	6,6	41	2,8	17	1
Swaziland	Countrywide	1995	Survey	44	35	79,5	9	20,5	6	13,6	4	9,1	2	4,5	7	15,9	4	9,1	1	2,3	0	0
Uganda	3 GLRA Zones *	1997	Survey	45	22	48,9	23	51,1	17	37,8	2	4,4	5	11,1	10	22,2	13	28,9	8	17,8	0	0
UR Tanzania (2)	Countrywide	2007	Survey	49	41	83,7	8	16,3	8	16,3	0	0,0	2	4,1	2	4,1	5	10,2	5	10,2	0	0
Zambia	Countrywide	2000	Survey	44	38	86,4	6	13,6	3	6,8	1	2,3	1	2,3	2	4,5	5	11,4	2	4,5	0	0
Zimbabwe	Nearly Countrywide	1995	Survey	36	31	86,1	5	13,9	5	13,9	3	8,3	0	0,0	1	2,8	2	5,6	2	5,6	0	0
AMERICAS																						
Argentina	Countrywide	2005	Survey	136	102	75,0	34	25,0	25	18,4	25	18,4	7	5,1	17	12,5	11	8,1	2	1,5	4	2
Bolivia	Countrywide	1996	Survey	107	63	58,9	44	41,1	11	10,3	20	18,7	8	7,5	16	15,0	35	32,7	4	3,7	13	12
Brazil	Nearly Countrywide	1996	Survey	793	679	85,6	114	14,4	89	11,2	48	6,1	2	0,3	43	5,4	58	7,3	33	4,2	5	0
Canada	Countrywide	2006	Surveillance	106	89	84,0	17	16,0	15	14,2	2	1,9	2	1,9	5	4,7	13	12,3	11	10,4	0	0
Chile	Countrywide	2001	Survey	291	233	80,1	58	19,9	33	11,3	17	5,8	10	3,4	37	12,7	37	12,7	12	4,1	6	3
Colombia	Countrywide	2000	Survey	new only																		
Costa Rica	Countrywide	2006	Survey	21	20	95,2	1	4,8	1	4,8	1	4,8	1	4,8	0	0,0	0	0,0	0	0,0	0	0
Cuba	Countrywide	2005	Sentinel	19	12	63,2	7	36,8	2	10,5	1	5,3	0	0,0	6	31,6	6	31,6	1	5,3	0	0
Dominican Republic	Countrywide	1995	Survey	117	56	47,9	61	52,1	43	36,8	37	31,6	15	12,8	30	25,6	26	22,2	12	10,3	10	0
Ecuador	Countrywide	2002	Survey	185	104	56,2	81	43,8	56	30,3	62	33,5	10	5,4	38	20,5	24	13,0	5	2,7	11	0
El Salvador	Countrywide	2001	Survey	100	78	78,0	22	22,0	12	12,0	13	13,0	3	3,0	9	9,0	12	12,0	3	3,0	5	0
Guatemala	Countrywide	2002	Survey	155	70	45,2	85	54,8	56	36,1	45	29,0	31	20,0	67	43,2	34	21,9	6	3,9	3	0
Honduras	Countrywide	2004	Survey	73	45	61,6	28	38,4	18	24,7	15	20,5	5	6,8	11	15,1	16	21,9	7	9,6	5	0
Mexico	Baja California, Sinaloa, Oaxaca	1997	Survey	107	63	58,9	44	41,1	35	32,7	30	28,0	15	14,0	20	18,7	16	15,0	11	10,3	2	0
Nicaragua	Countrywide	2006	Survey	103	66	64,1	37	35,9	30	29,1	9	8,7	9	8,7	21	20,4	18	17,5	11	10,7	1	0
Paraguay	Countrywide	2001	Survey	51	41	80,4	10	19,6	6	11,8	6	11,8	1	2,0	2	3,9	7	13,7	3	5,9	4	0
Peru	Countrywide	2006	Survey	360	210	58,3	150	41,7	109	30,3	95	26,4	33	9,2	107	29,7	52	14,4	13	3,6	8	0
Puerto Rico	Countrywide	2005	Surveillance	combined only																		
Uruguay	Countrywide	2005	Survey	33	30	90,9	3	9,1	2	6,1	2	6,1	0	0,0	1	3,0	1	3,0	0	0,0	0	0
USA	Countrywide	2005	Surveillance	combined only																		
Venezuela	Countrywide	1999	Survey	104	72	69,2	32	30,8	24	23,1	19	18,3	8	7,7	16	15,4	12	11,5	6	5,8	3	0
EASTERN MEDITERRANEAN																						
Egypt	Countrywide	2002	Survey	217	69	31,8	148	68,2	101	46,5	110	50,7	67	30,9	117	53,9	40	18,4	6	2,8	15	0
Iran	Countrywide	1998	Survey	56	24	42,9	32	57,1	28	50,0	28	50,0	18	32,1	22	39,3	4	7,1	1	1,8	0	0
Jordan	Countrywide	2004	Survey	30	5	16,7	25	83,3	17	56,7	14	46,7	11	36,7	21	70,0	5	16,7	0	0,0	0	0
Lebanon	Countrywide	2003	Survey	16	4	25,0	12	75,0	12	75,0	10	62,5	7	43,8	8	50,0	1	6,3	1	6,3	0	0
Morocco	Countrywide	2006	Survey	181	144	79,6	37	20,4	32	17,7	22	12,2	7	3,9	30	16,6	8	4,4	3	1,7	0	0
Oman	Countrywide	2006	Surveillance	14	8	57,1	6	42,9	5	35,7	5	35,7	5	35,7	6	42,9	1	7,1	0	0,0	0	0
Qatar	Countrywide	2006	Surveillance	combined only																		
Yemen	Countrywide	2004	Survey	53	42	79,2	11	20,8	7	13,2	6	11,3	4	7,5	11	20,8	4	7,5	0	0,0	0	0
EUROPE																						
Andorra	Countrywide	2005	Surveillance	0	0		0		0		0		0		0		0		0		0	
Armenia	Countrywide	2007	Survey	340	87	25,6	253	74,4	215	63,2	160	47,1	74	21,8	205	60,3	58	17,1	24	7,1	11	0
Austria	Countrywide	2005	Surveillance	16	14	87,5	2	12,5	2	12,5	2	12,5	1	6,3	1	6,3	0	0,0	0	0,0	0	0
Azerbaijan	Baku City	2007	Survey	552	86	15,6	466	84,4	440	79,7	309	56,0	171	31,0	416	75,4	61	11,1	36	6,5	0	0
Belgium	Countrywide	2005	Surveillance	41	37	90,2	4	9,8	4	9,8	3	7,3	3	7,3	0	0,0	1	2,4	1	2,4	0	0
Bosnia & Herzegovina	Countrywide	2005	Surveillance	106	80	75,5	26	24,5	14	13,2	14	13,2	5	4,7	9	8,5	15	14,2	5	4,7	5	0
Croatia	Countrywide	2005	Surveillance	61	56	91,8	5	8,2	3	4,9	3	4,9	3	4,9	5	8,2	2	3,3	0	0,0	0	0
Czech Republic	Countrywide	2005	Surveillance	20	12	60,0	8	40,0	7	35,0	6	30,0	5	25,0	8	40,0	1	5,0	0	0,0	0	0
Denmark	Countrywide	2005	Surveillance	18	14	77,8	4	22,2	3	16,7	0	0,0	1	5,6	0	0,0	4	22,2	3	16,7	0	0
Estonia	Countrywide	2005	Surveillance	71	26	36,6	45	63,4	43	60,6	37	52,1	35	49,3	41	57,7	5	7,0	3	4,2	0	0
Finland	Countrywide	2005	Surveillance	22	21	95,5	1	4,5	1	4,5	1	4,5	1	4,5	1	4,5	0	0,0	0	0,0	0	0
France	Countrywide	2005	Sentinel	112	88	78,6	24	21,4	16	14,3	9	8,0	3	2,7	16	14,3	13	11,6	5	4,5	1	0
Georgia	Countrywide	2006	Survey	515	175	34,0	340	66,0	243	47,2	147	28,5	56	10,9	299	58,1	123	23,9	28	5,4	4	0
Germany	Countrywide	2005	Surveillance	251	188	74,9	63	25,1	55	21,9	32	12,7	20	8,0	49	19,5	20	8,0	13	5,2	0	0

108

Mono E	%	Mono S	%	Mdr	%	Hr	%	Hre	%	Hrs	%	Hres	%	Poly	%	He	%	Hs	%	Hes	%	Re	%	Rs	%	Res	%	Es	%
2	1,9	5	4,7	11	10,4	3	2,8	2	1,9	1	0,9	5	4,7	6	5,7	0	0,0	4	3,8	0	0,0	0	0,0	2	1,9	0	0,0	0	0,0
0	0,0	1	3,0	6	18,2	0	0,0	3	9,1	2	6,1	1	3,0	2	6,1	1	3,0	0	0,0	0	0,0	1	3,0	0	0,0	0	0,0	0	0,0
0	0,0	16	21,1	9	11,8	0	0,0	3	3,9	0	0,0	6	7,9	7	9,2	0	0,0	5	6,6	1	1,3	0	0,0	0	0,0	1	1,3	0	0,0
0	0,0	0	0,0	0	0,0	0	0,0	0	0,0	0	0,0	0	0,0	0	0,0	0	0,0	0	0,0	0	0,0	0	0,0	0	0,0	0	0,0	0	0,0
0	0,0	0	0,0	9	28,1	1	3,1	1	3,1	3	9,4	4	12,5	4	12,5	0	0,0	3	9,4	1	3,1	0	0,0	0	0,0	0	0,0	0	0,0
0	0,0	0	0,0	0	0,0	0	0,0	0	0,0	0	0,0	0	0,0	3	6,5	0	0,0	3	6,5	0	0,0	0	0,0	0	0,0	0	0,0	0	0,0
0	0,0	2	3,8	3	5,7	0	0,0	0	0,0	2	3,8	1	1,9	4	7,5	0	0,0	3	5,7	1	1,9	0	0,0	0	0,0	0	0,0	0	0,0
0	0,0	0	0,0	2	3,9	2	3,9	0	0,0	0	0,0	0	0,0	2	3,9	0	0,0	1	2,0	0	0,0	0	0,0	1	2,0	0	0,0	0	0,0
0	0,0	4	3,3	4	3,3	2	1,6	0	0,0	1	0,8	1	0,8	24	19,7	0	0,0	24	19,7	0	0,0	0	0,0	0	0,0	0	0,0	0	0,0
2	2,4	7	8,2	8	9,4	0	0,0	0	0,0	0	0,0	0	0,0	8	9,4	1	1,2	0	0,0	1	1,2	0	0,0	0	0,0	0	0,0	0	0,0
0	0,0	3	7,1	7	16,7	0	0,0	0	0,0	1	2,4	6	14,3	2	4,8	0	0,0	1	2,4	1	2,4	0	0,0	0	0,0	0	0,0	0	0,0
0	0,0	0	0,0	3	23,1	0	0,0	0	0,0	3	23,1	0	0,0	1	7,7	1	7,7	0	0,0	0	0,0	0	0,0	0	0,0	0	0,0	0	0,0
1	0,1	38	2,6	98	6,7	38	2,6	9	0,6	26	1,8	25	1,7	35	2,4	3	0,2	29	2,0	2	0,1	1	0,1	0	0,0	0	0,0	0	0,0
0	0,0	3	6,8	4	9,1	1	2,3	0	0,0	1	2,3	2	4,5	1	2,3	0	0,0	1	2,3	0	0,0	0	0,0	0	0,0	0	0,0	0	0,0
3	6,7	2	4,4	2	4,4	1	2,2	0	0,0	1	2,2	0	0,0	8	17,8	1	2,2	6	13,3	0	0,0	0	0,0	0	0,0	0	0,0	1	2,2
0	0,0	0	0,0	0	0,0	0	0,0	0	0,0	0	0,0	0	0,0	3	6,1	1	2,0	1	2,0	1	2,0	0	0,0	0	0,0	0	0,0	0	0,0
1	2,3	2	4,5	1	2,3	1	2,3	0	0,0	0	0,0	0	0,0	0	0,0	0	0,0	0	0,0	0	0,0	0	0,0	0	0,0	0	0,0	0	0,0
0	0,0	0	0,0	3	8,3	2	5,6	0	0,0	1	2,8	0	0,0	0	0,0	0	0,0	0	0,0	0	0,0	0	0,0	0	0,0	0	0,0	0	0,0
0	0,0	5	3,7	21	15,4	8	5,9	3	2,2	6	4,4	4	2,9	2	1,5	0	0,0	2	1,5	0	0,0	0	0,0	0	0,0	0	0,0	0	0,0
5	4,7	13	12,1	5	4,7	4	3,7	0	0,0	0	0,0	1	0,9	4	3,7	2	1,9	0	0,0	0	0,0	0	0,0	2	1,9	0	0,0	0	0,0
1	0,1	19	2,4	43	5,4	31	3,9	1	0,1	11	1,4	0	0,0	13	1,6	0	0,0	13	1,6	0	0,0	0	0,0	0	0,0	0	0,0	0	0,0
0	0,0	2	1,9	2	1,9	1	0,9	0	0,0	0	0,0	1	0,9	2	1,9	0	0,0	1	0,9	1	0,9	0	0,0	0	0,0	0	0,0	0	0,0
0	0,0	19	6,5	11	3,8	0	0,0	3	1,0	1	0,3	7	2,4	10	3,4	0	0,0	10	3,4	0	0,0	0	0,0	0	0,0	0	0,0	0	0,0
0	0,0	0	0,0	1	4,8	0	0,0	1	4,8	0	0,0	0	0,0	0	0,0	0	0,0	0	0,0	0	0,0	0	0,0	0	0,0	0	0,0	0	0,0
0	0,0	5	26,3	1	5,3	0	0,0	0	0,0	1	5,3	0	0,0	0	0,0	0	0,0	0	0,0	0	0,0	0	0,0	0	0,0	0	0,0	0	0,0
0	0,0	4	3,4	23	19,7	3	2,6	3	2,6	10	8,5	7	6,0	12	10,3	2	1,7	4	3,4	2	1,7	1	0,9	3	2,6	0	0,0	0	0,0
0	0,0	8	4,3	45	24,3	23	12,4	3	1,6	16	8,6	3	1,6	12	6,5	0	0,0	3	1,6	3	1,6	1	0,5	5	2,7	0	0,0	0	0,0
1	1,0	3	3,0	7	7,0	3	3,0	1	1,0	2	2,0	1	1,0	3	3,0	0	0,0	2	2,0	0	0,0	0	0,0	1	1,0	0	0,0	0	0,0
3	1,9	22	14,2	41	26,5	3	1,9	2	1,3	11	7,1	25	16,1	10	6,5	0	0,0	9	5,8	0	0,0	1	0,6	0	0,0	0	0,0	0	0,0
0	0,0	4	5,5	9	12,3	3	4,1	1	1,4	2	2,7	3	4,1	3	4,1	1	1,4	1	1,4	0	0,0	0	0,0	1	1,4	0	0,0	0	0,0
0	0,0	3	2,8	24	22,4	9	8,4	2	1,9	1	0,9	12	11,2	4	3,7	0	0,0	0	0,0	0	0,0	0	0,0	3	2,8	1	0,9	0	0,0
1	1,0	5	4,9	8	7,8	1	1,0	1	1,0	1	1,0	5	4,9	11	10,7	1	1,0	9	8,7	1	1,0	0	0,0	0	0,0	0	0,0	0	0,0
0	0,0	0	0,0	2	3,9	1	2,0	0	0,0	0	0,0	1	2,0	1	2,0	0	0,0	1	2,0	0	0,0	0	0,0	0	0,0	0	0,0	0	0,0
0	0,0	31	8,6	85	23,6	18	5,0	4	1,1	37	10,3	26	7,2	13	3,6	0	0,0	10	2,8	1	0,3	0	0,0	0	0,0	2	0,6	0	0,0
0	0,0	1	3,0	2	6,1	2	6,1	0	0,0	0	0,0	0	0,0	0	0,0	0	0,0	0	0,0	0	0,0	0	0,0	0	0,0	0	0,0	0	0,0
0	0,0	3	2,9	14	13,5	4	3,8	2	1,9	5	4,8	3	2,9	6	5,8	1	1,0	3	2,9	0	0,0	0	0,0	0	0,0	2	1,9	0	0,0
2	0,9	17	7,8	83	38,2	5	2,3	2	0,9	21	9,7	55	25,3	25	11,5	1	0,5	7	3,2	4	1,8	0	0,0	10	4,6	2	0,9	1	0,5
0	0,0	0	0,0	3	5,4	27	48,2	7	12,5	2	3,6	2	3,6	16	28,6	1	1,8	0	0,0	0	0,0	0	0,0	1	1,8	0	0,0	0	0,0
0	0,0	5	16,7	12	40,0	2	6,7	2	6,7	1	3,3	7	23,3	8	26,7	0	0,0	4	13,3	1	3,3	0	0,0	2	6,7	0	0,0	1	3,3
0	0,0	0	0,0	10	62,5	2	12,5	1	6,3	2	12,5	5	31,3	1	6,3	0	0,0	0	0,0	1	6,3	0	0,0	0	0,0	0	0,0	0	0,0
0	0,0	5	2,8	22	12,2	2	1,1	1	0,6	14	7,7	5	2,8	7	3,9	1	0,6	6	3,3	0	0,0	0	0,0	0	0,0	0	0,0	0	0,0
0	0,0	1	7,1	5	35,7	0	0,0	0	0,0	0	0,0	5	35,7	0	0,0	0	0,0	0	0,0	0	0,0	0	0,0	0	0,0	0	0,0	0	0,0
0	0,0	4	7,5	6	11,3	0	0,0	0	0,0	2	3,8	4	7,5	1	1,9	0	0,0	1	1,9	0	0,0	0	0,0	0	0,0	0	0,0	0	0,0
0		0		0		0		0		0		0		0		0		0		0		0		0		0		0	
0	0,0	23	6,8	147	43,2	8	2,4	1	0,3	83	24,4	55	16,2	48	14,1	4	1,2	29	8,5	11	3,2	0	0,0	1	0,3	1	0,3	2	0,6
0	0,0	0	0,0	2	12,5	1	6,3	0	0,0	0	0,0	1	6,3	0	0,0	0	0,0	0	0,0	0	0,0	0	0,0	0	0,0	0	0,0	0	0,0
0	0,0	25	4,5	308	55,8	11	2,0	2	0,4	142	25,7	153	27,7	97	17,6	1	0,2	80	14,5	15	2,7	0	0,0	1	0,2	0	0,0	0	0,0
0	0,0	0	0,0	3	7,3	0	0,0	3	7,3	0	0,0	0	0,0	0	0,0	0	0,0	0	0,0	0	0,0	0	0,0	0	0,0	0	0,0	0	0,0
1	0,9	4	3,8	7	6,6	4	3,8	0	0,0	1	0,9	2	1,9	4	3,8	1	0,9	1	0,9	0	0,0	1	0,9	1	0,9	0	0,0	0	0,0
0	0,0	2	3,3	3	4,9	0	0,0	0	0,0	0	0,0	3	4,9	0	0,0	0	0,0	0	0,0	0	0,0	0	0,0	0	0,0	0	0,0	0	0,0
0	0,0	1	5,0	6	30,0	0	0,0	0	0,0	1	5,0	5	25,0	1	5,0	0	0,0	1	5,0	0	0,0	0	0,0	0	0,0	0	0,0	0	0,0
1	5,6	0	0,0	0	0,0	0	0,0	0	0,0	0	0,0	0	0,0	0	0,0	0	0,0	0	0,0	0	0,0	0	0,0	0	0,0	0	0,0	0	0,0
0	0,0	2	2,8	37	52,1	0	0,0	1	1,4	2	2,8	34	47,9	3	4,2	0	0,0	3	4,2	0	0,0	0	0,0	0	0,0	0	0,0	0	0,0
0	0,0	0	0,0	1	4,5	0	0,0	0	0,0	0	0,0	1	4,5	0	0,0	0	0,0	0	0,0	0	0,0	0	0,0	0	0,0	0	0,0	0	0,0
0	0,0	7	6,3	8	7,1	2	1,8	0	0,0	3	2,7	3	2,7	3	2,7	0	0,0	3	2,7	0	0,0	0	0,0	0	0,0	0	0,0	0	0,0
0	0,0	91	17,7	141	27,4	6	1,2	2	0,4	83	16,1	50	9,7	76	14,8	1	0,2	70	13,6	3	0,6	0	0,0	2	0,4	0	0,0	0	0,0
0	0,0	7	2,8	31	12,4	1	0,4	0	0,0	11	4,4	19	7,6	12	4,8	0	0,0	10	4,0	1	0,4	0	0,0	1	0,4	0	0,0	0	0,0

Annex 2

Country	Sub-National	Year	Method	Patients Tested	Susceptible	%	Any Res.	%	Any H	%	Any R	%	Any E	%	Any S	%	Mono H	%	Mono H	%	Mono R	%
Iceland	Countrywide	2005	Surveillance	1	1	100,0	0	0,0	0	0,0	0	0,0	0	0,0	0	0,0	0	0,0	0	0,0	0	0,
Ireland	Countrywide	2005	Surveillance	10	8	80,0	2	20,0	2	20,0	1	10,0	0	0,0	0	0,0	1	10,0	1	10,0	0	0,
Israel	Countrywide	2005	Surveillance	3	3	100,0	0	0,0	0	0,0	0	0,0	0	0,0	0	0,0	0	0,0	0	0,0	0	
Italy	Half of the country	2005	Surveillance	79	50	63,3	29	36,7	24	30,4	14	17,7	8	10,1	23	29,1	9	11,4	4	5,1	0	
Kazakhstan	Countrywide	2001	Survey	319	57	17,9	262	82,1	216	67,7	196	61,4	173	54,2	246	77,1	26	8,2	3	0,9	1	
Latvia	Countrywide	2005	Surveillance	182	86	47,3	96	52,7	90	49,5	66	36,3	63	34,6	93	51,1	9	4,9	3	1,6	0	0
Lithuania	Countrywide	2005	Surveillance	440	176	40,0	264	60,0	250	56,8	212	48,2	239	54,3	141	32,0	27	6,1	14	3,2	2	0
Luxembourg	Countrywide	2005	Surveillance	0	0		0		0		0		0		0		0		0		0	
Malta	Countrywide	2005	Surveillance	0	0		0		0		0		0		0		0		0		0	
Netherlands	Countrywide	2005	Surveillance	30	25	83,3	5	16,7	3	10,0	2	6,7	0	0,0	2	6,7	3	10,0	1	3,3	1	3
Norway	Countrywide	2005	Surveillance	8	8	100,0	0	0,0	0	0,0	0	0,0	0	0,0	0	0,0	0	0,0	0	0,0	0	
Poland	Countrywide	2004	Surveillance	522	428	82,0	94	18,0	71	13,6	51	9,8	12	2,3	55	10,5	39	7,5	17	3,3	7	
Portugal	Countrywide	2005	Surveillance	172	127	73,8	35	20,3	26	15,1	19	11,0	10	5,8	18	10,5	14	8,1	6	3,5	2	
Republic of Moldova	Countrywide	2006	Surveillance	2054	605	29,5	1.449	70,5	1.259	61,3	1.108	53,9	607	29,6	1.167	56,8	199	9,7	59	2,9	23	
Romania	Countrywide	2004	Surveillance	382	257	67,3	125	32,7	108	28,3	49	12,8	54	14,1	74	19,4	48	12,6	31	8,1	7	
Russian Federation	Ivanovo Oblast	2002	Surveillance	155	28	18,1	127	81,9	116	74,8	93	60,0	68	43,9	120	77,4	10	6,5	1	0,6	2	
Russian Federation	Orel Oblast	2006	Surveillance	30	16	53,3	14	46,7	14	46,7	5	16,7	6	20,0	11	36,7	2	6,7	2	6,7	0	
Russian Federation	Mary El oblast	2006	Surveillance	new only																		
Russian Federation	Tomsk Oblast	2005	Surveillance	new only																		
Serbia	Countrywide	2005	Surveillance	121	107	88,4	14	11,6	7	5,8	8	6,6	6	5,0	6	5,0	7	5,8	2	1,7	1	
Slovakia	Countrywide	2005	Surveillance	56	46	82,1	10	17,9	10	17,9	4	7,1	1	1,8	3	5,4	3	5,4	3	5,4	0	
Slovenia	Countrywide	2005	Surveillance	28	24	85,7	4	14,3	3	10,7	1	3,6	1	3,6	3	10,7	2	7,1	1	3,6	0	
Spain	Galicia	2005	Surveillance	68	59	86,8	9	13,2	5	7,4	1	1,5	1	1,5	6	8,8	6	8,8	2	2,9	0	
Spain	Aragon	2005	Surveillance	26	21	80,8	5	19,2	5	19,2	4	15,4	2	7,7	2	7,7	1	3,8	1	3,8	0	
Spain	Barcelona	2005	Surveillance	combined only																		
Sweden	Countrywide	2005	Surveillance	17	13	76,5	4	23,5	4	23,5	2	11,8	1	5,9	0	0,0	2	11,8	2	11,8	0	
Switzerland	Countrywide	2005	Surveillance	30	28	93,3	2	6,7	2	6,7	2	6,7	2	6,7	0	0,0	0	0,0	0	0,0	0	
Turkmenistan	Dashoguz Velayat (Aral Sea Region)	2002	Survey	98	37	37,8	61	62,2	47	48,0	19	19,4	15	15,3	50	51,0	23	23,5	9	9,2	1	
Ukraine	Donetsk	2006	Survey	494	147	29,8	347	70,2	298	60,3	241	48,8	40	8,1	253	51,2	67	13,6	32	6,5	8	
United Kingdom	Countrywide	2005	Surveillance	271	246	90,8	25	9,2	23	8,5	9	3,3	2	0,7	0	0,0	18	6,6	16	5,9	2	
Uzbekistan	Tashkent	2005	Survey	85	12	14,1	73	85,9	69	81,2	51	60,0	24	28,2	71	83,5	5	5,9	1	1,2	0	
SOUTH-EAST ASIA																						
India	Mayhurbhanj District, Orissa State	2001	Survey	new only																		
India	Wardha District, Maharashtra State	2001	Survey	new only																		
India	Delhi State	1995	Survey	combined only																		
India	Raichur District, Karnataka State	1999	Survey	new only																		
India	North Arcot District, Tamil Nadu State	1999	Survey	new only																		
India	Ernakulam district, Kerala State	2004	Survey	new only																		
India	Gujarat State	2006	Survey	1047	562	53,7	485	46,3	385	36,8	190	18,1	105	10,0	274	26,2	220	21,0	122	11,7	10	
India	Tamil Nadu State	1997	Survey	new only																		
India	Hoogli district, West Bengal State	2001	Survey	new only																		
Indonesia	Mimika district, Papua Province	2004	Survey	new only																		
Myanmar	Countrywide	2003	Survey	116	81	69,8	35	30,2	31	26,7	18	15,5	1	0,9	24	20,7	6	5,2	2	1,7	0	
Nepal	Countrywide	2007	Survey	162	121	74,7	41	25,3	37	22,8	19	11,7	14	8,6	31	19,1	10	6,2	6	3,7	0	
Sri Lanka	Countrywide	2006	Survey	34	31	91,2	3	8,8	2	5,9	0	0,0	0	0,0	1	2,9	3	8,8	2	5,9	0	
Thailand	Countrywide	2006	Survey	194	96	49,5	98	50,5	86	44,3	68	35,1	50	25,8	65	33,5	22	11,3	10	5,2	1	
WESTERN PACIFIC																						
Australia	Countrywide	2005	Surveillance	combined only																		
Cambodia	Countrywide	2001	Survey	96	79	82,3	17	17,7	16	16,7	3	3,1	0	0,0	7	7,3	10	10,4	9	9,4	0	
China	Guandong Province	1999	Survey	63	39	61,9	24	38,1	15	23,8	14	22,2	9	14,3	13	20,6	9	14,3	2	3,2	1	
China	Beijing Municipality	2004	Survey	154	100	64,9	54	35,1	38	24,7	23	14,9	14	9,1	33	21,4	17	11,0	7	4,5	2	
China	Shandong Province	1997	Survey	220	110	50,0	110	50,0	89	40,5	51	23,2	23	10,5	76	34,5	35	15,9	21	9,5	1	
China	Henan Province	2001	Survey	265	104	39,2	161	60,8	125	47,2	113	42,6	48	18,1	114	43,0	38	14,3	11	4,2	8	
China (3)	Liaoning Province	1999	Survey	86	38	44,2	48	55,8	36	41,9	25	29,1	12	14,0	36	41,9	13	15,1	2	2,3	3	
China	Heilongjiang Province	2005	Survey	421	137	32,5	284	67,5	202	48,0	170	40,4	103	24,5	136	32,3	101	24,0	37	8,8	24	
China	Hubei Province	1999	Survey	238	132	55,5	106	44,5	79	33,2	64	26,9	21	8,8	61	25,6	32	13,4	13	5,5	4	
China	Zhejiang Province	1999	Survey	140	57	40,7	83	59,3	62	44,3	63	45,0	25	17,9	39	27,9	26	18,6	10	7,1	9	
China	Shanghai Municipality	2005	Survey	200	145	72,5	55	27,5	43	21,5	30	15,0	20	10,0	25	12,5	19	9,5	11	5,5	2	
China	Inner Mongolia Autonomous region	2002	Survey	308	92	29,9	216	70,1	174	56,5	157	51,0	98	31,8	92	29,9	52	16,9	23	7,5	16	
China, Hong Kong SAR	Hong Kong	2005	Surveillance	163	125	76,7	38	23,3	28	17,2	16	9,8	9	5,5	25	15,3	15	9,2	7	4,3	1	
China, Macao SAR	Macao	2005	Surveillance	19	14	73,7	5	26,3	4	21,1	3	15,8	1	5,3	3	15,8	2	10,5	1	5,3	0	
Fiji	Countrywide	2006	Surveillance	combined only																		
Guam	Countrywide	2002	Survey	combined only																		

Mono E	%	Mono S	%	Mdr	%	Hr	%	Hre	%	Hrs	%	Hres	%	Poly	%	He	%	Hs	%	Hes	%	Re	%	Rs	%	Res	%	Es	%
0	0,0	0	0,0	0	0,0	0	0,0	0	0,0	0	0,0	0	0,0	0	0,0	0	0,0	0	0,0	0	0,0	0	0,0	0	0,0	0	0,0	0	0,0
0	0,0	0	0,0	1	10,0	1	10,0	0	0,0	0	0,0	0	0,0	0	0,0	0	0,0	0	0,0	0	0,0	0	0,0	0	0,0	0	0,0	0	0,0
0	0,0	0	0,0	0	0,0	0	0,0	0	0,0	0	0,0	0	0,0	0	0,0	0	0,0	0	0,0	0	0,0	0	0,0	0	0,0	0	0,0	0	0,0
0	0,0	5	6,3	14	17,7	2	2,5	0	0,0	5	6,3	7	8,9	6	7,6	0	0,0	5	6,3	1	1,3	0	0,0	0	0,0	0	0,0	0	0,0
4	1,3	18	5,6	180	56,4	6	1,9	1	0,3	39	12,2	134	42,0	56	17,6	0	0,0	18	5,6	15	4,7	1	0,3	4	1,3	10	3,1	8	2,5
0	0,0	6	3,3	66	36,3	0	0,0	0	0,0	8	4,4	58	31,9	21	11,5	0	0,0	16	8,8	5	2,7	0	0,0	0	0,0	0	0,0	0	0,0
11	2,5	0	0,0	209	47,5	5	1,1	67	15,2	3	0,7	134	30,5	28	6,4	23	5,2	1	0,2	3	0,7	0	0,0	1	0,2	0	0,0	0	0,0
0		0		0		0		0		0		0		0		0		0		0		0		0		0		0	
0		0		0		0		0		0		0		0		0		0		0		0		0		0		0	
0	0,0	1	3,3	1	3,3	1	3,3	0	0,0	0	0,0	0	0,0	1	3,3	0	0,0	1	3,3	0	0,0	0	0,0	0	0,0	0	0,0	0	0,0
0	0,0	0	0,0	0	0,0	0	0,0	0	0,0	0	0,0	0	0,0	0	0,0	0	0,0	0	0,0	0	0,0	0	0,0	0	0,0	0	0,0	0	0,0
1	0,2	14	2,7	43	8,2	11	2,1	2	0,4	23	4,4	7	1,3	12	2,3	1	0,2	9	1,7	1	0,2	0	0,0	1	0,2	0	0,0	0	0,0
2	1,2	4	2,3	16	9,3	5	2,9	1	0,6	5	2,9	5	2,9	5	2,9	1	0,6	3	1,7	0	0,0	0	0,0	0	0,0	1	0,6	0	0,0
32	1,6	85	4,1	1.044	50,8	137	6,7	407	19,8	12	0,6	488	23,8	206	10,0	14	0,7	107	5,2	35	1,7	5	0,2	24	1,2	12	0,6	9	0,4
0	0,0	10	2,6	42	11,0	4	1,0	3	0,8	5	1,3	30	7,9	35	9,2	6	1,6	14	3,7	15	3,9	0	0,0	0	0,0	0	0,0	0	0,0
1	0,6	6	3,9	90	58,1	2	1,3	0	0,0	28	18,1	60	38,7	27	17,4	1	0,6	19	12,3	5	3,2	0	0,0	1	0,6	0	0,0	1	0,6
0	0,0	0	0,0	5	16,7	0	0,0	0	0,0	1	3,3	4	13,3	7	23,3	1	3,3	5	16,7	1	3,3	0	0,0	0	0,0	0	0,0	0	0,0
1	0,8	3	2,5	5	4,1	0	0,0	2	1,7	2	1,7	1	0,8	2	1,7	0	0,0	0	0,0	2	1,7	0	0,0	0	0,0	0	0,0	0	0,0
0	0,0	0	0,0	4	7,1	3	5,4	0	0,0	1	1,8	0	0,0	3	5,4	1	1,8	2	3,6	0	0,0	0	0,0	0	0,0	0	0,0	0	0,0
0	0,0	1	3,6	1	3,6	0	0,0	0	0,0	1	3,6	0	0,0	1	3,6	0	0,0	0	0,0	1	3,6	0	0,0	0	0,0	0	0,0	0	0,0
1	1,5	3	4,4	1	1,5	0	0,0	0	0,0	1	1,5	0	0,0	2	2,9	0	0,0	2	2,9	0	0,0	0	0,0	0	0,0	0	0,0	0	0,0
0	0,0	0	0,0	4	15,4	2	7,7	0	0,0	0	0,0	2	7,7	0	0,0	0	0,0	0	0,0	0	0,0	0	0,0	0	0,0	0	0,0	0	0,0
0	0,0	0	0,0	2	11,8	1	5,9	1	5,9	0	0,0	0	0,0	0	0,0	0	0,0	0	0,0	0	0,0	0	0,0	0	0,0	0	0,0	0	0,0
0	0,0	0	0,0	2	6,7	0	0,0	2	6,7	0	0,0	0	0,0	0	0,0	0	0,0	0	0,0	0	0,0	0	0,0	0	0,0	0	0,0	0	0,0
0	0,0	13	13,3	18	18,4	0	0,0	0	0,0	10	10,2	8	8,2	20	20,4	1	1,0	13	13,3	6	6,1	0	0,0	0	0,0	0	0,0	0	0,0
0	0,0	27	5,5	219	44,3	48	9,7	5	1,0	136	27,5	30	6,1	61	12,3	1	0,2	42	8,5	4	0,8	0	0,0	14	2,8	0	0,0	0	0,0
0	0,0	0	0,0	7	2,6	5	1,8	2	0,7	0	0,0	0	0,0	0	0,0	0	0,0	0	0,0	0	0,0	0	0,0	0	0,0	0	0,0	0	0,0
0	0,0	4	4,7	51	60,0	1	1,2	0	0,0	27	31,8	23	27,1	17	20,0	0	0,0	16	18,8	1	1,2	0	0,0	0	0,0	0	0,0	0	0,0
0	0,0	88	8,4	182	17,4	49	4,7	21	2,0	43	4,1	69	6,6	83	7,9	7	0,7	66	6,3	10	1,0	0	0,0	0	0,0	0	0,0	0	0,0
0	0,0	4	3,4	18	15,5	9	7,8	0	0,0	8	6,9	1	0,9	11	9,5	0	0,0	11	9,5	0	0,0	0	0,0	0	0,0	0	0,0	0	0,0
0	0,0	4	2,5	19	11,7	3	1,9	1	0,6	4	2,5	11	6,8	12	7,4	0	0,0	10	6,2	2	1,2	0	0,0	0	0,0	0	0,0	0	0,0
0	0,0	1	2,9	0	0,0	0	0,0	0	0,0	0	0,0	0	0,0	0	0,0	0	0,0	0	0,0	0	0,0	0	0,0	0	0,0	0	0,0	0	0,0
0	0,0	11	5,7	67	34,5	12	6,2	9	4,6	8	4,1	38	19,6	9	4,6	1	0,5	6	3,1	2	1,0	0	0,0	0	0,0	0	0,0	0	0,0
0	0,0	1	1,0	3	3,1	1	1,0	0	0,0	2	2,1	0	0,0	4	4,2	0	0,0	4	4,2	0	0,0	0	0,0	0	0,0	0	0,0	0	0,0
0	0,0	6	9,5	11	17,5	4	6,3	3	4,8	0	0,0	4	6,3	4	6,3	0	0,0	1	1,6	1	1,6	1	1,6	1	1,6	0	0,0	0	0,0
0	0,0	8	5,2	18	11,7	6	3,9	2	1,3	7	4,5	3	1,9	19	12,3	3	1,9	8	5,2	2	1,3	1	0,6	2	1,3	0	0,0	3	1,9
0	0,0	13	5,9	43	19,5	7	3,2	4	1,8	16	7,3	16	7,3	32	14,5	1	0,5	22	10,0	2	0,9	0	0,0	7	3,2	0	0,0	0	0,0
4	1,5	15	5,7	97	36,6	20	7,5	2	0,8	41	15,5	34	12,8	26	9,8	0	0,0	13	4,9	4	1,5	2	0,8	5	1,9	1	0,4	1	0,4
0	0,0	8	9,3	21	24,4	6	7,0	0	0,0	6	7,0	9	10,5	14	16,3	1	1,2	11	12,8	1	1,2	0	0,0	0	0,0	1	1,2	0	0,0
0	0,0	40	9,5	128	30,4	25	5,9	58	13,8	6	1,4	39	9,3	55	13,1	3	0,7	32	7,6	2	0,5	1	0,2	17	4,0	0	0,0	0	0,0
0	0,0	15	6,3	52	21,8	19	8,0	5	2,1	18	7,6	10	4,2	22	9,2	1	0,4	11	4,6	2	0,8	3	1,3	5	2,1	0	0,0	0	0,0
1	0,7	6	4,3	49	35,0	20	14,3	1	0,7	10	7,1	18	12,9	8	5,7	1	0,7	0	0,0	2	1,4	2	1,4	3	2,1	0	0,0	0	0,0
1	0,5	5	2,5	25	12,5	6	3,0	10	5,0	2	1,0	7	3,5	11	5,5	0	0,0	7	3,5	0	0,0	0	0,0	2	1,0	1	0,5	1	0,5
0	0,0	13	4,2	129	41,9	34	11,0	48	15,6	6	1,9	41	13,3	35	11,4	2	0,6	17	5,5	3	1,0	1	0,3	9	2,9	2	0,6	1	0,3
1	0,6	6	3,7	13	8,0	3	1,8	0	0,0	4	2,5	6	3,7	10	6,1	0	0,0	8	4,9	0	0,0	1	0,6	0	0,0	1	0,6	0	0,0
0	0,0	1	5,3	3	15,8	1	5,3	0	0,0	1	5,3	1	5,3	1	5,3	0	0,0	0	0,0	0	0,0	0	0,0	0	0,0	0	0,0	0	0,0

Annex 2

Country	Sub-National	Year	Method	Patients Tested	Susceptible	%	Any Res.	%	Any H	%	Any R	%	Any E	%	Any S	%	Mono	%	Mono H	%	Mono R	%
Japan	Countrywide	2002	Surveillance	417	312	74,8	105	25,2	79	18,9	46	11,0	35	8,4	60	14,4	49	11,8	26	6,2	2	0,
Malaysia	Peninsular Malaysia	1997	Survey	16	13	81,3	3	18,8	0	0,0	1	6,3	0	0,0	2	12,5	3	18,8	0	0,0	1	6,
Mongolia	Countrywide	1999	Survey	new only																		
New Caledonia	Countrywide	2005	Survey	combined only																		
New Zealand	Countrywide	2006	Surveillance	16	15	93,8	1	6,3	1	6,3	0	0,0	0	0,0	0	0,0	1	6,3	1	6,3	0	0,
Northern Mariana Is	Countrywide	2006	Surveillance	new only																		
Philippines	Countrywide	2004	Survey	129	81	62,8	48	37,2	40	31,0	33	25,6	12	9,3	22	17,1	17	13,2	10	7,8	5	3,
Rep. Korea	Countrywide	2004	Survey	278	201	72,3	77	27,7	67	24,1	47	16,9	27	9,7	16	5,8	29	10,4	20	7,2	7	2,
Singapore	Countrywide	2005	Surveillance	105	94	89,5	11	10,5	4	3,8	3	2,9	1	1,0	7	6,7	9	8,6	2	1,9	2	1,
Solomon Islands	Countrywide	2004	Survey	combined only																		
Vanuatu	Countrywide	2006	Surveillance	new only																		
Viet Nam	Countrywide	2006	Survey	207	85	41,1	122	58,9	90	43,5	44	21,3	30	14,5	105	50,7	38	18,4	8	3,9	2	1,

(1) Several countries conducting routine diagnostic surveillance do not routinely test for streptomycin. Where this is the case the proportion tested is indicated in a footnote.
(2) Data from UR Tanzania and Madagascar are preliminary
(3) Based on patient re-interviews it is expected that between 20-30% of resistant cases may have been classified as new when in fact they had been treated previously. Therefore, among new cases could be reduced from 10% to 8%. The reduction would be

Mono E	%	Mono S	%	Mdr	%	Hr	%	Hre	%	Hrs	%	Hres	%	Poly	%	He	%	Hs	%	Hes	%	Re	%	Rs	%	Res	%	Es	%
1	0,2	20	4,8	41	9,8	6	1,4	6	1,4	10	2,4	19	4,6	15	3,6	3	0,7	6	1,4	3	0,7	1	0,2	0	0,0	2	0,5	0	0,0
0	0,0	2	12,5	0	0,0	0	0,0	0	0,0	0	0,0	0	0,0	0	0,0	0	0,0	0	0,0	0	0,0	0	0,0	0	0,0	0	0,0	0	0,0
.	.	.	.	.	.	.	.	.	.	.	.	.	.	.	.	.	.	.	.	.	.	.	.	.	.	.	.	.	.
0	0,0	0	0,0	0	0,0	0	0,0	0	0,0	0	0,0	0	0,0	0	0,0	0	0,0	0	0,0	0	0,0	0	0,0	0	0,0	0	0,0	0	0,0
.	.	.	.	.	.	.	.	.	.	.	.	.	.	.	.	.	.	.	.	.	.	.	.	.	.	.	.	.	.
0	0,0	2	1,6	27	20,9	7	5,4	4	3,1	8	6,2	8	6,2	4	3,1	0	0,0	3	2,3	0	0,0	0	0,0	1	0,8	0	0,0	0	0,0
0	0,0	2	0,7	39	14,0	14	5,0	16	5,8	4	1,4	5	1,8	9	3,2	4	1,4	3	1,1	1	0,4	0	0,0	0	0,0	1	0,4	0	0,0
0	0,0	5	4,8	1	1,0	0	0,0	0	0,0	0	0,0	1	1,0	1	1,0	0	0,0	1	1,0	0	0,0	0	0,0	0	0,0	0	0,0	0	0,0
.	.	.	.	.	.	.	.	.	.	.	.	.	.	.	.	.	.	.	.	.	.	.	.	.	.	.	.	.	.
2	1,0	26	12,6	40	19,3	5	2,4	0	0,0	15	7,2	20	9,7	44	21,3	0	0,0	34	16,4	8	3,9	0	0,0	2	1,0	0	0,0	0	0,0

Annex 3: Notified prevalence of resistance to specific drugs among all TB cases tested for resistance to at least INH and RIF (1) 1994-2007

Country	Sub-National	Year	Method	Patients Tested	Susceptible	%	Any Res.	%	Any H	%	Any R	%	Any E	%	Any S	%	Mono	%	Mono H	%	Mono R	%
AFRICA																						
Algeria	Countrywide	2001	Survey	new only																		
Benin	Countrywide	1997	Survey	new only																		
Botswana	Countrywide	2002	Survey	1288	1.141	88,6	147	11,4	68	5,3	37	2,9	24	1,9	99	7,7	93	7,2	22	1,7	10	0,8
Central African Republic	Bangui	1998	Survey	497	409	82,3	88	17,7	54	10,9	13	2,6	17	3,4	55	11,1	54	10,9	22	4,4	1	0,2
Côte d'Ivoire	Countrywide	2006	Survey	new only																		
DR Congo	Kinshasa	1999	Survey	710	433	61,0	277	39,0	163	23,0	44	6,2	109	15,4	200	28,2	131	18,5	31	4,4	1	0,1
Ethiopia	Countrywide	2005	Survey	880	627	71,3	253	28,8	81	9,2	33	3,8	30	3,4	216	24,5	186	21,1	20	2,3	9	1,0
Gambia	Countrywide	2000	Survey	225	216	96,0	9	4,0	5	2,2	2	0,9	0	0,0	3	1,3	8	3,6	4	1,8	1	0,4
Guinea	Sentinel sites	1998	Survey	571	476	83,4	95	16,6	66	11,6	13	2,3	9	1,6	62	10,9	56	9,8	27	4,7	1	0,2
Kenya	Nearly Countrywide	1995	Survey	491	446	90,8	45	9,2	45	9,2	0	0,0	0	0,0	0	0,0	7	1,4	38	7,7	38	7,7	0	0,0
Lesotho	Countrywide	1995	Survey	383	336	87,7	47	12,3	42	11,0	6	1,6	2	0,5	19	5,0	31	8,1	26	6,8	0	0,0
Madagascar (2)	Countrywide	2007	Survey	865	808	93,4	57	6,6	42	4,9	7	0,8	4	0,5	28	3,2	44	5,1	30	3,5	0	0,0
Mozambique	Countrywide	1999	Survey	1150	881	76,6	269	23,4	220	19,1	59	5,1	6	0,5	138	12,0	152	13,2	103	9,0	19	1,7
Rwanda	Countrywide	2005	Survey	701	618	88,2	83	11,8	47	6,7	33	4,7	42	6,0	62	8,8	43	6,1	7	1,0	1	0,
Senegal	Countrywide	2006	Survey	279	241	86,4	38	13,6	20	7,2	12	4,3	15	5,4	30	10,8	22	7,9	4	1,4	0	0,0
Sierra Leone	Nearly Countrywide	1997	Survey	130	93	71,5	37	28,5	20	15,4	4	3,1	1	0,8	28	21,5	25	19,2	8	6,2	0	0,
South Africa	Countrywide	2002	Survey	5708	5.141	90,1	567	9,9	422	7,4	207	3,6	79	1,4	298	5,2	294	5,2	150	2,6	31	0,5
Swaziland	Countrywide	1995	Survey	378	330	87,3	48	12,7	36	9,5	7	1,9	5	1,3	31	8,2	26	6,9	14	3,7	0	0,0
Uganda	3 GLRA Zones *	1997	Survey	419	322	76,8	97	23,2	42	10,0	5	1,2	28	6,7	60	14,3	61	14,6	20	4,8	1	0,2
UR Tanzania (2)	Countrywide	2007	Survey	418	387	92,6	31	7,4	24	5,7	4	1,0	5	1,2	15	3,6	20	4,8	13	3,1	0	0,
Zambia	Countrywide	2000	Survey	489	432	88,3	57	11,7	31	6,3	9	1,8	10	2,0	26	5,3	43	8,8	17	3,5	0	0,0
Zimbabwe	Nearly Countrywide	1995	Survey	712	685	96,2	27	3,8	27	3,8	16	2,2	4	0,6	6	0,8	11	1,5	11	1,5	0	0,0
AMERICAS																						
Argentina	Countrywide	2005	Survey	819	717	87,5	102	12,5	64	7,8	41	5,0	11	1,3	61	7,4	54	6,6	16	2,0	5	0,
Bolivia	Countrywide	1996	Survey	605	434	71,7	171	28,3	62	10,2	50	8,3	33	5,5	65	10,7	135	22,3	38	6,3	27	4,
Brazil	Nearly Countrywide	1996	Survey	2888	2.594	89,8	294	10,2	213	7,4	71	2,5	5	0,2	119	4,1	193	6,7	112	3,9	9	0,
Canada	Countrywide	2006	Surveillance	1241	1.132	91,2	109	8,8	91	7,3	16	1,3	13	1,0	34	2,7	80	6,4	62	5,0	4	0,
Chile	Countrywide	2001	Survey	1158	1.009	87,1	149	12,9	72	6,2	24	2,1	12	1,0	115	9,9	101	8,7	24	2,1	7	0,
Colombia	Countrywide	2000	Survey	new only																		
Costa Rica	Countrywide	2006	Survey	284	264	93,0	20	7,0	10	3,5	6	2,1	14	4,9	0	0,0	7	2,5	5	1,8	1	0,
Cuba	Countrywide	2005	Sentinel	198	177	89,4	21	10,6	3	1,5	2	1,0	0	0,0	19	9,6	19	9,6	1	0,5	1	0,
Dominican Republic	Countrywide	1995	Survey	420	236	56,2	184	43,8	103	24,5	86	20,5	26	6,2	94	22,4	104	24,8	38	9,0	31	7
Ecuador	Countrywide	2002	Survey	997	753	75,5	244	24,5	145	14,5	121	12,1	20	2,0	130	13,0	123	12,3	34	3,4	26	2
El Salvador	Countrywide	2001	Survey	711	654	92,0	57	8,0	20	2,8	20	2,8	5	0,7	32	4,5	42	5,9	6	0,8	10	1
Guatemala	Countrywide	2002	Survey	823	505	61,4	318	38,6	128	15,6	73	8,9	83	10,1	260	31,6	190	23,1	14	1,7	8	1
Honduras	Countrywide	2004	Survey	530	447	84,3	83	15,7	45	8,5	25	4,7	13	2,5	49	9,2	55	10,4	18	3,4	7	1,
Mexico	Baja California, Sinaloa, Oaxaca	1997	Survey	441	350	79,4	91	20,6	59	13,4	42	9,5	25	5,7	44	10,0	51	11,6	25	5,7	4	0
Nicaragua	Countrywide	2006	Survey	423	344	81,3	79	18,7	51	12,1	12	2,8	13	3,1	46	10,9	51	12,1	24	5,7	2	0,
Paraguay	Countrywide	2001	Survey	286	250	87,4	36	12,6	21	7,3	14	4,9	7	2,4	14	4,9	23	8,0	10	3,5	7	2
Peru	Countrywide	2006	Survey	2169	1.599	73,7	570	26,3	318	14,7	200	9,2	69	3,2	449	20,7	306	14,1	58	2,7	17	0
Puerto Rico	Countrywide	2005	Surveillance	94	91	96,8	3	3,2	2	2,1	0	0,0	1	1,1	2	2,1	1	1,1	0	0,0	0	0
Uruguay	Countrywide	2005	Survey	368	358	97,3	10	2,7	6	1,6	3	0,8	1	0,3	2	0,5	8	2,2	4	1,1	1	0
USA	Countrywide	2005	Surveillance	10584	9.329	88,1	1.255	11,9	836	7,9	168	1,6	127	1,2	675	6,4	874	8,3	472	4,5	38	0
Venezuela	Countrywide	1999	Survey	873	783	89,7	90	10,3	54	6,2	27	3,1	16	1,8	52	6,0	50	5,7	19	2,2	6	0
EASTERN MEDITERRANEAN																						
Egypt	Countrywide	2002	Survey	849	508	59,8	341	40,2	163	19,2	154	18,1	85	10,0	266	31,3	177	20,8	23	2,7	37	4
Iran	Countrywide	1998	Survey	722	584	80,9	138	19,1	93	12,9	69	9,6	49	6,8	87	12,0	58	8,0	19	2,6	6	0
Jordan	Countrywide	2004	Survey	141	80	56,7	61	43,3	27	19,1	27	19,1	22	15,6	46	32,6	28	19,9	1	0,7	4	2
Lebanon	Countrywide	2003	Survey	206	157	76,2	49	23,8	35	17,0	15	7,3	14	6,8	31	15,0	20	9,7	8	3,9	2	1
Morocco	Countrywide	2006	Survey	1238	1.125	90,9	113	9,1	78	6,3	31	2,5	10	0,8	88	7,1	52	4,2	18	1,5	2	0
Oman	Countrywide	2006	Surveillance	164	148	90,2	16	9,8	12	7,3	7	4,3	6	3,7	11	6,7	8	4,9	4	2,4	0	0
Qatar	Countrywide	2006	Surveillance	278	250	89,9	28	10,1	25	9,0	3	1,1	1	0,4	5	1,8	22	7,9	18	6,5	0	0
Yemen	Countrywide	2004	Survey	563	503	89,3	60	10,7	27	4,8	21	3,7	19	3,4	51	9,1	37	6,6	4	0,7	0	0
EUROPE																						
Andorra	Countrywide	2005	Surveillance	9	8	88,9	1	11,1	1	11,1	0	0,0	0	0,0	1	11,1	0	0,0	0	0,0	0	0
Armenia	Countrywide	2007	Survey	892	432	48,4	460	51,6	365	40,9	220	24,7	98	11,0	365	40,9	148	16,6	58	6,5	18	2
Austria	Countrywide	2005	Surveillance	609	537	88,2	72	11,8	57	9,4	16	2,6	10	1,6	41	6,7	40	6,6	27	4,4	2	0
Azerbaijan	Baku City	2007	Survey	1103	327	29,6	776	70,4	665	60,3	434	39,3	239	21,7	697	63,2	170	15,4	61	5,5	1	0
Belgium	Countrywide	2005	Surveillance	758	710	93,7	48	6,3	42	5,5	13	1,7	14	1,8	0	0,0	33	4,4	27	3,6	2	0
Bosnia & Herzegovina	Countrywide	2005	Surveillance	1141	1.100	96,4	41	3,6	22	1,9	21	1,8	8	0,7	13	1,1	25	2,2	8	0,7	8	0
Croatia	Countrywide	2005	Surveillance	647	625	96,6	22	3,4	15	2,3	9	1,4	6	0,9	13	2,0	12	1,9	8	1,2	0	
Czech Republic	Countrywide	2005	Surveillance	582	531	91,2	51	8,8	28	4,8	14	2,4	9	1,5	42	7,2	30	5,2	8	1,4	0	
Denmark	Countrywide	2005	Surveillance	325	304	93,5	21	6,5	18	5,5	5	1,5	7	2,2	0	0,0	16	4,9	13	4,0	0	
Estonia	Countrywide	2005	Surveillance	387	251	64,9	136	35,1	108	27,9	79	20,4	77	19,9	124	32,0	39	10,1	11	2,8	0	
Finland	Countrywide	2005	Surveillance	315	301	95,6	14	4,4	11	3,5	4	1,3	4	1,3	3	1,0	10	3,2	7	2,2	1	
France	Countrywide	2005	Sentinel	1501	1.358	90,5	143	9,5	94	6,3	26	1,7	13	0,9	80	5,3	96	6,4	47	3,1	2	
Georgia	Countrywide	2006	Survey	1422	617	43,4	805	56,6	474	33,3	233	16,4	106	7,5	691	48,6	408	28,7	85	6,0	9	
Germany	Countrywide	2005	Surveillance	3886	3.408	87,7	478	12,3	327	8,4	118	3,0	92	2,4	329	8,5	263	6,8	118	3,0	9	

Mono E	%	Mono S	%	Mdr	%	Hr	%	Hre	%	Hrs	%	Hres	%	Poly	%	He	%	Hs	%	Hes	%	Re	%	Rs	%	Res	%	Es	%
4	0,3	57	4,4	21	1,6	6	0,5	4	0,3	4	0,3	7	0,5	33	2,6	2	0,2	19	1,5	4	0,3	0	0,0	5	0,4	1	0,1	2	0,2
0	0,0	31	6,2	11	2,2	2	0,4	5	1,0	2	0,4	2	0,4	23	4,6	2	0,4	13	2,6	6	1,2	1	0,2	0	0,0	0	0,0	1	0,2
36	5,1	63	8,9	41	5,8	2	0,3	4	0,6	5	0,7	30	4,2	105	14,8	3	0,4	66	9,3	22	3,1	0	0,0	0	0,0	2	0,3	12	1,7
1	0,1	156	17,7	22	2,5	3	0,3	3	0,3	1	0,1	15	1,7	45	5,1	1	0,1	33	3,8	5	0,6	0	0,0	1	0,1	1	0,1	4	0,5
0	0,0	3	1,3	1	0,4	1	0,4	0	0,0	0	0,0	0	0,0	0	0,0	0	0,0	0	0,0	0	0,0	0	0,0	0	0,0	0	0,0	0	0,0
0	0,0	28	4,9	12	2,1	2	0,4	1	0,2	5	0,9	4	0,7	27	4,7	2	0,4	23	4,0	2	0,4	0	0,0	0	0,0	0	0,0	0	0,0
0	0,0	0	0,0	0	0,0	0	0,0	0	0,0	0	0,0	0	0,0	7	1,4	0	0,0	7	1,4	0	0,0	0	0,0	0	0,0	0	0,0	0	0,0
0	0,0	5	1,3	6	1,6	2	0,5	0	0,0	3	0,8	1	0,3	10	2,6	0	0,0	9	2,3	1	0,3	0	0,0	0	0,0	0	0,0	0	0,0
0	0,0	20	2,3	6	0,7	3	0,3	1	0,1	0	0,0	2	0,2	7	0,8	1	0,1	5	0,6	0	0,0	0	0,0	1	0,1	0	0,0	0	0,0
0	0,0	30	2,6	40	3,5	9	0,8	0	0,0	25	2,2	6	0,5	77	6,7	0	0,0	77	6,7	0	0,0	0	0,0	0	0,0	0	0,0	0	0,0
12	1,7	23	3,3	32	4,6	1	0,1	0	0,0	2	0,3	29	4,1	8	1,1	0	0,0	7	1,0	1	0,1	0	0,0	0	0,0	0	0,0	0	0,0
3	1,1	15	5,4	12	4,3	0	0,0	1	0,4	2	0,7	9	3,2	4	1,4	0	0,0	2	0,7	2	0,7	0	0,0	0	0,0	0	0,0	0	0,0
0	0,0	17	13,1	4	3,1	0	0,0	0	0,0	4	3,1	0	0,0	8	6,2	1	0,8	7	5,4	0	0,0	0	0,0	0	0,0	0	0,0	0	0,0
1	0,0	112	2,0	175	3,1	59	1,0	19	0,3	52	0,9	45	0,8	98	1,7	8	0,1	84	1,5	5	0,1	1	0,0	0	0,0	0	0,0	0	0,0
1	0,3	11	2,9	7	1,9	1	0,3	1	0,3	3	0,8	2	0,5	15	4,0	0	0,0	14	3,7	1	0,3	0	0,0	0	0,0	0	0,0	0	0,0
12	2,9	28	6,7	4	1,0	2	0,5	1	0,2	1	0,2	0	0,0	32	7,6	1	0,2	17	4,1	0	0,0	0	0,0	0	0,0	0	0,0	14	3,3
0	0,0	7	1,7	4	1,0	0	0,0	1	0,2	2	0,5	1	0,2	7	1,7	2	0,5	4	1,0	1	0,2	0	0,0	0	0,0	0	0,0	0	0,0
4	0,8	22	4,5	9	1,8	5	1,0	3	0,6	0	0,0	1	0,2	5	1,0	2	0,4	3	0,6	0	0,0	0	0,0	0	0,0	0	0,0	0	0,0
0	0,0	0	0,0	16	2,2	10	1,4	0	0,0	2	0,3	4	0,6	0	0,0	0	0,0	0	0,0	0	0,0	0	0,0	0	0,0	0	0,0	0	0,0
1	0,1	32	3,9	36	4,4	15	1,8	4	0,5	11	1,3	6	0,7	12	1,5	0	0,0	12	1,5	0	0,0	0	0,0	0	0,0	0	0,0	0	0,0
23	3,8	47	7,8	11	1,8	9	1,5	0	0,0	1	0,2	1	0,2	25	4,1	4	0,7	9	1,5	0	0,0	5	0,8	7	1,2	0	0,0	0	0,0
3	0,1	69	2,4	62	2,1	49	1,7	1	0,0	12	0,4	0	0,0	39	1,4	1	0,0	38	1,3	0	0,0	0	0,0	0	0,0	0	0,0	0	0,0
3	0,2	11	0,9	12	1,0	4	0,3	1	0,1	4	0,3	3	0,2	17	1,4	1	0,1	11	0,9	5	0,4	0	0,0	0	0,0	0	0,0	0	0,0
0	0,0	70	6,0	17	1,5	0	0,0	3	0,3	5	0,4	9	0,8	31	2,7	0	0,0	31	2,7	0	0,0	0	0,0	0	0,0	0	0,0	0	0,0
9	3,2	0	0,0	5	1,8	0	0,0	5	1,8	0	0,0	0	0,0	8	2,8	0	0,0	0	0,0	0	0,0	0	0,0	0	0,0	0	0,0	0	0,0
0	0,0	17	8,6	1	0,5	0	0,0	0	0,0	1	0,5	0	0,0	1	0,5	0	0,0	1	0,5	0	0,0	0	0,0	0	0,0	0	0,0	0	0,0
1	0,2	34	8,1	43	10,2	12	2,9	4	1,0	16	3,8	11	2,6	37	8,8	2	0,5	17	4,0	3	0,7	2	0,5	10	2,4	0	0,0	3	0,7
2	0,2	61	6,1	85	8,5	43	4,3	7	0,7	30	3,0	5	0,5	36	3,6	0	0,0	23	2,3	3	0,3	2	0,2	7	0,7	1	0,1	0	0,0
3	0,4	23	3,2	9	1,3	5	0,7	1	0,1	2	0,3	1	0,1	6	0,8	0	0,0	5	0,7	0	0,0	0	0,0	1	0,1	0	0,0	0	0,0
26	3,2	142	17,3	61	7,4	5	0,6	3	0,4	18	2,2	35	4,3	67	8,1	1	0,1	46	5,6	6	0,7	1	0,1	2	0,2	1	0,1	10	1,2
0	0,0	30	5,7	17	3,2	4	0,8	3	0,6	2	0,4	8	1,5	11	2,1	2	0,4	8	1,5	0	0,0	1	0,2	0	0,0	0	0,0	0	0,0
1	0,2	21	4,8	32	7,3	10	2,3	3	0,7	3	0,7	16	3,6	8	1,8	2	0,5	0	0,0	0	0,0	2	0,5	3	0,7	1	0,2	0	0,0
2	0,5	23	5,4	10	2,4	1	0,2	3	0,7	1	0,2	5	1,2	18	4,3	1	0,2	15	3,5	1	0,2	0	0,0	0	0,0	1	0,0	1	0,2
0	0,0	6	2,1	7	2,4	2	0,7	2	0,7	1	0,3	2	0,7	6	2,1	1	0,3	3	1,0	0	0,0	0	0,0	0	0,0	0	0,0	2	0,7
0	0,0	231	10,7	180	8,3	35	1,6	10	0,5	82	3,8	53	2,4	84	3,9	1	0,0	77	3,6	2	0,1	0	0,0	1	0,0	2	0,1	1	0,0
1	1,1	0	0,0	0	0,0	0	0,0	0	0,0	0	0,0	0	0,0	2	2,1	0	0,0	2	2,1	0	0,0	0	0,0	0	0,0	0	0,0	0	0,0
1	0,3	2	0,5	2	0,5	2	0,5	0	0,0	0	0,0	0	0,0	0	0,0	0	0,0	0	0,0	0	0,0	0	0,0	0	0,0	0	0,0	0	0,0
15	0,1	349	3,3	124	1,2	28	0,3	13	0,1	28	0,3	55	0,5	257	2,4	12	0,1	209	2,0	19	0,2	2	0,0	4	0,0	0	0,0	11	0,1
1	0,1	24	2,7	18	2,1	6	0,7	2	0,2	6	0,7	4	0,5	22	2,5	3	0,3	13	1,5	1	0,1	1	0,1	0	0,0	2	0,2	2	0,2
5	0,6	112	13,2	97	11,4	5	0,6	2	0,2	26	3,1	64	7,5	67	7,9	3	0,4	35	4,1	5	0,6	0	0,0	18	2,1	2	0,2	4	0,5
2	0,3	31	4,3	60	8,3	15	2,1	3	0,4	8	1,1	34	4,7	20	2,8	5	0,7	8	1,1	1	0,1	1	0,1	2	0,3	0	0,0	3	0,4
2	1,4	21	14,9	18	12,8	3	2,1	3	2,1	2	1,4	10	7,1	15	10,6	1	0,7	5	3,5	2	1,4	1	0,7	3	2,1	1	0,7	2	1,4
3	1,5	7	3,4	12	5,8	2	1,0	2	1,0	2	1,0	6	2,9	17	8,3	0	0,0	14	6,8	1	0,5	1	0,5	0	0,0	0	0,0	1	0,5
0	0,0	32	2,6	28	2,3	2	0,2	1	0,1	18	1,5	6	0,5	33	2,7	1	0,1	29	2,3	2	0,2	0	0,0	1	0,1	0	0,0	0	0,0
0	0,0	4	2,4	7	4,3	1	0,6	0	0,0	0	0,0	6	3,7	1	0,6	0	0,0	1	0,6	0	0,0	0	0,0	0	0,0	0	0,0	0	0,0
1	0,4	3	1,1	3	1,1	2	0,7	0	0,0	1	0,4	0	0,0	3	1,1	2	0,7	1	0,4	0	0,0	0	0,0	0	0,0	0	0,0	0	0,0
2	0,4	31	5,5	21	3,7	1	0,2	1	0,2	4	0,7	15	2,7	2	0,4	1	0,2	1	0,2	0	0,0	0	0,0	0	0,0	0	0,0	0	0,0
0	0,0	0	0,0	0	0,0	0	0,0	0	0,0	0	0,0	0	0,0	1	11,1	0	0,0	1	11,1	0	0,0	0	0,0	0	0,0	0	0,0	0	0,0
1	0,1	71	8,0	199	22,3	12	1,3	1	0,1	120	13,5	66	7,4	113	12,7	5	0,6	81	9,1	22	2,5	0	0,0	2	0,2	1	0,1	2	0,2
0	0,0	11	1,8	13	2,1	1	0,2	1	0,2	4	0,7	7	1,1	19	3,1	0	0,0	16	2,6	2	0,3	0	0,0	1	0,2	0	0,0	0	0,0
0	0,0	108	9,8	431	39,1	13	1,2	3	0,3	205	18,6	210	19,0	175	15,9	1	0,1	147	13,3	25	2,3	0	0,0	2	0,2	0	0,0	0	0,0
4	0,5	0	0,0	11	1,5	5	0,7	6	0,8	0	0,0	0	0,0	4	0,5	4	0,5	0	0,0	0	0,0	0	0,0	0	0,0	0	0,0	0	0,0
2	0,2	7	0,6	11	1,0	7	0,6	0	0,0	1	0,1	3	0,3	5	0,4	2	0,2	1	0,1	0	0,0	1	0,1	1	0,1	0	0,0	0	0,0
0	0,0	4	0,6	6	0,9	0	0,0	1	0,2	2	0,3	3	0,5	4	0,6	0	0,0	1	0,2	0	0,0	0	0,0	1	0,2	2	0,3	0	0,0
1	0,2	21	3,6	13	2,2	0	0,0	0	0,0	5	0,9	8	1,4	8	1,4	0	0,0	7	1,2	0	0,0	0	0,0	1	0,2	0	0,0	0	0,0
3	0,9	0	0,0	5	1,5	1	0,3	4	1,2	0	0,0	0	0,0	0	0,0	0	0,0	0	0,0	0	0,0	0	0,0	0	0,0	0	0,0	0	0,0
0	0,0	28	7,2	79	20,4	0	0,0	1	0,3	5	1,3	73	18,9	18	4,7	0	0,0	15	3,9	3	0,8	0	0,0	0	0,0	0	0,0	0	0,0
1	0,3	1	0,3	3	1,0	1	0,3	0	0,0	0	0,0	2	0,6	1	0,3	1	0,3	0	0,0	0	0,0	0	0,0	0	0,0	0	0,0	0	0,0
3	0,2	44	2,9	24	1,6	8	0,5	2	0,1	8	0,5	6	0,4	23	1,5	1	0,1	21	1,4	1	0,1	0	0,0	0	0,0	0	0,0	0	0,0
3	0,2	311	21,9	219	15,4	13	0,9	2	0,1	116	8,2	88	6,2	178	12,5	2	0,1	160	11,3	8	0,6	0	0,0	5	0,4	0	0,0	3	0,2
7	0,2	129	3,3	105	2,7	9	0,2	3	0,1	33	0,8	60	1,5	110	2,8	1	0,0	86	2,2	17	0,4	2	0,1	1	0,0	0	0,0	2	0,1

Annex 3

Country	Sub-National	Year	Method	Patients Tested	Susceptible	%	Any Res.	%	Any H	%	Any R	%	Any E	%	Any S	%	Mono H	%	Mono H	%	Mono R	%
Iceland	Countrywide	2005	Surveillance	8	8	100,0	0	0,0	0	0,0	0	0,0	0	0,0	0	0,0	0	0,0	0	0,0	0	0,0
Ireland	Countrywide	2005	Surveillance	273	260	95,2	13	4,8	13	4,8	3	1,1	2	0,7	3	1,1	9	3,3	9	3,3	0	0,0
Israel	Countrywide	2005	Surveillance	217	171	78,8	46	21,2	32	14,7	12	5,5	13	6,0	41	18,9	15	6,9	2	0,9	0	0,
Italy	Half of the country	2005	Surveillance	585	504	86,2	81	13,8	57	9,7	26	4,4	13	2,2	52	8,9	44	7,5	22	3,8	2	0,
Kazakhstan	Countrywide	2001	Survey	678	211	31,1	467	68,9	369	54,4	252	37,2	262	38,6	431	63,6	76	11,2	14	2,1	2	0,
Latvia	Countrywide	2005	Surveillance	1055	646	61,2	409	38,8	360	34,1	160	15,2	155	14,7	366	34,7	89	8,4	40	3,8	0	0,
Lithuania	Countrywide	2005	Surveillance	1739	1.159	66,6	580	33,4	514	29,6	342	19,7	475	27,3	204	11,7	137	7,9	74	4,3	2	0,
Luxembourg	Countrywide	2005	Surveillance	37	33	89,2	4	10,8	3	8,1	0	0,0	0	0,0	2	5,4	3	8,1	2	5,4	0	0,
Malta	Countrywide	2005	Surveillance	11	9	81,8	2	18,2	0	0,0	0	0,0	0	0,0	2	18,2	2	18,2	0	0,0	0	0,
Netherlands	Countrywide	2005	Surveillance	841	767	91,2	74	8,8	55	6,5	13	1,5	3	0,4	35	4,2	49	5,8	30	3,6	6	0,
Norway	Countrywide	2005	Surveillance	214	170	79,4	44	20,6	21	9,8	3	1,4	4	1,9	31	14,5	33	15,4	10	4,7	0	0,
Poland	Countrywide	2004	Surveillance	3239	2.993	92,4	246	7,6	162	5,0	66	2,0	16	0,5	131	4,0	164	5,1	82	2,5	13	0,
Portugal	Countrywide	2005	Surveillance	1579	1.331	84,3	238	15,1	117	7,4	33	2,1	28	1,8	163	10,3	165	10,4	48	3,0	3	0,
Republic of Moldova	Countrywide	2006	Surveillance	2879	1.076	37,4	1.803	62,6	1.516	52,7	1.279	44,4	714	24,8	1.447	50,3	317	11,0	89	3,1	29	1,
Romania	Countrywide	2004	Surveillance	1251	1.002	80,1	249	19,9	180	14,4	91	7,3	74	5,9	140	11,2	125	10,0	62	5,0	20	1,
Russian Federation	Ivanovo Oblast	2002	Surveillance	505	225	44,6	280	55,4	225	44,6	140	27,7	109	21,6	264	52,3	51	10,1	6	1,2	3	0,
Russian Federation	Orel Oblast	2006	Surveillance	347	246	70,9	101	29,1	78	22,5	35	10,1	20	5,8	87	25,1	29	8,4	7	2,0	1	0,
Russian Federation	Mary El oblast	2006	Surveillance	new only																		
Russian Federation	Tomsk Oblast	2005	Surveillance	new only																		
Serbia	Countrywide	2005	Surveillance	1233	1.186	96,2	47	3,8	16	1,3	17	1,4	13	1,1	28	2,3	30	2,4	5	0,4	4	0,
Slovakia	Countrywide	2005	Surveillance	311	282	90,7	29	9,3	23	7,4	11	3,5	1	0,3	13	4,2	13	4,2	9	2,9	1	0,
Slovenia	Countrywide	2005	Surveillance	245	231	94,3	14	5,7	10	4,1	1	0,4	1	0,4	7	2,9	11	4,5	7	2,9	0	0,
Spain	Galicia	2005	Surveillance	634	588	92,7	46	7,3	25	3,9	2	0,3	1	0,2	28	4,4	37	5,8	16	2,5	0	0,
Spain	Aragon	2005	Surveillance	226	208	92,0	18	8,0	16	7,1	5	2,2	3	1,3	4	1,8	12	5,3	10	4,4	1	0,
Spain	Barcelona	2005	Surveillance	538	485	90,1	53	9,9	28	5,2	5	0,9	1	0,2	33	6,1	42	7,8	17	3,2	1	0,
Sweden	Countrywide	2005	Surveillance	442	386	87,3	56	12,7	46	10,4	5	1,1	3	0,7	9	2,0	52	11,8	42	9,5	1	0,
Switzerland	Countrywide	2005	Surveillance	457	433	94,7	24	5,3	23	5,0	6	1,3	2	0,4	0	0,0	19	4,2	18	3,9	1	0,
Turkmenistan	Dashoguz Velayat (Aral Sea Region)	2002	Survey	203	110	54,2	93	45,8	63	31,0	23	11,3	17	8,4	76	37,4	45	22,2	15	7,4	1	0,
Ukraine	Donetsk	2006	Survey	1497	751	50,2	746	49,8	609	40,7	421	28,1	70	4,7	537	35,9	215	14,4	101	6,7	20	1,
United Kingdom	Countrywide	2005	Surveillance	4800	4.459	92,9	341	7,1	322	6,7	54	1,1	16	0,3	3	0,1	297	6,2	278	5,8	15	0,
Uzbekistan	Tashkent	2005	Survey	292	112	38,4	180	61,6	158	54,1	85	29,1	50	17,1	162	55,5	36	12,3	15	5,1	1	0,
SOUTH-EAST ASIA																						
India	Mayhurbhanj District, Orissa State	2001	Survey	new only																		
India	Wardha District, Maharashtra State	2001	Survey	new only																		
India	Delhi State	1995	Survey	2240	1.514	67,6	726	32,4	646	28,8	314	14,0	156	7,0	406	18,1	245	10,9	181	8,1	7	0,
India	Raichur District, Karnataka State	1999	Survey	new only																		
India	North Arcot District, Tamil Nadu State	1999	Survey	new only																		
India	Ernakulam district, Kerala State	2004	Survey	new only																		
India	Gujarat State	2006	Survey	2618	1.798	68,7	820	31,3	558	21,3	230	8,8	135	5,2	502	19,2	466	17,8	206	7,9	13	0,
India	Tamil Nadu State	1997	Survey	new only																		
India	Hoogli district, West Bengal State	2001	Survey	new only																		
Indonesia	Mimika district, Papua Province	2004	Survey	new only																		
Myanmar	Countrywide	2003	Survey	849	741	87,3	108	12,7	79	9,3	52	6,1	10	1,2	74	8,7	33	3,9	9	1,1	0	0,
Nepal	Countrywide	2007	Survey	930	776	83,4	154	16,6	101	10,9	41	4,4	43	4,6	113	12,2	80	8,6	27	2,9	0	0,
Sri Lanka	Countrywide	2006	Survey	624	613	98,2	11	1,8	6	1,0	3	0,5	1	0,2	5	0,8	9	1,4	4	0,6	2	0,
Thailand	Countrywide	2006	Survey	1344	1.066	79,3	278	20,7	197	14,7	98	7,3	70	5,2	156	11,6	154	11,5	75	5,6	11	0,
WESTERN PACIFIC																						
Australia	Countrywide	2005	Surveillance	808	726	89,9	82	10,1	71	8,8	14	1,7	7	0,9	35	4,3	53	6,6	43	5,3	1	0,
Cambodia	Countrywide	2001	Survey	734	651	88,7	83	11,3	57	7,8	7	1,0	1	0,1	39	5,3	64	8,7	39	5,3	3	0,
China	Guandong Province	1999	Survey	524	440	84,0	84	16,0	58	11,1	30	5,7	20	3,8	41	7,8	46	8,8	24	4,6	3	0,
China	Beijing Municipality	2004	Survey	1197	956	79,9	241	20,1	129	10,8	67	5,6	57	4,8	128	10,7	130	10,9	42	3,5	13	0,
China	Shandong Province	1997	Survey	1229	941	76,6	288	23,4	203	16,5	89	7,2	40	3,3	199	16,2	134	10,9	59	4,8	7	0,
China	Henan Province	2001	Survey	1487	962	64,7	525	35,3	333	22,4	230	15,5	101	6,8	385	25,9	228	15,3	51	3,4	25	0,
China (3)	Liaoning Province	1999	Survey	904	512	56,6	392	43,4	243	26,9	118	13,1	43	4,8	315	34,8	190	21,0	46	5,1	7	0,
China	Heilongjiang Province	2005	Survey	1995	1.142	57,2	853	42,8	470	23,6	337	16,9	196	9,8	519	26,0	441	22,1	98	4,9	58	0,
China	Hubei Province	1999	Survey	1097	841	76,7	256	23,3	162	14,8	97	8,8	26	2,4	159	14,5	126	11,5	45	4,1	14	0,
China	Zhejiang Province	1999	Survey	942	740	78,6	202	21,4	133	14,1	115	12,2	37	3,9	111	11,8	93	9,9	32	3,4	22	0,
China	Shanghai Municipality	2005	Survey	964	791	82,1	173	17,9	128	13,3	67	7,0	43	4,5	87	9,0	76	7,9	36	3,7	8	0,
China	Inner Mongolia Autonomous region	2002	Survey	1114	616	55,3	498	44,7	338	30,3	236	21,2	170	15,3	264	23,7	200	18,0	63	5,7	29	0,
China, Hong Kong SAR	Hong Kong	2005	Surveillance	4350	3.873	89,0	477	11,0	228	5,2	57	1,3	36	0,8	353	8,1	336	7,7	92	2,1	12	0,
China, Macao SAR	Macao	2005	Surveillance	284	237	83,5	47	16,5	32	11,3	10	3,5	5	1,8	30	10,6	30	10,6	15	5,3	1	0,
Fiji	Countrywide	2006	Surveillance	38	38	100,0	0	0,0	0	0,0	0	0,0	0	0,0	0	0,0	0	0,0	0	0,0	0	0,
Guam	Countrywide	2002	Survey	47	45	95,7	2	4,3	4	8,5	2	4,3	1	2,1	2	4,3	0	0,0	0	0,0	0	0,

Mono E	%	Mono S	%	Mdr	%	Hr	%	Hre	%	Hrs	%	Hres	%	Poly	%	He	%	Hs	%	Hes	%	Re	%	Rs	%	Res	%	Es	%
0	0,0	0	0,0	0	0,0	0	0,0	0	0,0	0	0,0	0	0,0	0	0,0	0	0,0	0	0,0	0	0,0	0	0,0	0	0,0	0	0,0	0	0,0
0	0,0	0	0,0	3	1,1	1	0,4	1	0,4	0	0,0	1	0,4	1	0,4	0	0,0	1	0,4	0	0,0	0	0,0	0	0,0	0	0,0	0	0,0
1	0,5	12	5,5	12	5,5	1	0,5	1	0,5	2	0,9	8	3,7	19	8,8	0	0,0	16	7,4	2	0,9	0	0,0	0	0,0	0	0,0	1	0,5
1	0,2	19	3,2	22	3,8	4	0,7	0	0,0	8	1,4	10	1,7	15	2,6	0	0,0	11	1,9	2	0,3	0	0,0	2	0,3	0	0,0	0	0,0
7	1,0	53	7,8	231	34,1	8	1,2	1	0,1	56	8,3	166	24,5	160	23,6	2	0,3	68	10,0	54	8,0	2	0,3	4	0,6	13	1,9	17	2,5
1	0,1	48	4,5	160	15,2	1	0,1	1	0,1	18	1,7	140	13,3	160	15,2	0	0,0	147	13,9	13	1,2	0	0,0	0	0,0	0	0,0	0	0,0
61	3,5	0	0,0	338	19,4	20	1,2	127	7,3	5	0,3	186	10,7	105	6,0	91	5,2	4	0,2	7	0,4	1	0,1	0	0,0	1	0,1	1	0,1
0	0,0	1	2,7	0	0,0	0	0,0	0	0,0	0	0,0	0	0,0	1	2,7	0	0,0	1	2,7	0	0,0	0	0,0	0	0,0	0	0,0	0	0,0
0	0,0	2	18,2	0	0,0	0	0,0	0	0,0	0	0,0	0	0,0	0	0,0	0	0,0	0	0,0	0	0,0	0	0,0	0	0,0	0	0,0	0	0,0
0	0,0	13	1,5	7	0,8	2	0,2	1	0,1	2	0,2	2	0,2	18	2,1	0	0,0	18	2,1	0	0,0	0	0,0	0	0,0	0	0,0	0	0,0
3	1,4	20	9,3	3	1,4	0	0,0	0	0,0	3	1,4	0	0,0	8	3,7	0	0,0	7	3,3	1	0,5	0	0,0	0	0,0	0	0,0	0	0,0
3	0,1	66	2,0	51	1,6	14	0,4	2	0,1	26	0,8	9	0,3	31	1,0	1	0,0	27	0,8	1	0,0	0	0,0	2	0,1	0	0,0	0	0,0
11	0,7	103	6,5	28	1,8	8	0,5	3	0,2	9	0,6	8	0,5	45	2,8	2	0,1	38	2,4	1	0,1	0	0,0	1	0,1	1	0,1	2	0,1
45	1,6	154	5,3	1.204	41,8	151	5,2	482	16,7	14	0,5	557	19,3	282	9,8	23	0,8	155	5,4	45	1,6	5	0,2	29	1,0	12	0,4	13	0,5
2	0,2	41	3,3	67	5,4	13	1,0	5	0,4	9	0,7	40	3,2	57	4,6	7	0,6	27	2,2	17	1,4	0	0,0	3	0,2	1	0,1	2	0,2
1	0,2	41	8,1	133	26,3	2	0,4	1	0,2	43	8,5	87	17,2	96	19,0	3	0,6	73	14,5	12	2,4	0	0,0	3	0,6	1	0,2	4	0,8
0	0,0	21	6,1	33	9,5	3	0,9	1	0,3	15	4,3	14	4,0	39	11,2	2	0,6	33	9,5	3	0,9	0	0,0	1	0,3	0	0,0	0	0,0
1	0,1	20	1,6	9	0,7	2	0,2	3	0,2	2	0,2	2	0,2	8	0,6	2	0,2	0	0,0	0	0,0	2	0,2	1	0,1	1	0,1	2	0,2
0	0,0	3	1,0	8	2,6	5	1,6	0	0,0	3	1,0	0	0,0	8	2,6	1	0,3	5	1,6	0	0,0	0	0,0	2	0,6	0	0,0	0	0,0
0	0,0	4	1,6	1	0,4	0	0,0	0	0,0	1	0,4	0	0,0	2	0,8	0	0,0	1	0,4	1	0,4	0	0,0	0	0,0	0	0,0	0	0,0
1	0,2	20	3,2	2	0,3	1	0,2	0	0,0	1	0,2	0	0,0	7	1,1	0	0,0	7	1,1	0	0,0	0	0,0	0	0,0	0	0,0	0	0,0
0	0,0	1	0,4	4	1,8	2	0,9	0	0,0	0	0,0	2	0,9	2	0,9	1	0,4	1	0,4	0	0,0	0	0,0	0	0,0	0	0,0	0	0,0
0	0,0	24	4,5	4	0,7	2	0,4	0	0,0	1	0,2	1	0,2	7	1,3	0	0,0	7	1,3	0	0,0	0	0,0	0	0,0	0	0,0	0	0,0
1	0,2	8	1,8	4	0,9	2	0,5	1	0,2	0	0,0	1	0,2	0	0,0	0	0,0	0	0,0	0	0,0	0	0,0	0	0,0	0	0,0	0	0,0
0	0,0	0	0,0	5	1,1	3	0,7	2	0,4	0	0,0	0	0,0	0	0,0	0	0,0	0	0,0	0	0,0	0	0,0	0	0,0	0	0,0	0	0,0
0	0,0	29	14,3	22	10,8	0	0,0	0	0,0	13	6,4	9	4,4	26	12,8	1	0,5	18	8,9	7	3,4	0	0,0	0	0,0	0	0,0	0	0,0
1	0,1	93	6,2	379	25,3	72	4,8	11	0,7	251	16,8	45	3,0	152	10,2	4	0,3	117	7,8	8	0,5	0	0,0	22	1,5	0	0,0	1	0,1
3	0,1	1	0,0	39	0,8	29	0,6	10	0,2	0	0,0	0	0,0	5	0,1	3	0,1	2	0,0	0	0,0	0	0,0	0	0,0	0	0,0	0	0,0
0	0,0	20	6,8	83	28,4	2	0,7	0	0,0	38	13,0	43	14,7	61	20,9	0	0,0	53	18,2	7	2,4	0	0,0	1	0,3	0	0,0	0	0,0
4	0,2	53	2,4	298	13,3	94	4,2	22	1,0	104	4,6	78	3,5	183	8,2	12	0,5	123	5,5	32	1,4	0	0,0	8	0,4	1	0,0	7	0,3
3	0,1	244	9,3	219	8,4	56	2,1	28	1,1	53	2,0	82	3,1	135	5,2	10	0,4	111	4,2	14	0,5	0	0,0	0	0,0	0	0,0	0	0,0
0	0,0	24	2,8	47	5,5	20	2,4	3	0,4	19	2,2	5	0,6	28	3,3	1	0,1	22	2,6	0	0,0	1	0,1	4	0,5	0	0,0	0	0,0
4	0,4	49	5,3	41	4,4	4	0,4	4	0,4	8	0,9	25	2,7	33	3,5	2	0,2	23	2,5	8	0,9	0	0,0	0	0,0	0	0,0	0	0,0
0	0,0	3	0,5	1	0,2	0	0,0	0	0,0	0	0,0	0	0,0	1	0,2	0	0,0	1	0,2	0	0,0	0	0,0	0	0,0	0	0,0	0	0,0
5	0,4	63	4,7	86	6,4	15	1,1	12	0,9	14	1,0	45	3,3	38	2,8	4	0,3	29	2,2	3	0,2	0	0,0	1	0,1	0	0,0	1	0,1
0	0,0	9	1,1	12	1,5	1	0,1	1	0,1	5	0,6	5	0,6	17	2,1	1	0,1	15	1,9	0	0,0	0	0,0	1	0,1	0	0,0	0	0,0
0	0,0	22	3,0	3	0,4	1	0,1	0	0,0	2	0,3	0	0,0	16	2,2	1	0,1	14	1,9	0	0,0	0	0,0	1	0,1	0	0,0	0	0,0
0	0,0	19	3,6	24	4,6	8	1,5	5	1,0	2	0,4	9	1,7	14	2,7	1	0,2	7	1,3	2	0,4	2	0,4	1	0,2	0	0,0	1	0,2
14	1,2	61	5,1	42	3,5	21	1,8	3	0,3	12	1,0	6	0,5	69	5,8	14	1,2	29	2,4	2	0,2	6	0,5	6	0,5	0	0,0	12	1,0
1	0,1	67	5,5	72	5,9	11	0,9	6	0,5	30	2,4	25	2,0	82	6,7	4	0,3	65	5,3	3	0,2	1	0,1	9	0,7	0	0,0	0	0,0
14	0,9	138	9,3	192	12,9	38	2,6	7	0,5	88	5,9	59	4,0	105	7,1	2	0,1	75	5,0	13	0,9	3	0,2	9	0,6	1	0,1	2	0,1
2	0,2	135	14,9	106	11,7	16	1,8	2	0,2	60	6,6	28	3,1	96	10,6	3	0,3	82	9,1	6	0,7	1	0,1	3	0,3	1	0,1	0	0,0
3	0,2	282	14,1	241	12,1	49	2,5	121	6,1	10	0,5	61	3,1	171	8,6	3	0,2	125	6,3	3	0,2	2	0,1	35	1,8	1	0,1	2	0,1
1	0,1	66	6,0	70	6,4	25	2,3	7	0,6	27	2,5	11	1,0	60	5,5	2	0,2	43	3,9	2	0,2	3	0,3	10	0,9	0	0,0	0	0,0
3	0,3	36	3,8	85	9,0	30	3,2	1	0,1	27	2,9	27	2,9	24	2,5	1	0,1	12	1,3	3	0,3	2	0,2	6	0,6	0	0,0	0	0,0
1	0,1	31	3,2	55	5,7	13	1,3	27	2,8	3	0,3	12	1,2	42	4,4	1	0,1	36	3,7	0	0,0	0	0,0	3	0,3	1	0,1	1	0,1
5	0,4	103	9,2	188	16,9	47	4,2	77	6,9	10	0,9	54	4,8	110	9,9	11	1,0	61	5,5	15	1,3	2	0,2	15	1,3	2	0,2	4	0,4
2	0,0	230	5,3	41	0,9	8	0,2	3	0,1	13	0,3	17	0,4	100	2,3	5	0,1	85	2,0	5	0,1	2	0,0	1	0,0	1	0,0	1	0,0
0	0,0	14	4,9	9	3,2	1	0,4	0	0,0	4	1,4	4	1,4	8	2,8	0	0,0	7	2,5	1	0,4	0	0,0	1	0,4	0	0,0	0	0,0
0	0,0	0	0,0	0	0,0	0	0,0	0	0,0	0	0,0	0	0,0	0	0,0	0	0,0	0	0,0	0	0,0	0	0,0	0	0,0	0	0,0	0	0,0
0	0,0	0	0,0	2	4,3	0	0,0	0	0,0	0	0,0	0	0,0	0	0,0	0	0,0	0	0,0	0	0,0	0	0,0	0	0,0	0	0,0	0	0,0

Annex 3

Country	Sub-National	Year	Method	Patients Tested	Susceptible	%	Any Res.	%	Any H	%	Any R	%	Any E	%	Any S	%	Mono H	%	Mono H	%	Mono R	%
Japan	Countrywide	2002	Surveillance	3122	2.784	89,2	338	10,8	156	5,0	74	2,4	58	1,9	248	7,9	233	7,5	59	1,9	7	0,2
Malaysia	Peninsular Malaysia	1997	Survey	1017	966	95,0	51	5,0	16	1,6	6	0,6	5	0,5	32	3,1	45	4,4	10	1,0	5	0,5
Mongolia	Countrywide	1999	Survey	new only																		
New Caledonia	Countrywide	2005	Survey	5	4	80,0	1	20,0	1	20,0	0	0,0	0	0,0	1	20,0	0	0,0	0	0,0	0	0,0
New Zealand	Countrywide	2006	Surveillance	266	239	89,8	27	10,2	18	6,8	1	0,4	1	0,4	18	6,8	18	6,8	9	3,4	0	0,0
Northern Mariana Is	Countrywide	2006	Surveillance	new only																		
Philippines	Countrywide	2004	Survey	1094	848	77,5	246	22,5	170	15,5	77	7,0	53	4,8	137	12,5	139	12,7	67	6,1	9	0,
Rep. Korea	Countrywide	2004	Survey	2914	2.516	86,3	398	13,7	328	11,3	145	5,0	97	3,3	86	3,0	232	8,0	165	5,7	32	1,
Singapore	Countrywide	2005	Surveillance	1000	931	93,1	69	6,9	34	3,4	8	0,8	8	0,8	42	4,2	53	5,3	18	1,8	5	0,
Solomon Islands	Countrywide	2004	Survey	84	84	100,0	0	0,0	0	0,0	0	0,0	0	0,0	0	0,0	0	0,0	0	0,0	0	0,
Vanuatu	Countrywide	2006	Surveillance	new only																		
Viet Nam	Countrywide	2006	Survey	1826	1.207	66,1	619	33,9	400	21,9	97	5,3	72	3,9	480	26,3	329	18,0	122	6,7	7	0,

(1) Several countries conducting routine diagnostic surveillance do not routinely test for streptomycin. Where this is the case the proportion tested is indicated in a footnote.
(2) Data from UR Tanzania and Madagascar are preliminary
(3) Based on patient re-interviews it is expected that between 20-30% of resistant cases may have been classified as new when in fact they had been treated previously. Therefore, M among new cases could be reduced from 10% to 8%. The reduction would be

Mono E	%	Mono S	%	Mdr	%	Hr	%	Hre	%	Hrs	%	Hres	%	Poly	%	He	%	Hs	%	Hes	%	Re	%	Rs	%	Res	%	Es	%
3	0,1	164	5,3	60	1,9	8	0,3	9	0,3	13	0,4	30	1,0	45	1,4	3	0,1	27	0,9	7	0,2	1	0,0	2	0,1	4	0,1	1	0,0
4	0,4	26	2,6	1	0,1	0	0,0	0	0,0	0	0,0	1	0,1	5	0,5	0	0,0	5	0,5	0	0,0	0	0,0	0	0,0	0	0,0	0	0,0
.	.	.	.	.	.	.	.	.	.	.	.	.	.	.	.	.	.	.	.	.	.	.	.	.	.	.	.	.	.
0	0,0	0	0,0	0	0,0	0	0,0	0	0,0	0	0,0	0	0,0	1	20,0	0	0,0	1	20,0	0	0,0	0	0,0	0	0,0	0	0,0	0	0,0
0	0,0	9	3,4	1	0,4	0	0,0	0	0,0	0	0,0	1	0,4	8	3,0	0	0,0	8	3,0	0	0,0	0	0,0	0	0,0	0	0,0	0	0,0
.	.	.	.	.	.	.	.	.	.	.	.	.	.	.	.	.	.	.	.	.	.	.	.	.	.	.	.	.	.
1	0,1	62	5,7	66	6,0	17	1,6	9	0,8	13	1,2	27	2,5	41	3,7	5	0,5	24	2,2	8	0,7	1	0,1	1	0,1	0	0,0	2	0,2
7	0,2	28	1,0	110	3,8	38	1,3	49	1,7	8	0,3	15	0,5	56	1,9	20	0,7	29	1,0	4	0,1	1	0,0	1	0,0	1	0,0	0	0,0
2	0,2	28	2,8	3	0,3	0	0,0	0	0,0	0	0,0	3	0,3	13	1,3	2	0,2	10	1,0	1	0,1	0	0,0	0	0,0	0	0,0	0	0,0
0	0,0	0	0,0	0	0,0	0	0,0	0	0,0	0	0,0	0	0,0	0	0,0	0	0,0	0	0,0	0	0,0	0	0,0	0	0,0	0	0,0	0	0,0
.	.	.	.	.	.	.	.	.	.	.	.	.	.	.	.	.	.	.	.	.	.	.	.	.	.	.	.	.	.
5	0,3	195	10,7	84	4,6	5	0,3	0	0,0	35	1,9	44	2,4	206	11,3	0	0,0	177	9,7	17	0,9	0	0,0	6	0,3	0	0,0	6	0,3

Annex 4: Survey methods 1994–2007

Country	Sub-national	Year	Report	Population in area surveyed	TB patients notified in area surveyed	sm+ TB patients notified in area surveyed	Patients tested	Method	Survey duration (months)	Medical record/ TB register cross check	Patient interview	Re-interview	Sample target complete	Software
AFRICA														
Algeria	Countrywide	2001	3	32.853.798	21.501	8.654	713	Proportionate cluster	12		Structured questionnaire		Yes	
Benin	Countrywide	1997	1	8.438.853	3.457	2.739	337	Proportionate cluster	24			No	Yes	
Botswana	Countrywide	2002	3	1.764.926	10.104	3.170	548	100% diagnostic units	8		Structured questionnaire	No	Yes	
Central African Republic	Bangui	1998	2	620.000	3.338	2.153	291	100% diagnostic units	3			No	Yes	
Côte d'Ivoire	Countrywide	2006	4	18.153.867	20.026	12.496	980	Proportionate cluster			Structured questionnaire		Yes	
DR Congo	Kinshasa	1999	3		18.207	10.710	1.338	Proportionate cluster			Structured questionnaire	No		
Ethiopia	Countrywide	2005	4	77.430.702	125.135	38.525	3.119	Proportionate cluster	12		Structured questionnaire		Slightly under target	
Gambia	Countrywide	2000	3	1.517.079	2.120	1.127	166	100% diagnostic units	7			No	Yes	
Guinea	Sentinel sites	1998	2	7.164.893	7.000	3.362	120	Random cluster	10			No	Yes	
Kenya	Nearly Countrywide	1995	1	34.255.722	108.401	40.389	8.975	Proportionate cluster	5			No		
Lesotho	Countrywide	1995	1	1.794.769	11.404	4.280	1.041	Proportionate cluster	18			No	Yes	
Madagascar	Countrywide	2007	4	18.605.921	19.475	13.056	1.498	Proportionate cluster	23	Yes	Structured questionnaire	Yes	Yes	Epi Info
Mozambique	Countrywide	1999	2	19.792.295	33.718	17.877	1.886	Proportionate cluster	9		Structured questionnaire	No	Yes	
Rwanda	Countrywide	2005	4	9.037.690	7.680	4.166	831	100% diagnostic units	4	Yes	Structured questionnaire	Yes	Yes	SPSS
Senegal	Countrywide	2006	4	11.658.172	10.120	6.722	920	Proportionate cluster	16	Yes	Structured questionnaire	Yes	Yes	SDRTB4
Sierra Leone	Nearly Countrywide	1997	2	5.525.478	6.930	4.370	330	Random cluster	6			No	Yes	
South Africa	Countrywide	2002	3	47.431.829	302.467	125.460	60.588	Proportionate cluster	12		Structured questionnaire	No	Yes	
Swaziland	Countrywide	1995	1	1.032.438	8.864	2.187	470	Proportionate cluster	18			No	Yes	
Uganda	3 GLRA Zones *	1997	2	9.919.700	16.000	5.405	5.405	Proportionate cluster	18			No	Yes	
UR Tanzania	Countrywide	2007	4	38.328.809	64.200	25.264	5.032	Proportionate cluster	16		Structured questionnaire	Yes	Unfinished	MS Excel and Epi Info
Zambia	Countrywide	2000	3	11.668.457	53.267	14.857	5.496	Proportionate cluster	14		Structured questionnaire	No	Yes	
Zimbabwe	Nearly Countrywide	1995	1	13.009.534	54.891	13.155	5.941	All diagnostic centers	30		Structured questionnaire	No	Yes	
AMERICAS														
Argentina	Countrywide	2005	4	38.747.148	11.242	4.709	809	Proportionate cluster	12	Yes	Structured questionnaire	Yes	Slightly under target	SDRTB4 Epi Info
Bolivia	Countrywide	1996	1	9.182.015	9.973	6.278	772	Proportionate cluster	11			No	Yes	
Brazil	Nearly Countrywide	1996	1	186.404.913	87.223	42.093	9.637	Proportionate cluster	14					
Canada	Countrywide	2006	4	32.299.496	1.616	433	104	All bacteriologically confirmed cases (100%)	12	Yes	Routine	Yes	Yes	Oracle and MS Access
Chile	Countrywide	2001	3	16.295.102	2.225	1.186	232	Proportionate cluster	6		Structured questionnaire	No	Yes	
Colombia	Countrywide	2000	3	45.600.244	10.360	6.870	443	Proportionate cluster	12			No	Yes	
Costa Rica	Countrywide	2006	4	4.327.228	560	330	45	100% diagnostic units	16	Yes	Structured questionnaire	Yes	No	SDRTB4
Cuba	Countrywide	2005	4	11.269.400	781	467	49	Proportionate cluster	12	Yes	Routine	Yes	Yes	MS Excel
Dominican Republic	Countrywide	1995	1	8.894.907	5.312	2.949	729	Proportionate cluster	21			No	Yes	
Ecuador	Countrywide	2002	3	13.228.423	4.808	3.048	795	100% diagnostic units	18		Structured questionnaire	No	Yes	
El Salvador	Countrywide	2001	3	6.880.951	1.830	1.059	114	100% diagnostic units	12		Structured questionnaire		Yes	
Guatemala	Countrywide	2002	4	12.599.059	3.861	2.420	159	Proportionate cluster	10		Structured questionnaire	Yes	Yes	MS Excel
Honduras	Countrywide	2004	3	7.204.723	3.333	2.069	181	Proportionate cluster	30	Yes	Structured questionnaire	Yes	Yes	SDRTB4
Mexico	Baja California, Sinaloa, Oaxaca	1997	2	94.732.320	19.932	11.997	2.026	100% diagnostic units	7			No		
Nicaragua	Countrywide	2006	4				-	Proportionate cluster	17	Yes	Structured questionnaire	Yes	Yes	SDRTB4 and Epi Info
Paraguay	Countrywide	2001	4	6.158.259	2.348	1.260	273	Proportionate cluster			Structured questionnaire		Yes	
Peru	Countrywide	2006	4	27.968.244	35.541	18.490	4.989	Proportionate cluster	8	Yes	Structured questionnaire	Yes	Yes	SDRTB4 National surveillance system
Puerto Rico	Countrywide	2005	4	3.954.584	113	60	-	All bacteriologically confirmed cases (100%)	12	No	Not collected at National level	No	NA	TIMS and SAS

Country	Sub-national	Year	Report	Population in area surveyed	TB patients notified in area surveyed	sm+ TB patients notified in area surveyed	Patients tested	Method	Survey duration (months)	Medical record/ TB register cross check	Patient interview	Re-interview	Sample target complete	Software
Uruguay	Countrywide	2005	4	3.463.197	626	355	19		12		Structured questionnaire		Yes	
USA	Countrywide	2005	4	298.212.895	14.097	5.089		All bacteriologically confirmed cases (100%)	12		Not collected at National level	No	NA	TIMS and SAS
Venezuela	Countrywide	1999	3	26.749.114	6.950	3.653	350	Proportionate cluster	9		Structured questionnaire	No	Yes	
EASTERN MEDITERRANEAN														
Egypt	Countrywide	2002	3	74.032.884	11.735	5.217	738	Proportionate cluster	12		Structured questionnaire	No	Yes	
Iran	Countrywide	1998	2	69.515.206	9.608	4.686	474	Random cluster	18			No	Yes	
Jordan	Countrywide	2004	4	5.702.776	371	86	10	100% diagnostic units	12	Yes	Structured questionnaire	Yes	Yes	MS Excel
Lebanon	Countrywide	2003	4	3.576.818	391	131	4	100% diagnostic units	22	Yes	Structured questionnaire	Yes	Yes	MS Excel
Morocco	Countrywide	2006	4	31.478.460	26.269	12.757		Proportionate cluster	22	Yes	Structured questionnaire	Yes	Yes	Epi Info
Oman	Countrywide	2006	4	2.566.981	261	131	4	All bacteriologically confirmed cases (100%)	12		Routine		NA	
Qatar	Countrywide	2006	4	812.842	325	96	-	All bacteriologically confirmed cases (100%)	12	Yes	Routine		NA	
Yemen	Countrywide	2004	4	20.974.655	9.063	3.379	351	100% diagnostic units	12		Structured questionnaire		Yes	MS Excel
EUROPE														
Andorra	Countrywide	2005	4	67.151	10	5	-	All bacteriologically confirmed cases (100%)	12		Routine		NA	
Armenia	Countrywide	2007	4	3.016.312	2.322	581	327	100% diagnostic units	13	Yes	Structured questionnaire	Yes	Yes	
Austria	Countrywide	2005	4	8.189.444	954	234	26	All bacteriologically confirmed cases (100%)	12		Routine		NA	SDRTB4
Azerbaijan	Baku City	2007	4	1.827.500	3.960	781	-	100% diagnostic units	11	Yes	Structured questionnaire	Yes	Yes	
Belgium	Countrywide	2005	4	10.419.049	1.144	380	68	All bacteriologically confirmed cases (100%)	12		Routine		NA	SDRTB4 and MS Excel
Bosnia & Herzegovina	Countrywide	2005	4	3.907.074	2.160	640	156	All bacteriologically confirmed cases (100%)	12		Routine		NA	
Croatia	Countrywide	2005	4	4.551.338	1.144	372	94	All bacteriologically confirmed cases (100%)	12		Routine		NA	
Czech Republic	Countrywide	2005	4	10.219.603	1.007	308	34	All bacteriologically confirmed cases (100%)	12		Routine		NA	
Denmark	Countrywide	2005	4	5.430.590	424	129	29	All bacteriologically confirmed cases (100%)	12		Routine		NA	
Estonia	Countrywide	2005	4	1.329.697	519	162	94	All bacteriologically confirmed cases (100%)	12		Routine		NA	
Finland	Countrywide	2005	4	5.249.060	361	130	22	All bacteriologically confirmed cases (100%)	12		Routine		NA	
France	Countrywide	2005	4	60.495.537	5.374	1.941	371	All bacteriologically confirmed cases (100%)	12		Routine		NA	
Georgia	Countrywide	2006	4	4.474.404	6.448	1.509	2.152	100% diagnostic units	12	Yes	Structured questionnaire	Yes	Yes	
Germany	Countrywide	2005	4	82.689.210	6.045	1.379	493	All bacteriologically confirmed cases (100%)	12		Routine		NA	SDRTB3
Iceland	Countrywide	2005	4	294.561	11	2	1	All bacteriologically confirmed cases (100%)	12		Routine		NA	
Ireland	Countrywide	2005	4	4.147.901	461	130	40	All bacteriologically confirmed cases (100%)	12		Routine		NA	
Israel	Countrywide	2005	4	6.724.564	406	98	7	All bacteriologically confirmed cases (100%)	12		Routine		NA	
Italy	Half of the country	2005	4				-	All bacteriologically confirmed cases (100%)	12		Routine		NA	
Kazakhstan	Countrywide	2001	3	14.825.105	31.187	6.911	8.884	100% diagnostic units	2		Structured questionnaire	No	Yes	
Latvia	Countrywide	2005	4	2.306.988	1.443	536	205	All bacteriologically confirmed cases (100%)	12		Routine		NA	
Lithuania	Countrywide	2005	4	3.431.033	2.574	964	460	All bacteriologically confirmed cases (100%)	12		Routine		NA	
Luxembourg	Countrywide	2005	4	464.904	37	14	-	All bacteriologically confirmed cases (100%)	12		Routine		NA	
Malta	Countrywide	2005	4	401.630	23	5	1	All bacteriologically confirmed cases (100%)	12		Routine		NA	
Netherlands	Countrywide	2005	4	16.299.173	1.157	237	44	All bacteriologically confirmed cases (100%)	12		Routine		NA	
Norway	Countrywide	2005	4	4.620.275	290	48	14	All bacteriologically confirmed cases (100%)	12		Routine		NA	
Poland	Countrywide	2004	4	38.529.562	9.280	2.823	1.077	100% diagnostic units	12	Yes	Routine		Yes	
Portugal	Countrywide	2005	4	10.494.502	3.536	1.302	350							
Republic of Moldova	Countrywide	2006	4	4.205.747	6.278	1.696	1.777	100% diagnostic units	12	Yes	Routine	Yes	Yes	
Romania	Countrywide	2004	4	21.711.472	29.347	10.801	6.938	100% diagnostic units	12		Structured questionnaire		Yes	
Russian Federation	Ivanovo Oblast	2002	3	1.114.925	1.363	684		All bacteriologically confirmed cases (100%)	12			No	NA	
Russian Federation	Orel Oblast	2006	4	842.351	486	286	-	All bacteriologically confirmed cases (100%)	12		Routine		NA	

Annex 4

Country	Sub-national	Year	Report	Population in area surveyed	TB patients notified in area surveyed	sm+ TB patients notified in area surveyed	Patients tested	Method	Survey duration (months)	Medical record/ TB register cross check	Patient interview	Re-interview	Sample target complete	Software
Russian Federation	Mary El oblast	2006	4	716.850	588	480	-	All bacteriologically confirmed cases (100%)	12		Routine		NA	
Russian Federation	Tomsk Oblast	2005	4	1.036.500	990	968	215	All bacteriologically confirmed cases (100%)	12		Routine		NA	
Serbia	Countrywide	2005	4				-	All bacteriologically confirmed cases (100%)	12		Routine		NA	
Slovakia	Countrywide	2005	4	5.400.908	760	162	108	All bacteriologically confirmed cases (100%)	12		Routine		NA	
Slovenia	Countrywide	2005	4	1.966.814	278	109	29	All bacteriologically confirmed cases (100%)	12		Routine		NA	MS Exc
Spain	Galicia	2005	4	2.750.985	1.053	361	96	All bacteriologically confirmed cases (100%)	12	Yes	Structured questionaire	Yes	NA	MS Access
Spain	Aragon	2005	4	1.230.090	255	121	26	All bacteriologically confirmed cases (100%)	12	Yes	Structured questionaire	No	NA	
Spain	Barcelona	2005	4	2.736.589	410	109	-	All bacteriologically confirmed cases (100%)	12		Structured questionaire	Yes	NA	
Sweden	Countrywide	2005	4	9.041.262	569	134	30	All bacteriologically confirmed cases (100%)	12		Routine		NA	
Switzerland	Countrywide	2005	4	7.252.331	626	108	118	All bacteriologically confirmed cases (100%)	12		Routine		NA	
Turkmenistan	Dashoguz Velayat (Aral Sea Region)	2002	3	1.141.900	1.300	366	425	100% diagnostic units	9			No	Yes	
Ukraine	Donetsk	2006	4	4.659.018	6.346	1.283	1.764	100% diagnostic units	12	Yes	Structured questionaire	Yes	Yes (civilian only)	
United Kingdom	Countrywide	2005	4	59.667.844	8.633	1.821	460	All bacteriologically confirmed cases (100%)	12		Routine		NA	
Uzbekistan	Tashkent	2005	4		4.839	2.847	-	100% diagnostic units	12		Structured questionaire		Yes	
SOUTH-EAST ASIA														
India	Mayhurbhanj District, Orissa State	2001	4	2.400.000	4.412	2.130	155	100% diagnostic units	9	Yes	Structured questionaire	Yes	Slightly under target	
India	Wardha District, Maharashtra State	2001	3	1.300.000	1.826	726	183	100% diagnostic units	10		Structured questionaire	No	Yes	MS Ex and SP
India	Delhi State	1995	1	16.000.000	45.717	12.703	6.008	100% diagnostic units	6		Structured questionaire	No	Yes	
India	Raichur District, Karnataka State	1999	3	1.800.000	3.047	1.289	492	100% diagnostic units	6		Structured questionaire	No	Yes	
India	North Arcot District, Tamil Nadu State	1999	3	5.664.823	5.600	2.000	952	100% diagnostic units	3		Structured questionaire	No	Yes	
India	Ernakulam district, Kerala State	2004	4	3.200.000	2.598	1.117	262	100% diagnostic units	4	Yes	Structured questionaire	Yes	Yes	
India	Gujarat State	2006	4	54.900.000	77.087	30.289	15.986	Proportionate cluster	10	Yes	Structured questionaire	Yes	Yes	
India	Tamil Nadu State	1997	2	64.800.000	92.725	37.254	7.602	Proportionate cluster	2		Structured questionaire	No	Yes	
India	Hoogli district, West Bengal State	2001	4	5.400.000	6.996	2.958	608	100% diagnostic units	11	Yes	Structured questionaire	Yes	Slightly under target	MS Exce Acce and STA
Indonesia	Mimika district, Papua Province	2004	4	131.715	410	194	-	100% diagnostic units	10	Yes	Structured questionaire	Yes	Yes	Epi In
Myanmar	Countrywide	2003	4	50.519.492	107.991	36.541	5.597	Proportionate cluster	11	Yes	Structured questionaire	Yes	Yes	SDR and Acce
Nepal	Countrywide	2007	4	27.132.629	34.077	14.617	2.973	Proportionate cluster	12	Yes	Structured questionaire	Yes	Yes	
Sri Lanka	Countrywide	2006	4	20.742.905	9.695	4.868	510	All bacteriologically confirmed cases (100%)	12		Structured questionaire		Yes	SDRT
Thailand	Countrywide	2006	4	64.232.758	57.895	29.762	1.795	Proportionate cluster	19	Yes	Structured questionaire	Yes	Yes	
WESTERN PACIFIC														
Australia	Countrywide	2005	4	20.155.129	1.072	244	31	All bacteriologically confirmed cases (100%)	12			No	NA	
Cambodia	Countrywide	2001	3	14.071.014	36.123	21.001	1.306	Proportionate cluster	7	Yes	Structured questionaire	No	Yes	
China	Guandong Province	1999	2	88.890.000	54.609	32.268	7.645	Proportionate cluster	12		Structured questionaire		Yes	MS E
China	Beijing Municipality	2004	4	15.380.000	2.866	1.015	433	100% diagnostic units	12	Yes	Structured questionaire	Yes	Yes	
China	Shandong Province	1997	2	92.840.000	38.880	30.234	5.443	Proportionate cluster	12		Structured questionaire		Yes	
China	Henan Province	2001	3	97.170.000	80.827	42.075	1.201	Proportionate cluster	12		Structured questionaire		Yes	
China	Liaoning Province	1999	3	42.280.000	23.390	12.013	1.465	Proportionate cluster	12		Structured questionaire		Yes	
China	Heilongjiang Province	2005	4	38.160.000	37.925	19.214	4.630	Proportionate cluster	12	No	Structured questionaire	Yes	Yes	SDR
China	Hubei Province	1999	3	60.310.000	51.109	33.218	5.868	Proportionate cluster	10		Structured questionaire		Yes	
China	Zhejiang Province	1999	2	47.200.000	37.568	14.658	5.259	Proportionate cluster	12		Structured questionaire		Yes	SDR
China	Shanghai Municipality	2005	4	17.780.000	7.224	3.123	942	100% diagnostic units	12		Structured questionaire	Yes	Yes	

Country	Sub-national	Year	Report	Population in area surveyed	TB patients notified in area surveyed	sm+ TB patients notified in area surveyed	Patients tested	Method	Survey duration (months)	Medical record/ TB register cross check	Patient interview	Re-interview	Sample target complete	Software
China	Inner Mongolia Autonomous region	2002	4	23.850.000	20.478	11.574	3.204	Proportionate cluster	13		Structured questionaire	Yes	Yes	Visual Foxpro and MS Excel
China, Hong Kong SAR	Hong Kong	2005	4				-	All bacteriologically confirmed cases (100%)	12		Routine	Yes	NA	MS Access
China, Macao SAR	Macao	2005	4	460.162	415	136	31	All bacteriologically confirmed cases (100%)	12		Routine		NA	
Fiji	Countrywide	2006	4				-	Random cluster	12					
Guam	Countrywide	2002	4				-	Random cluster						MS Excel
Japan	Countrywide	2002	4	128.084.652	28.319	10.931	1.992	100% diagnostic units	11	Yes	Routine	Yes	Yes	
Malaysia	Peninsular Malaysia	1997	2	16.489.355	16.066	8.446	983	Proportionate cluster	17			No	Yes	
Mongolia	Countrywide	1999	3	2.646.487	4.743	1.868	341	100% diagnostic units	7		Structured questionaire	No	Yes	
New Caledonia	Countrywide	2005	4				-	Random cluster					Yes	SAS
New Zealand	Countrywide	2006	4	4.027.947	355	140	19	All bacteriologically confirmed cases (100%)	12	Yes	Routine	Yes	NA	
Northern Mariana Is	Countrywide	2006	4				-	ll bacteriologically confirmed cases (100%)	12	Yes				
Philippines	Countrywide	2004	4	83.054.478	137.100	81.647	3.957	Proportionate cluster	12		Structured questionaire		Yes	
Rep. Korea	Countrywide	2004	4	47.816.936	46.969	11.638	7.098	Proportionate cluster			Routine			National Surveillance system
Singapore	Countrywide	2005	4	4.325.539	1.469	552	153	All bacteriologically confirmed cases (100%)	12		Routine	Yes	NA	
Solomon Islands	Countrywide	2004	4	477.742	397	169	5	Random cluster						
Vanuatu	Countrywide	2006	4	211.367	81	35	8	Random cluster					Yes	
Viet Nam	Countrywide	2006	4	84.238.231	95.970	55.570	7.301	Proportionate cluster			Structured questionaire			

Annex 5: Laboratory methods 1994-2007

Country	Sub-national	Year	Supranational Laboratory	Culture method	DST method	Number of culture labs used in survey	Number of DST labs used in survey	H	R	E	S	PZA	Km	Amk	Cap	Cip	Ofl	% agreement H	% agreement R	Retesting
AFRICA																				
Algeria	Countrywide	2001	Laboratoire de la Tuberculose, Institut Pasteur d'Algérie, Alger, ALGERIA	Löwenstein-Jensen	Proportion method	1	1													Yes
Benin	Countrywide	1997	Laboratoire de la Tuberculose, Institut Pasteur d'Algérie, Alger, ALGERIA	Löwenstein-Jensen	Proportion method															Yes
Botswana	Countrywide	2002	Centers for Disease Control and Prevention, Mycobacteriology/Tuberculosis Laboratory, Georgia, USA	BACTEC 460	Resistance ratio method															
Central African Republic	Bangui	1998	Institut Pasteur, Centre National de Référence des Mycobactéries, Paris, FRANCE	Löwenstein-Jensen	Proportion method															
Côte d'Ivoire	Countrywide	2006	Institut Pasteur, Centre National de Référence des Mycobactéries, Paris, FRANCE		Proportion method															Yes
DR Congo	Kinshasa	1999	Département de Microbiologie – Unité de Mycobactériologie Institut de Médecine Tropicale, Antwerp, BELGIUM																	Yes
Ethiopia	Countrywide	2005	National Institute of Public Health and the Environment (RIVM), Bilthoven, NETHERLANDS	Löwenstein-Jensen	Proportion method	1	1													Yes
Gambia	Countrywide	2000	Health Protection Agency, National Mycobacterium Reference Unit, Department of Infectious Diseases, UNITED KINGDOM	Löwenstein-Jensen and BACTEC 460	Resistance ratio method	1														Yes
Guinea	Sentinel sites	1998	Institut Pasteur, Centre National de Référence des Mycobactéries, Paris, FRANCE	Löwenstein-Jensen	Proportion method															Yes
Kenya	Nearly Countrywide	1995	Health Protection Agency, National Mycobacterium Reference Unit, Department of Infectious Diseases, UNITED KINGDOM	Löwenstein-Jensen	Resistance ratio method															
Lesotho	Countrywide	1995	The Medical Research Council, TB Research Lead Programme, Pretoria, SOUTH AFRICA	Löwenstein-Jensen	Proportion method															
Madagascar	Countrywide	2007	Health Protection Agency, National Mycobacterium Reference Unit, Department of Infectious Diseases, UNITED KINGDOM	Löwenstein-Jensen	Proportion method	1	1	0.1	40.0	2.0	4.0									Yes
Mozambique	Countrywide	1999	Swedish Institute for Infectious Disease Control (SIDC), Solna, SWEDEN	Löwenstein-Jensen	Proportion method															
Rwanda	Countrywide	2005	Département de Microbiologie – Unité de Mycobactériologie Institut de Médecine Tropicale, Antwerp, BELGIUM	Various	Proportion method	1	1	0.2	40.0	2.0	4.0		6		10		2	100	100	Yes
Senegal	Countrywide	2006	Département de Microbiologie – Unité de Mycobactériologie Institut de Médecine Tropicale, Antwerp, BELGIUM	Löwenstein-Jensen	Proportion method	1	1	0.2	40.0	2.0	4.0									Yes
Sierra Leone	Nearly Countrywide	1997	Armauer Hansen Institut, Wuertzburg, GERMANY	Löwenstein-Jensen	Proportion method															Yes
South Africa	Countrywide	2002	The Medical Research Council, TB Research Lead Programme, Pretoria, SOUTH AFRICA	Löwenstein-Jensen	Proportion method															NA
Swaziland	Countrywide	1995	The Medical Research Council, TB Research Lead Programme, Pretoria, SOUTH AFRICA	Löwenstein-Jensen	Proportion method															
Uganda	3 GLRA Zones *	1997	Armauer Hansen Institut, Wuertzburg, Germany	Löwenstein-Jensen	Proportion method															Yes
UR Tanzania	Countrywide	2007	Département de Microbiologie Unité de Mycobactériologie Institut de Médecine Tropicale, Antwerp, BELGIUM	Löwenstein-Jensen	Proportion method	1	1	1.0	40.0	2.0	5.0							100	100	Yes
Zambia	Countrywide	2000	The Medical Research Council, TB Research Lead Programme, Pretoria, SOUTH AFRICA	Löwenstein-Jensen	Proportion method															
Zimbabwe	Nearly Countrywide	1995	National Reference Center for Mycobacteria, Borstel, GERMANY	Löwenstein-Jensen	Various															
AMERICAS																				
Argentina	Countrywide	2005	Mycobacteria Laboratory, National Institute of Infectious Diseases, ANLIS "Dr Carlos G. Malbran", Buenos Aires, ARGENTINA	Löwenstein-Jensen and BACTEC 460	Proportion method	45	8	0.2	40.0	2.0	4.0	100	20	MIC	40	MIC	2	100	100	Yes
Bolivia	Countrywide	1996	Mycobacteria Laboratory, National Institute of Infectious Diseases, ANLIS "Dr Carlos G. Malbran", Buenos Aires, ARGENTINA	Löwenstein-Jensen	Proportion method															
Brazil	Nearly Countrywide	1996	Mycobacteria Laboratory, National Institute of Infectious Diseases, ANLIS "Dr Carlos G. Malbran", Buenos Aires, ARGENTINA	Löwenstein-Jensen	Proportion method															Yes

Country	Sub-national	Year	Supranational Laboratory	Culture method	DST method	Number of culture labs used in survey	Number of DST labs used in survey	H	R	E	S	PZA	Km	Amk	Cap	Cip	Ofl	% agreement H	% agreement R	Restesting
Canada	Countrywide	2006	Centers for Disease Control and Prevention, Mycobacteriology/ Tuberculosis Laboratory, Georgia, USA	Various	Proportion method	10	10	0.1	2.0	2.5	2.0	100.0	5.0	1.0	1.3		2	100	100	NA
Chile	Countrywide	2001	Instituto de Salud Publica de Chile, Santiago, CHILE	Löwenstein-Jensen	Proportion method															NA
Colombia	Countrywide	2000	Instituto de Salud Publica de Chile, Santiago, CHILE	Ogawa	Proportion method															Yes
Costa Rica	Countrywide	2006	Departamento de Micobacterias, Instituto de Diagnostico y, Referencia Epidemiológicos (INDRE), MEXICO	Löwenstein-Jensen	Proportion method	1	1	0.2	40.0	2.0	4.0							96	96	Yes
Cuba	Countrywide	2005	Mycobacteria Laboratory, National Institute of Infectious Diseases, ANLIS "Dr Carlos G. Malbran," Buenos Aires, ARGENTINA	Löwenstein-Jensen	Proportion method	46	1	0.2	40.0	2.0	4.0							100	100	NA
Dominican Republic	Countrywide	1995	Laboratory Centre for Disease Control, Ottawa, CANADA (historical)	Löwenstein-Jensen	Proportion method															Yes
Ecuador	Countrywide	2002	Instituto de Salud Publica de Chile, Santiago, CHILE	Löwenstein-Jensen	Proportion method															Yes
El Salvador	Countrywide	2001	Instituto de Salud Publica de Chile, Santiago, CHILE	Löwenstein-Jensen	Proportion method															Yes
Guatemala	Countrywide	2002	Instituto de Salud Publica de Chile, Santiago, CHILE	Löwenstein-Jensen	Proportion method	8	1	0.2	40.0	2.0	4.0							99	100	Yes
Honduras	Countrywide	2004	Instituto de Salud Publica de Chile, Santiago, CHILE	Löwenstein-Jensen	Proportion method	4	1	0.2	40.0	2.0	4.0							96	100	Yes
Mexico	Baja California, Sinaloa, Oaxaca	1997	Centers for Disease Control and Prevention, Mycobacteriology/ Tuberculosis Laboratory, Georgia, USA	Löwenstein-Jensen	Proportion method															
Nicaragua	Countrywide	2006	Instituto de Salud Publica de Chile, Santiago, CHILE	Löwenstein-Jensen	Proportion method	2	1	0.2	40.0	2.0	4.0							100	90	Yes
Paraguay	Countrywide	2001	Mycobacteria Laboratory, National Institute of Infectious Diseases, ANLIS "Dr Carlos G. Malbran," Buenos Aires, ARGENTINA	Löwenstein-Jensen	Proportion method															
Peru	Countrywide	2006	Instituto de Salud Publica de Chile, Santiago, CHILE	Ogawa	Proportion method			0.2	40.0	0.2	4.0							100	100	Yes
Puerto Rico	Countrywide	2005	Centers for Disease Control and Prevention, Mycobacteriology/ Tuberculosis Laboratory, Georgia, USA	Various	Various								5	4	10		2			NA
Uruguay	Countrywide	2005	Mycobacteria Laboratory, National Institute of Infectious Diseases, ANLIS "Dr Carlos G. Malbran," Buenos Aires, ARGENTINA	Löwenstein-Jensen	Proportion method	1	1	0.2	40.0	2.0	4.0					0.5		100	100	
USA	Countrywide	2005	Centers for Disease Control and Prevention, Mycobacteriology/ Tuberculosis Laboratory, Georgia, USA	Various	Various								5	4	10		2			NA
Venezuela	Countrywide	1999	Instituto de Salud Publica de Chile, Santiago, CHILE	Löwenstein-Jensen	Proportion method															
EASTERN MEDITERRANEAN																				
Egypt	Countrywide	2002	Laboratoire de la Tuberculose, Institut Pasteur d'Algerie, Alger, ALGERIA	Löwenstein-Jensen	Proportion method															Yes
Iran	Countrywide	1998	Research Institute of Tuberculosis, Japan Anti-Tuberculosis Association, Tokyo, JAPAN	Löwenstein-Jensen	Proportion method															No
Jordan	Countrywide	2004	Laboratoire de la Tuberculose, Institut Pasteur d'Algerie, Alger, ALGERIA		Proportion method	1	1	0.2	40.0	2.0	4.0							73	93	Yes
Lebanon	Countrywide	2003	Institut Pasteur, Centre National de Référence des Mycobacteries, Paris, FRANCE	Various	Proportion method	1	1	0.1	2.0	2.5	2.0							100	100	Yes
Morocco	Countrywide	2006	Laboratoire de la Tuberculose, Institut Pasteur d'Algerie, Alger, ALGERIA	Löwenstein-Jensen	Proportion method	12	1	0.2	40.0	2.0	4.0	0.2						100	100	Yes
Oman	Countrywide	2006	Istituto Superiore di Sanità Dipartimento di Malattie Infettive, Parassitarie e Immunomediate, Rome, ITALY and Laboratory of Bacteriology & Medical Mycology and San Raffaele del Monte Tabor Foundation (hSR), Milan, ITALY		Proportion method	10	1													NA
Qatar	Countrywide	2006	Istituto Superiore di Sanità Dipartimento di Malattie Infettive, Parassitarie e Immunomediate, Rome, ITALY and Laboratory of Bacteriology & Medical Mycology and San Raffaele del Monte Tabor Foundation (hSR), Milan, ITALY		Proportion method	1													100	100	NA

Annex 5

Country	Sub-national	Year	Supranational Laboratory	Culture method	DST method	Number of culture labs used in survey	Number of DST labs used in survey	H	R	E	S	PZA	Km	Amk	Cap	Cip	Ofl	% agreement H	% agreement R	Rechecking
Yemen	Countrywide	2004	Research Institute of Tuberculosis, Japan Anti-Tuberculosis Association, Tokyo, JAPAN		Proportion method	4	1													Yes
EUROPE																				
Andorra	Countrywide	2005				1	0													NA
Armenia	Countrywide	2007	National Reference Center for Mycobacteria, Borstel, GERMANY	Löwenstein-Jensen or Middlebrook	Proportion method	1	1											100	100	Yes
Austria	Countrywide	2005	National Reference Center for Mycobacteria, Borstel, GERMANY			11	9											100	100	NA
Azerbaijan	Baku City	2007	National Reference Center for Mycobacteria, Borstel, GERMANY		Proportion method	1	1													Yes
Belgium	Countrywide	2005	Health Protection Agency, National Mycobacterium Reference Unit, Department of Infectious Diseases, UNITED KINGDOM		Proportion method	155	25											100	100	NA
Bosnia & Herzegovina	Countrywide	2005	National Reference Center for Mycobacteria, Borstel, GERMANY		Proportion method	8	8													NA
Croatia	Countrywide	2005	National Reference Center for Mycobacteria, Borstel, GERMANY		Proportion method	15	8													NA
Czech Republic	Countrywide	2005	National Institute of Public Health, Prague, CZECH REPUBLIC		Proportion method	45	14											100	100	NA
Denmark	Countrywide	2005	Swedish Institute for Infectious Disease Control (SIDC), Solna, SWEDEN		Proportion method	1	1											95	100	NA
Estonia	Countrywide	2005	Swedish Institute for Infectious Disease Control (SIDC), Solna, SWEDEN		Absolute concentration method	3	2											90	95	NA
Finland	Countrywide	2005	Swedish Institute for Infectious Disease Control (SIDC), Solna, SWEDEN		Proportion method	15	2											100	90	NA
France	Countrywide	2005	Health Protection Agency, National Mycobacterium Reference Unit, Department of Infectious Diseases, UNITED KINGDOM		Proportion method	310	110											100	100	NA
Georgia	Countrywide	2006	Département de Microbiologie Unité de Mycobactériologie Institut de Médecine Tropicale, Antwerp, Belgium	Löwenstein-Jensen	Absolute concentration method	1	1	0.2	40.0	2.0	4.0							100	100	Yes
Germany	Countrywide	2005	National Reference Center for Mycobacteria, Borstel, GERMANY	Various	Proportion method	200	63													NA
Iceland	Countrywide	2005	Swedish Institute for Infectious Disease Control (SIDC), Solna, SWEDEN		Proportion method	1	0													NA
Ireland	Countrywide	2005	Health Protection Agency, National Mycobacterium Reference Unit, Department of Infectious Diseases, UNITED KINGDOM		Proportion method	13	4											100	100	NA
Israel	Countrywide	2005	Health Protection Agency, National Mycobacterium Reference Unit, Department of Infectious Diseases, UNITED KINGDOM		Proportion method	19	2											100	100	NA
Italy	Half of the country	2005	Istituto Superiore di Sanità Dipartimento di Malattie Infettive, Parassitarie e Immunomediate. Rome, ITALY and Laboratory of Bacteriology & Medical Mycology and San Raffaele del Monte Tabor Foundation (hSR), Milan, ITALY		Proportion method	9	1											100	100	NA
Kazakhstan	Countrywide	2001	National Reference Center for Mycobacteria, Borstel, GERMANY	Löwenstein-Jensen	Absolute concentration method													100	100	Yes
Latvia	Countrywide	2005	Swedish Institute for Infectious Disease Control (SIDC), Solna, SWEDEN		Absolute concentration method	9	1											95	100	NA
Lithuania	Countrywide	2005	Swedish Institute for Infectious Disease Control (SIDC), Solna, SWEDEN		Absolute concentration method	5	5											100	95	NA
Luxembourg	Countrywide	2005			Proportion method	1	1													NA
Malta	Countrywide	2005	Health Protection Agency, National Mycobacterium Reference Unit, Department of Infectious Diseases, UNITED KINGDOM		Proportion method	1	1													NA
Netherlands	Countrywide	2005	National Institute of Public Health and the Environment (RIVM), Bilthoven,			43	15													NA

Country	Sub-national	Year	Supranational Laboratory	Culture method	DST method	Number of culture labs used in survey	Number of DST labs used in survey	H	R	E	S	PZA	Km	Amk	Cap	Cip	Ofl	% agreement H	% agreement R	Restesting
Norway	Countrywide	2005	Swedish Institute for Infectious Disease Control (SIDC), Solna, SWEDEN		Proportion method	13	3													NA
Poland	Countrywide	2004	National Institute of Public Health and the Environment (RIVM), Bilthoven, NETHERLANDS			72	72													NA
Portugal	Countrywide	2005																		
Republic of Moldova	Countrywide	2006	National Reference Center for Mycobacteria, Borstel, GERMANY	Löwenstein-Jensen	Absolute concentration method	4	4	1.0	40.0	2.0	5.0		30.0		30.0	2.0	2.0	95	95	Yes
Romania	Countrywide	2004	Swedish Institute for Infectious Disease Control (SIDC), Solna, SWEDEN	Löwenstein-Jensen		110	65													Yes
Russian Federation	Ivanovo Oblast	2002			Proportion method															
Russian Federation	Orel Oblast	2006	Swedish Institute for Infectious Disease Control (SIDC), Solna, SWEDEN		Absolute concentration method														95	NA
Russian Federation	Mary El oblast	2006	Swedish Institute for Infectious Disease Control (SIDC), Solna, SWEDEN		Absolute concentration method															NA
Russian Federation	Tomsk Oblast	2005	Massachusetts State Laboratory, Massachusetts, USA		Absolute concentration method														95	Yes
Serbia	Countrywide	2005	National Reference Center for Mycobacteria, Borstel, GERMANY		Proportion method	45	10													NA
Slovakia	Countrywide	2005	National Reference Center for Mycobacteria, Borstel, GERMANY		Proportion method	14	6											90	90	NA
Slovenia	Countrywide	2005	National Reference Center for Mycobacteria, Borstel, GERMANY		Proportion method	5	1											100	100	NA
Spain	Galicia	2005	Servicio de Microbiologia Hospital Universitaris, Vall d'Hebron, Barcelona, SPAIN	Various	Proportion method	13	1	0.1	1.0	5.0	1.0	100 ug/ml	5	1	1.25		2	100	100	No
Spain	Aragon	2005	Servicio de Microbiologia Hospital Universitaris, Vall d'Hebron, Barcelona, SPAIN	Various	Proportion method	7	7	1	1	5.0	1	100						100	100	Yes
Spain	Barcelona	2005	Servicio de Microbiologia Hospital Universitaris, Vall d'Hebron, Barcelona, SPAIN	Various	Proportion method	3	3											100	100	NA
Sweden	Countrywide	2005	Swedish Institute for Infectious Disease Control (SIDC), Solna, SWEDEN		Proportion method	5	5											100	100	NA
Switzerland	Countrywide	2005	Health Protection Agency, National Mycobacterium Reference Unit, Department of Infectious Diseases, UNITED KINGDOM		Proportion method	28	28											100	100	NA
Turkmenistan	Dashoguz Velayat (Aral Sea Region)	2002	National Reference Center for Mycobacteria, Borstel, GERMANY	Löwenstein-Jensen	Absolute concentration method															Yes
Ukraine	Donetsk	2006	Kuratorium Tuberkulose in der Welt e.V.IML (Institut für Mikrobiologie und Laboratoriumsdiagnostik) Gauting, GERMANY	Löwenstein-Jensen, Finn- 2	Absolute concentration method	14	1	1	40.0	2.0	10.0									Yes
United Kingdom	Countrywide	2005	Health Protection Agency, National Mycobacterium Reference Unit, Department of Infectious Diseases, UNITED KINGDOM		Resistance ratio method	268	10													NA
Uzbekistan	Tashkent	2005	Kuratorium Tuberkulose in der Welt e.V.IML (Institut für Mikrobiologie und Laboratoriumsdiagnostik) Gauting, GERMANY		Absolute concentration method	1	1													Yes
SOUTH-EAST ASIA																				
India	Mayurbhanj District, Orissa State	2001	TB Research Centre (TRC), Indian Council of Medical Research, Chennai, INDIA	Löwenstein-Jensen	Proportion method	1	1	0.2	40.0	2.0	4.0							100	100	NA
India	Wardha District, Maharashtra State	2001	TB Research Centre (TRC), Indian Council of Medical Research, Chennai, INDIA	Löwenstein-Jensen	Proportion method															NA
India	Delhi State	1995	Queensland Mycobacterium Reference Laboratory, Brisbane, AUSTRALIA	Löwenstein-Jensen	Proportion method															NA

Annex 5

Country	Sub-national	Year	Supranational Laboratory	Culture method	DST method	Number of culture labs used in survey	Number of DST labs used in survey	H	R	E	S	PZA	Km	Amk	Cap	Cip	Ofl	% agreement H	% agreement R	Retesting
India	Raichur District, Karnataka State	1999	TB Research Centre (TRC), Indian Council of Medical Research, Chennai, INDIA	Löwenstein-Jensen	Proportion method															NA
India	North Arcot District, Tamil Nadu State	1999	TB Research Centre (TRC), Indian Council of Medical Research, Chennai, INDIA	Löwenstein-Jensen	Proportion method															NA
India	Ernakulam district, Kerala State	2004	TB Research Centre (TRC), Indian Council of Medical Research, Chennai, INDIA	Löwenstein-Jensen	Proportion method	1	1	0.2	40.0	2.0	4.0							100	100	NA
India	Gujarat State	2006	TB Research Centre (TRC), Indian Council of Medical Research, Chennai, INDIA	Löwenstein-Jensen	Proportion method	1	1	0.2	40.0	2.0	4.0									NA
India	Tamil Nadu State	1997	Queensland Mycobacterium Reference Laboratory, Brisbane, AUSTRALIA	Löwenstein-Jensen	Resistance ratio method															NA
India	Hoogli district, West Bengal State	2001	TB Research Centre (TRC), Indian Council of Medical Research, Chennai, INDIA	Löwenstein-Jensen	Proportion method	1	1	0.2	40.0	2.0	4.0							100	100	NA
Indonesia	Mimika district, Papua Province	2004	Mycobacterium Reference Laboratory, Institute of Medical and Veterinary Science, Adelaide, AUSTRALIA	BACTEC 460	Proportion method	1	1	0.1; 0.4	2.0	2.5	2.0			1.0	2.5	1.0		100	100	Yes
Myanmar	Countrywide	2003	TB Research Centre (TRC), Indian Council of Medical Research, Chennai, INDIA	Löwenstein-Jensen and Ogawa	Proportion method	1	1	0.2	40.0	2.0	4.0							100	95	Yes
Nepal	Countrywide	2007	Kuratorium Tuberkulose in der Welt e.V./NRL (Institut für Mikrobiologie und Laboratoriumsdiagnostik) Gauting, GERMANY		Proportion method	1	1	0.2	40.0	2.0	4.0									Yes
Sri Lanka	Countrywide	2006	TB Research Centre (TRC), Indian Council of Medical Research, Chennai, INDIA		Proportion method	1	1													Planned
Thailand	Countrywide	2006	Département de Microbiologie Unité de Mycobactériologie Institut de Médecine Tropicale, Antwerp, BELGIUM	Löwenstein-Jensen	Proportion method	8	1	0.2	40.0	2.0	4.0							97	100	NA
WESTERN PACIFIC																				
Australia	Countrywide	2005	Mycobacterium Reference Laboratory, Institute of Medical and Veterinary Science, Adelaide, AUSTRALIA	Various	Proportion method	60	5													NA
Cambodia	Countrywide	2001	Research Institute of Tuberculosis, Japan Anti-Tuberculosis Association, Tokyo, JAPAN	Various	Proportion method	40	1													Yes
China	Guandong Province	1999	Korean Institute of Tuberculosis, Seoul, REPUBLIC OF KOREA	Löwenstein-Jensen	Proportion method	18	1	0.2	40.0	2.0	4.0							100	100	No
China	Beijing Municipality	2004	TB Reference Laboratory Department of Health, SAR Hong Kong, CHINA	Löwenstein-Jensen	Proportion method	30	1													No
China	Shandong Province	1997	Korean Institute of Tuberculosis, Seoul, REPUBLIC OF KOREA	Löwenstein-Jensen	Proportion method	30	1													No
China	Henan Province	2001	Korean Institute of Tuberculosis, Seoul, REPUBLIC OF KOREA	Löwenstein-Jensen	Proportion method	30	1	0.2	40.0	2.0	4.0							100	93	No
China	Liaoning Province	1999	TB Reference Laboratory Department of Health, SAR Hong Kong, CHINA	Löwenstein-Jensen	Proportion method	30	1													No
China	Heilongjiang Province	2005	TB Reference Laboratory Department of Health, SAR Hong Kong, CHINA	Löwenstein-Jensen	Proportion method	30	1	0.2	40.0	2.0	4.0							100	93	No
China	Hubei Province	1999	Korean Institute of Tuberculosis, Seoul, REPUBLIC OF KOREA	Löwenstein-Jensen	Proportion method	30	1													No
China	Zhejiang Province	1999	Korean Institute of Tuberculosis, Seoul, REPUBLIC OF KOREA	Löwenstein-Jensen	Proportion method	30	1													No
China	Shanghai Municipality	2005	TB Reference Laboratory Department of Health, SAR Hong Kong, CHINA	Löwenstein-Jensen	Proportion method	19	1	0.2	40.0	2.0	4.0							93	97	No
China	Inner Mongolia Autonomous region	2002	TB Reference Laboratory Department of Health, SAR Hong Kong, CHINA	Löwenstein-Jensen	Proportion method	30	1	0.2	40.0	2.0	4.0							93	97	No
China, Hong Kong SAR	Hong Kong	2005	TB Reference Laboratory Department of Health, SAR Hong Kong, CHINA	Löwenstein-Jensen	Absolute concentration method	1	1	0.2	32.0	2.8	16.0	50.0	16.0	8.0	32.0		2.4	100	100	NA
China, Macao SAR	Macao	2005	TB Reference Laboratory Department of Health, SAR Hong Kong, CHINA	Löwenstein-Jensen and BactALERT MP	1% Proportion Method-Bactec MGIT 960	1	1	0.1	1.0	5.0	1.0									NA
Fiji	Countrywide	2006	Queensland Mycobacterium Reference Laboratory, Brisbane, AUSTRALIA																	NA

Country	Sub-national	Year	Supranational Laboratory	Culture method	DST method	Number of culture labs used in survey	Number of DST labs used in survey	H	R	E	S	PZA	Km	Amk	Cap	Cip	Ofl	% agreement H	% agreement R	Retesting
Japan	Countrywide	2002	Research Institute of Tuberculosis, Japan Anti-Tuberculosis Association, Tokyo, JAPAN	MGIT and Ogawa	Proportion method			0.2, 1.0	40.0	2.5	10.0	100	20					100	100	NA
Malaysia	Peninsular Malaysia	1997	Research Institute of Tuberculosis, Japan Anti-Tuberculosis Association, Tokyo, JAPAN	Ogawa	Absolute concentration method	1	1													
Mongolia	Countrywide	1999	Research Institute of Tuberculosis, Japan Anti-Tuberculosis Association, Tokyo, JAPAN	Various	Proportion method	1	1													Yes
New Caledonia	Countrywide	2005																		NA
New Zealand	Countrywide	2006	Queensland Mycobacterium Reference Laboratory, Brisbane, AUSTRALIA	Various	Proportion method	30	3	0.1, 0.4	1.0	5.0	1.0	100		1.0	2.5	1.0				NA
Northern Mariana Is	Countrywide	2006	Hawaii State Laboratory under Centers for Disease Control and Prevention, Mycobacteriology/Tuberculosis Laboratory, Georgia, USA	Löwenstein-Jensen	Proportion method	1	1													NA
Philippines	Countrywide	2004	Research Institute of Tuberculosis, Japan Anti-Tuberculosis Association, Tokyo, JAPAN		Proportion method															Yes
Rep. Korea	Countrywide	2004	Korean Institute of Tuberculosis, Seoul, REPUBLIC OF KOREA		Proportion method	12	1													NA
Singapore	Countrywide	2005		Various	Proportion method	2	2	0.1, 1.0	1.0, 2.0	2.5, 5.0	2.0, 10.0	100 ug/ml	5.0		1.25		2.0	100	100	NA
Solomon Islands	Countrywide	2004	Mycobacterium Reference Laboratory, Institute of Medical and Veterinary Science, Adelaide, AUSTRALIA																	
Vanuatu	Countrywide	2006	Queensland Mycobacterium Reference Laboratory, Brisbane, AUSTRALIA																	NA
Viet Nam	Countrywide	2006	National Institute of Public Health and the Environment (RIVM), Bilthoven, NETHERLANDS																	NA

Annex 6: Trends in drug resistance among new TB cases 1994-2007

COUNTRY	METHOD	1994 tot	any	%	mdr	%	1995 tot	any	%	mdr	%	1996 tot	any	%	mdr	%	1997 tot	any	%	mdr	%	1998 tot	any	%	mdr	%	1999 tot	any	%	mdr	%
AFRICA																															
Botswana	Survey											407	15	3,7	1	0,2											638	40	6,3	3	0,
Sierra Leone	Survey											463	130	28,1	5	1,1	117	29	24,8	1	0,9										
South Africa, Mpumalanga Province	Survey																661	53	8,0	10	1,5										
AMERICAS																															
Argentina	Survey																										679	69	10,2	12	1,8
Canada	Surveillance	1325	146	11,0	10	0,8	1242	0	0,0	8	0,6	1203	0	0,0	9	0,7	1366	0	0,0	12	0,9	1206	0	0,0	7	0,6	1268	0	0,0	7	0,
Chile	Survey																732	67	9,2	3	0,4										
Cuba	Surveillance						337	28	8,3	1	0,3	426	35	8,2	4	0,9	241	21	8,7	0	0,0	284	13	4,6	0	0,0	321	27	8,4	3	0,
Nicaragua	Survey																					564	88	15,6	7	1,2					
Puerto Rico	Combined cases only																														
Uruguay	Survey																484	8	1,7	0	0,0						315	10	3,2	1	0,
USA	Combined cases only																														
EASTERN MEDITERRANEAN																															
Oman	Surveillance																										133	6	4,5	1	0,
Qatar	Combined cases only																														
EUROPE																															
Andorra	Surveillance																										6	0	0,0	0	0,
Austria	Surveillance																										703	36	5,1	2	0,
Belgium	Surveillance																0	0		0											
Bosnia & Herzegovina	Surveillance																										1154	25	2,2	3	0,
Croatia	Surveillance																										761	20	2,6	2	0,
Czech Republic	Surveillance	199	4	2,0	2	1,0																					628	17	2,7	2	0,
Denmark	Surveillance																					412	54	13,1	2	0,5	392	60	15,3	0	0,
Estonia	Surveillance																					377	139	36,9	53	14,1	428	143	33,4	75	17
Finland	Surveillance																410	20	4,9	0	0,0						371	8	2,2	0	0,
France	Surveillance											1491	123	8,2	8	0,5	787	73	9,3	0	0,0						910	84	9,2	6	0,
Germany	Surveillance																														
Iceland	Surveillance																										7	0	0,0	0	0,
Ireland	Surveillance																										101	2	2,0	1	1,
Israel	Surveillance																0	0		0							0	0		0	
Italy	Surveillance																										683	84	12,3	8	1,
Latvia	Surveillance																					789	236	29,9	71	9,0	825	254	30,8	86	10
Lithuania	Surveillance																										819	230	28,1	64	7,
Luxembourg	Surveillance																														
Malta	Surveillance																										13	0	0,0	0	0,
Netherlands	Surveillance											1042	96	9,2	6	0,6											899	79	8,8	4	0,
Norway	Surveillance											138	15	10,9	3	2,2											144	23	16,0	3	2,
Poland	Surveillance																2976	106	3,6	18	0,6										
Russian Federation, Ivanovo Oblast	Surveillance											248	70	28,2	10	4,0						222	72	32,4	20	9,0					
Russian Federation, Orel Oblast	Surveillance																														
Russian Federation, Tomsk Oblast	Surveillance																					417	121	29,0	27	6,					
Serbia & Montenegro, Belgrade	Surveillance																										290	13	4,5	0	0,
Slovakia	Surveillance																					589	16	2,7	2	0,3	456	13	2,9	3	0,
Slovenia	Surveillance																290	7	2,4	2	0,7						304	9	3,0	0	0,
Spain, Barcelona	Combined cases only											218	21	9,6	1	0,5						315	11	3,5	1	0,3	128	8	6,3	0	0,
Spain, Galicia	Surveillance																														
Sweden	Surveillance																356	28	7,9	2	0,6						377	44	11,7	3	0,
Switzerland	Surveillance																322	10	3,1	0	0,0						428	26	6,1	3	0,
United Kingdom	Surveillance																														
SOUTH-EASTERN ASIA																															
Nepal	Survey											787	77	9,8	9	1,1											668	89	13,3	25	
Thailand	Survey																1137	290	25,5	24	2,1										
WESTERN PACIFIC																															
Australia	Combined cases only																														
China, Henan Province	Survey											646	226	35,0	70	10,8															
China, Hong Kong SAR	Surveillance											4424	541	12,2	62	1,4	3432	406	11,8	39	1,1	3753	450	12,0	49	1,3	3460	442	12,8	35	
Guam	Combined cases only																														
Japan	Surveillance																1374	141	10,3	12	0,9										
New Caledonia	Survey											93	2	2,2	0	0,0											0	0		0	
New Zealand	Surveillance						144	8	5,5	2	1,4	136	6	4,4	0	0,0	123	16	13,0	1	0,8	155	20	12,9	2	1,3	228	19	8,3	2	
Northern Mariana Is	Surveillance																														
Rep. Korea	Survey	2486	258	10,4	39	1,6																					2370	251	10,6	52	
Singapore	Surveillance											980	47	4,8	3	0,3															
Viet Nam	Survey																640	208	32,5	15	2,3										

2000 New					2001 New					2002 New					2003 New					2004 New					2005 New					2006 New					2007 New				
ot	any	%	mdr	%	tot	any	%	mdr	%	tot	any	%	mdr	%	tot	any	%	mdr	%	tot	any	%	mdr	%	tot	any	%	mdr	%	tot	any	%	mdr	%	tot	any	%	mdr	%
.	.	.	.	.	.	.	.	.	.	1182	123	10,4	10	0,8	.	.	.	.	.	.	.	.	.	.	.	.	.	.	.	.	.	.	.	.	.	.	.	.	.
.	.	.	.	.	.	.	.	.	.	.	.	.	.	.	.	.	.	.	.	.	.	.	.	.	.	.	.	.	.	.	.	.	.	.	.	.	.	.	.
.	.	.	.	.	.	.	.	.	.	702	66	9,4	18	2,6	.	.	.	.	.	.	.	.	.	.	.	.	.	.	.	.	.	.	.	.	.	.	.	.	.
.	.	.	.	.	.	.	.	.	.	.	.	.	.	.	.	.	.	.	.	.	.	.	.	.	683	68	10,0	15	2,2	.	.	.	.	.	.	.	.	.	.
62	0	0,0	7	0,6	1262	0	0,0	9	0,7	1172	0	0,0	12	1,0	1153	0	0,0	6	0,5	1154	0	0,0	5	0,4	1087	130	12,0	13	1,2	1058	81	7,7	8	0,8	.	.	.	.	.
.	.	.	.	.	867	91	10,5	6	0,7	.	.	.	.	.	.	.	.	.	.	.	.	.	.	.	.	.	.	.	.	.	.	.	.	.	.	.	.	.	.
77	19	5,0	1	0,3	.	.	.	.	.	195	12	6,2	1	0,5	193	22	11,4	1	0,5	177	26	14,7	0	0,0	169	12	7,1	0	0,0	.	.	.	.	.	.	.	.	.	.
.	.	.	.	.	.	.	.	.	.	.	.	.	.	.	.	.	.	.	.	.	.	.	.	.	.	.	.	.	.	320	42	13,1	2	0,6	.	.	.	.	.
.	.	.	.	.	.	.	.	.	.	.	.	.	.	.	.	.	.	.	.	.	.	.	.	.	.	.	.	.	.	.	.	.	.	.	.	.	.	.	.
.	.	.	.	.	.	.	.	.	.	.	.	.	.	.	.	.	.	.	.	.	.	.	.	.	335	7	2,1	0	0,0	.	.	.	.	.	.	.	.	.	.
.	.	.	.	.	.	.	.	.	.	.	.	.	.	.	.	.	.	.	.	.	.	.	.	.	.	.	.	.	.	.	.	.	.	.	.	.	.	.	.
73	15	8,7	6	3,5	171	9	5,3	0	0,0	.	.	.	.	.	.	.	.	.	.	.	.	.	.	.	125	5	4,0	0	0,0	150	10	6,7	2	1,3	.	.	.	.	.
.	.	.	.	.	.	.	.	.	.	.	.	.	.	.	.	.	.	.	.	.	.	.	.	.	.	.	.	.	.	.	.	.	.	.	.	.	.	.	.
4	1	25,0	0	0,0	.	.	.	.	.	.	.	.	.	.	2	0	0,0	0	0,0	5	0	0,0	0	0,0	9	1	11,1	0	0,0	.	.	.	.	.	.	.	.	.	.
4	31	4,5	3	0,4	589	32	5,4	4	0,7	633	26	4,1	2	0,3	554	42	7,6	8	1,4	600	65	10,8	17	2,8	570	69	12,1	11	1,9	.	.	.	.	.	.	.	.	.	.
52	34	6,1	7	1,2	562	42	7,5	13	2,3	629	47	7,5	15	2,4	510	36	7,1	3	0,6	622	30	4,8	3	0,5	588	34	5,8	7	1,2	.	.	.	.	.	.	.	.	.	.
93	24	2,4	1	0,1	1132	13	1,1	0	0,0	933	4	0,4	2	0,2	951	16	1,7	1	0,1	1048	8	0,8	4	0,4	1035	15	1,4	4	0,4	.	.	.	.	.	.	.	.	.	.
30	14	1,8	1	0,1	713	18	2,5	2	0,3	747	14	1,9	4	0,5	732	30	4,1	4	0,5	669	11	1,6	3	0,4	586	17	2,9	3	0,5	.	.	.	.	.	.	.	.	.	.
6	27	4,4	7	1,1	663	27	4,1	8	1,2	488	27	5,5	9	1,8	610	28	4,6	1	0,2	480	26	5,4	4	0,8	562	43	7,7	7	1,2	.	.	.	.	.	.	.	.	.	.
2	47	12,0	1	0,3	356	45	12,6	0	0,0	273	36	13,2	1	0,4	283	22	7,8	0	0,0	267	20	7,5	0	0,0	307	17	5,5	5	1,6	.	.	.	.	.	.	.	.	.	.
0	117	28,5	50	12,2	375	125	33,3	53	14,1	373	110	29,5	63	16,9	361	112	31,0	51	14,1	358	105	29,3	51	14,2	316	91	28,8	42	13,3	.	.	.	.	.	.	.	.	.	.
4	17	4,5	1	0,3	348	23	6,6	3	0,9	325	18	5,5	3	0,9	271	11	4,1	2	0,7	200	12	6,0	0	0,0	198	8	4,0	2	1,0	.	.	.	.	.	.	.	.	.	.
7	88	9,3	8	0,8	1056	78	7,4	10	0,9	1255	105	8,4	11	0,9	1485	147	9,9	13	0,9	1431	115	8,0	14	1,0	1291	112	8,7	14	1,1	.	.	.	.	.	.	.	.	.	.
.	.	.	.	.	2354	198	8,4	43	1,8	3013	315	10,5	43	1,4	3041	323	10,6	35	1,2	3194	339	10,6	46	1,4	3094	339	11,0	57	1,8	.	.	.	.	.	.	.	.	.	.
8	0	0,0	0	0,0	11	1	9,1	0	0,0	6	0	0,0	0	0,0	4	1	25,0	1	25,0	7	2	28,6	0	0,0	7	0	0,0	0	0,0	.	.	.	.	.	.	.	.	.	.
6	4	2,9	1	0,7	67	3	4,5	0	0,0	186	9	4,8	0	0,0	191	8	4,2	1	0,5	197	15	7,6	2	1,0	200	6	3,0	1	0,5	.	.	.	.	.	.	.	.	.	.
3	79	31,2	36	14,2	294	69	23,5	17	5,8	305	57	18,7	6	2,0	296	56	18,9	16	5,4	250	55	22,0	11	4,4	211	46	21,8	12	5,7	.	.	.	.	.	.	.	.	.	.
8	78	11,3	8	1,2	746	108	14,5	7	0,9	196	41	20,9	12	6,1	390	65	16,7	11	2,8	510	72	14,1	6	1,2	485	47	9,7	8	1,6	.	.	.	.	.	.	.	.	.	.
7	284	31,7	83	9,3	911	287	31,5	99	10,9	953	285	29,9	91	9,5	965	267	27,7	80	8,3	895	280	31,3	114	12,7	873	313	35,9	94	10,8	.	.	.	.	.	.	.	.	.	.
1	194	27,7	61	8,7	972	237	24,4	75	7,7	925	253	27,4	84	9,1	955	254	26,6	86	9,0	1128	287	25,4	104	9,2	1293	313	24,2	127	9,8	.	.	.	.	.	.	.	.	.	.
)	3	7,7	0	0,0	28	2	7,1	0	0,0	31	3	9,7	0	0,0	53	7	13,2	1	1,9	31	2	6,5	1	3,2	36	4	11,1	0	0,0	.	.	.	.	.	.	.	.	.	.
9	0	0,0	0	0,0	9	0	0,0	0	0,0	13	1	7,7	0	0,0	2	0	0,0	0	0,0	7	0	0,0	0	0,0	11	2	18,2	0	0,0	.	.	.	.	.	.	.	.	.	.
8	82	10,7	7	0,9	484	34	7,0	2	0,4	636	33	5,2	2	0,3	518	57	11,0	6	1,2	636	48	7,5	1	0,2	709	59	8,3	5	0,7	.	.	.	.	.	.	.	.	.	.
0	39	24,4	3	1,9	182	31	17,0	2	1,1	181	30	16,6	7	3,9	219	35	16,0	0	0,0	223	37	16,6	4	1,8	193	43	22,3	3	1,6	.	.	.	.	.	.	.	.	.	.
.	.	.	.	.	3037	186	6,1	35	1,2	.	.	.	.	.	.	.	.	.	.	2716	152	5,6	8	0,3	.	.	.	.	.	.	.	.	.	.	.	.	.	.	.
.	.	.	.	.	.	.	.	.	.	350	153	43,7	43	12,3	.	.	.	.	.	.	.	.	.	.	.	.	.	.	.	.	.	.	.	.	.	.	.	.	.
.	.	.	.	.	.	.	.	.	.	379	80	21,1	10	2,6	330	53	16,1	11	3,3	328	86	26,2	19	5,8	311	82	26,4	23	7,4	317	87	27,4	28	8,8	.	.	.	.	.
1	198	35,3	48	8,6	532	196	36,8	57	10,7	533	199	37,3	73	13,7	527	176	33,4	59	11,2	565	227	40,2	95	16,8	515	182	35,3	77	15,0	.	.	.	.	.	.	.	.	.	.
9	14	5,6	1	0,4						320	21	6,6	4	1,3	292	19	6,5	3	1,0	264	19	7,2	1	0,4	.	.	.	.	.	.	.	.	.	.	.	.	.	.	.
	19	4,1	5	1,1	464	12	2,6	1	0,2	407	9	2,2	2	0,5	350	21	6,0	4	1,1	292	15	5,1	1	0,3	248	18	7,3	4	1,6	.	.	.	.	.	.	.	.	.	.
	7	2,5	0	0,0	281	15	5,3	3	1,1	262	9	3,4	1	0,4	226	9	4,0	1	0,4	202	5	2,5	0	0,0	217	10	4,6	0	0,0	.	.	.	.	.	.	.	.	.	.
	12	8,9	3	2,2	133	14	10,5	1	0,8	0	0	.	0	.	0	0	.	0	.	0	0	.	0	.	0	0	.	0	.	.	.	.	.	.	.	.	.	.	.
.	.	.	.	.	.	.	.	.	.	360	42	11,7	5	1,4	.	.	.	.	.	.	.	.	.	.	566	37	6,5	1	0,2	.	.	.	.	.	.	.	.	.	.
	36	11,2	4	1,2	338	35	10,4	2	0,6	319	36	11,3	4	1,3	322	34	10,6	6	1,9	347	31	8,9	5	1,4	425	52	12,2	2	0,5	.	.	.	.	.	.	.	.	.	.
	18	5,5	0	0,0	342	16	4,7	3	0,9	368	13	3,5	3	0,8	336	24	7,1	8	2,4	340	19	5,6	3	0,9	326	15	4,6	2	0,6	.	.	.	.	.	.	.	.	.	.
.	.	.	.	.	2752	200	7,3	23	0,8	3110	206	6,6	22	0,7	2919	216	7,4	28	1,0	3105	227	7,3	22	0,7	3428	245	7,1	23	0,7	.	.	.	.	.	.	.	.	.	.
.	.	.	.	.	755	83	11,0	10	1,3	.	.	.	.	.	.	.	.	.	.	.	.	.	.	.	.	.	.	.	.	.	.	.	.	.	766	113	14,8	22	2,9
.	.	.	.	.	1505	223	14,8	14	0,9	.	.	.	.	.	.	.	.	.	.	.	.	.	.	.	.	.	.	.	.	1150	180	15,7	19	1,7	.	.	.	.	.
.	.	.	.	.	.	.	.	.	.	.	.	.	.	.	.	.	.	.	.	.	.	.	.	.	.	.	.	.	.	.	.	.	.	.	.	.	.	.	.
.	.	.	.	.	1222	364	29,8	95	7,8	.	.	.	.	.	.	.	.	.	.	.	.	.	.	.	.	.	.	.	.	.	.	.	.	.	.	.	.	.	.
	400	11,5	37	1,1	3470	355	10,2	27	0,8	.	.	.	.	.	.	.	.	.	.	.	.	.	.	.	3271	362	11,1	28	0,9	.	.	.	.	.	.	.	.	.	.
.	.	.	.	.	.	.	.	.	.	.	.	.	.	.	.	.	.	.	.	.	.	.	.	.	.	.	.	.	.	.	.	.	.	.	.	.	.	.	.
.	.	.	.	.	.	.	.	.	.	2705	233	8,6	19	0,7	.	.	.	.	.	.	.	.	.	.	.	.	.	.	.	.	.	.	.	.	.	.	.	.	.
	0	.	0	.	0	0	.	0	.	0	0	.	0	.	0	0	.	0	.	.	.	.	.	.	0	0	.	0	.	.	.	.	.	.	.	.	.	.	.
	31	13,4	1	0,4	272	31	11,4	0	0,0	263	36	13,7	3	1,1	304	39	12,8	1	0,3	278	43	15,5	2	0,7	247	33	13,4	1	0,4	250	26	10,4	1	0,4	.	.	.	.	.
.	.	.	.	.	.	.	.	.	.	29	4	13,8	0	0,0	27	5	18,5	1	3,7	21	4	19,1	1	4,8	24	5	20,8	2	8,3	18	4	22,2	2	11,1	.	.	.	.	.
.	.	.	.	.	.	.	.	.	.	.	.	.	.	.	1348	165	12,2	32	2,4	2636	321	12,2	71	2,7	.	.	.	.	.	.	.	.	.	.	.	.	.	.	.
.	.	.	.	.	823	41	5,0	4	0,5	785	35	4,5	2	0,3	862	60	7,0	1	0,1	838	33	3,9	2	0,2	895	58	6,5	2	0,2	.	.	.	.	.	.	.	.	.	.
.	.	.	.	.	.	.	.	.	.	.	.	.	.	.	.	.	.	.	.	.	.	.	.	.	.	.	.	.	.	1619	497	30,7	44	2,7	1619	.	.	44	2,7

Annex 7: Trends in drug resistance among all TB cases 1994-2007

COUNTRY	METHOD	1994 Combined tot	any	%	mdr	%	1995 Combined tot	any	%	mdr	%	1996 Combined tot	any	%	mdr	%	1997 Combined tot	any	%	mdr	%	1998 Combined tot	any	%	mdr	%	1999 Combined tot	any	%	mdr	%
AFRICA																															
Botswana	Survey											521	32	6,1	8	1,5											783	73	9,3	16	2,0
Sierra Leone	Survey											635	221	34,8	27	4,3	130	37	28,5	4	3,1										
South Africa, Mpumalanga Province	Survey																761	75	9,9	18	2,4										
AMERICAS																															
Argentina	Survey																										828	103	12,4	26	3,
Canada	Surveillance	1.520	170	11,2	13	0,9	1.419	0	0,0	13	0,9	1.368	0	0,0	16	1,2	1.540	0	0,0	16	1,0	1.359	0	0,0	10	0,7	1.410	0	0,0	10	0,
Chile	Survey																881	94	10,7	10	1,1										
Cuba	Surveillance						349	40	11,5	3	0,9	437	44	10,1	5	1,1	266	30	11,3	6	2,3	327	27	8,3	3	0,9	369	36	9,8	5	1,
Nicaragua	Survey																					564	88	15,6	7	1,2					
Puerto Rico	Surveillance	132	18	13,6	3	2,3	158	19	12,0	8	5,1	166	18	10,8	3	1,8	193	26	13,5	5	2,6	165	15	9,1	3	1,8	175	13	7,4	1	0,
Uruguay	Survey																500	23	4,6	1	0,2						315	10	3,2	1	0,
USA	Surveillance	17.622	2.200	12,5	431	2,4	17.092	2.073	12,1	327	1,9	16.326	2.046	12,5	249	1,5	15.266	1.776	11,6	201	1,3	14.273	1.629	11,4	155	1,1	13.476	1.495	11,1	157	1,
EASTERN MEDITERRANEAN																															
Oman	Surveillance																										133	6	4,5	1	0,
Qatar	Surveillance																														
EUROPE																															
Andorra	Surveillance																										6	0	0,0	0	0,
Austria	Surveillance																										756	43	5,7	5	0,
Belgium	Surveillance																791	87	11,0	16	2,0										
Bosnia & Herzegovina	Surveillance																										1.275	38	3,0	6	0,
Croatia	Surveillance																										854	24	2,8	4	0,
Czech Republic	Surveillance						215	6	2,8	3	1,4																698	23	3,3	4	0,
Denmark	Surveillance																					444	58	13,1	3	0,7	416	64	15,4	0	0,
Estonia	Surveillance																					459	188	41,0	84	18,3	517	192	37,1	118	22,
Finland	Surveillance																412	20	4,9	0	0,0						398	9	2,3	0	0,
France	Surveillance											1.686	165	9,8	16	0,9	852	86	10,1	2	0,2						1.016	101	9,9	15	1,
Germany	Surveillance																														
Iceland	Surveillance																										8	0	0,0	0	0,
Ireland	Surveillance																										123	2	1,6	1	0,
Israel	Surveillance																					307	59	19,2	25	8,1	331	55	16,6	26	7
Italy	Surveillance																										810	162	20,0	51	6,
Latvia	Surveillance																					1.013	305	30,1	124	12,2	1.015	318	31,3	137	13,
Lithuania	Surveillance																										986	333	33,8	135	13,
Luxembourg	Surveillance																														
Malta	Surveillance																										13	0	0,0	0	0,
Netherlands	Surveillance						1.104	156	14,1	12	1,1	1.214	123	10,1	7	0,6											941	83	8,8	4	0,
Norway	Surveillance											144	16	11,1	4	2,8											184	24	13,0	3	1,
Poland	Surveillance																3.970	275	6,9	88	2,2										
Russian Federation, Ivanovo Oblast	Surveillance											281	103	36,7	19	6,8						276	109	39,5	34	12,3					
Russian Federation, Orel Oblast	Surveillance																														
Russian Federation, Tomsk Oblast	Surveillance																										649	255	39,3	89	13,
Serbia & Montenegro	Surveillance																										331	18	5,4	2	0,
Slovakia	Surveillance																					746	41	5,5	15	2,0	578	21	3,6	6	1,
Slovenia	Surveillance																326	10	3,1	3	0,9						339	11	3,2	2	0,
Spain, Barcelona	Surveillance											262	34	13,0	10	3,8						384	27	7,0	9	2,3	172	23	13,4	9	5
Spain, Galicia	Surveillance																														
Sweden	Surveillance																380	32	8,4	4	1,1						408	52	12,7	7	1,
Switzerland	Surveillance																362	21	5,8	5	1,4						485	38	7,8	9	1,
United Kingdom	Surveillance																														
SOUTH-EASTERN ASIA																															
Nepal	Survey											787	77	9,8	9	1,1											785	122	15,5	39	5
Thailand	Survey																1.137	290	25,5	24	2,1										
WESTERN PACIFIC																															
Australia	Surveillance						705	67	9,5	5	0,7	750	79	10,5	15	2,0						699	91	13,0	6	0,9	760	81	10,7	4	0
China, Henan Province	Survey											1.372	705	51,4	320	23,3															
China, Hong Kong SAR	Surveillance											5.207	752	14,4	137	2,6	3.746	491	13,1	63	1,7	4.019	518	12,9	79	2,0	3.680	500	13,6	52	
Guam	Survey						52	2	3,8	2	3,8	49	1	2,0	1	2,0	51	3	5,9	3	5,9	63	1	1,6	1	1,6	45	1	2,2	0	
Japan	Surveillance																1.638	253	15,4	64	3,9										
New Caledonia	Survey											105	3	2,9	0	0,0											8	3	37,5	0	
New Zealand	Surveillance						150	8	5,3	2	1,3	151	7	4,6	0	0,0	137	19	13,9	1	0,7	166	23	13,9	3	1,8	251	23	9,2	2	
Northern Mariana Is	Surveillance																														
Rep. Korea	Survey	2.675	358	13,4	91	3,4																					2.653	313	11,8	72	
Singapore	Surveillance											1.131	67	5,9	9	0,8															
Viet Nam	Survey																640	208	32,5	15	2,3										

	2000 Combined				2001 Combined				2002 Combined				2003 Combined				2004 Combined				2005 Combined				2006 Combined				2007 Combined			
tot	any	%	mdr	%	tot	any	%	mdr	%	tot	any	%	mdr	%	tot	any	%	mdr	%	tot	any	%	mdr	%	tot	any	%	mdr	%	tot	any	%	mdr	%	tot	any	%	mdr	%
										1.288	147	11,4	21	1,6																				
										877	107	12,2	42	4,8																				
																									819	102	12,5	36	4,4					
299	0	0,0	10	0,8	1.413	0	0,0	16	1,1	1.301	0	0,0	19	1,5	1.268	0	0,0	13	1,0	1.265	0	0,0	8	0,6	1.203	146	12,1	23	1,9	1.241	109	8,8	12	1,0
					1.158	149	12,9	17	1,5																									
15	25	6,0	2	0,5						231	23	10,0	2	0,9	241	34	14,1	5	2,1	205	36	17,6	4	2,0	198	21	10,6	1	0,5					
																														423	79	18,7	10	2,4
42	12	8,5	1	0,7	102	12	11,8	2	2,0	108	14	13,0	1	0,9	104	7	6,7	1	1,0	110	11	10,0	0	0,0	94	3	3,2	0	0,0					
																									368	10	2,7	2	0,5					
549	1.518	12,1	145	1,2	12.263	1.446	11,8	150	1,2	11.475	1.386	12,1	151	1,3	11.275	1.326	11,8	115	1,0	11.091	1.315	11,9	129	1,2	10.584	1.255	11,9	124	1,2					
80	22	12,2	13	7,2	183	16	8,7	7	3,8																136	11	8,1	5	3,7	164	16	9,8	7	4,3
79	34	12,2	2	0,7	284	28	9,9	1	0,4																223	34	15,2	5	2,2	278	28	10,1	3	1,1
5	2	40,0	0	0,0											2	0	0,0	0	0,0	5	0	0,0	0	0,0	9	1	11,1	0	0,0					
61	37	4,9	4	0,5	630	38	6,0	5	0,8	678	29	4,3	3	0,4	596	53	8,9	12	2,0	634	68	10,7	19	3,0	609	72	11,8	13	2,1					
30	52	7,1	11	1,5	749	63	8,4	18	2,4	806	66	8,2	21	2,6	796	63	7,9	9	1,1	857	51	6,0	12	1,4	758	48	6,3	11	1,5					
53	46	4,0	5	0,4	1.296	18	1,4	2	0,2	1.033	6	0,6	4	0,4	1.042	41	3,9	2	0,2	1.125	23	2,0	10	0,9	1.141	41	3,6	11	1,0					
79	20	2,3	2	0,2	808	25	3,1	5	0,6	844	22	2,6	6	0,7	837	42	5,0	8	1,0	757	13	1,7	3	0,4	647	22	3,4	6	0,9					
38	30	4,7	9	1,4	678	28	4,1	9	1,3	504	29	5,8	10	2,0	629	30	4,8	2	0,3	490	28	5,7	6	1,2	582	51	8,8	13	2,2					
25	56	13,2	2	0,5	380	49	12,9	0	0,0	297	39	13,1	1	0,3	299	22	7,4	0	0,0	289	21	7,3	0	0,0	325	21	6,5	5	1,5					
27	185	35,1	103	19,5	580	260	44,8	158	27,2	532	209	39,3	138	25,9	464	180	38,8	106	22,8	452	158	35,0	90	19,9	387	136	35,1	79	20,4					
47	22	5,0	2	0,5	410	27	6,6	4	1,0	384	19	4,9	3	0,8	340	15	4,4	3	0,9	286	14	4,9	0	0,0	315	14	4,4	3	1,0					
91	130	10,9	15	1,3	1.313	109	8,3	15	1,1	1.511	142	9,4	23	1,5	1.727	186	10,8	25	1,4	1.699	151	8,9	26	1,5	1.501	143	9,5	24	1,6					
					3.881	412	10,6	105	2,7	4.693	524	11,2	95	2,0	4.459	515	11,5	93	2,1	4.057	503	12,4	101	2,5	3.886	478	12,3	105	2,7					
9	0	0,0	0	0,0	12	1	8,3	0	0,0	6	0	0,0	0	0,0	4	1	25,0	1	25,0	8	2	25,0	0	0,0	8	0	0,0	0	0,0					
16	7	3,2	3	1,4	104	5	4,8	1	1,0	237	10	4,2	0	0,0	253	13	5,1	1	0,4	263	21	8,0	2	0,8	273	13	4,8	3	1,1					
31	90	32,0	41	14,6	317	82	25,9	22	6,9	344	75	21,8	17	4,9	316	65	20,6	20	6,3	265	56	21,1	12	4,5	217	46	21,2	12	5,5					
06	132	16,4	35	4,3	910	160	17,6	38	4,2	509	112	22,0	33	6,5	788	129	16,4	42	5,3	763	128	16,8	24	3,1	585	81	13,8	22	3,8					
14	378	33,0	150	13,1	1.098	347	31,6	150	13,7	1.241	473	38,1	226	18,2	1.191	410	34,4	174	14,6	1.101	389	35,3	195	17,7	1.055	409	38,8	160	15,2					
21	330	35,8	156	16,9	1.452	508	35,0	266	18,3	1.343	517	38,5	297	22,1	1.398	551	39,4	312	22,3	1.592	571	35,9	318	20,0	1.739	580	33,4	338	19,4					
14	3	6,8	0	0,0	29	2	6,9	0	0,0	32	3	9,4	0	0,0	54	7	13,0	1	1,9	31	2	6,5	1	3,2	37	4	10,8	0	0,0					
	0		0	0,0	19	0	0,0	0	0,0	13	1	7,7	0	0,0	7	0	0,0	0	0,0						11	2	18,2	0	0,0					
53	90	10,4	8	0,9	503	34	6,8	2	0,4	768	48	6,3	2	0,3	619	66	10,7	8	1,3	759	59	7,8	3	0,4	841	74	8,8	7	0,8					
70	40	23,5	3	1,8	214	37	17,3	5	2,3	192	32	16,7	7	3,6	272	46	16,9	3	1,1	246	39	15,9	4	1,6	214	44	20,6	3	1,4					
					3.705	297	8,0	92	2,5											3.239	246	7,6	51	1,6										
										505	280	55,4	133	26,3																				
										589	234	39,7	99	16,8	371	70	18,9	18	4,9	379	111	29,3	32	8,4	347	101	29,1	32	9,2	347	101	29,1	33	9,5
2	273	40,0	87	12,8	671	290	43,2	116	17,3	650	270	41,5	124	19,1	660	262	39,7	119	18,0	677	306	45,2	148	21,9	707	332	47,0	201	28,4					
79	19	6,8	1	0,4						357	23	6,4	5	1,4	334	23	6,9	3	0,9	297	20	6,7	2	0,7										
5	34	5,9	7	1,2	575	22	3,8	6	1,0	497	18	3,6	3	0,6	406	28	6,9	6	1,5	344	18	5,2	1	0,3	311	29	9,3	8	2,6					
0	11	3,4	0	0,0	307	18	5,9	3	1,0	292	16	5,5	2	0,7	257	11	4,3	1	0,4	230	7	3,0	0	0,0	245	14	5,7	1	0,4					
2	18	11,1	6	3,7	165	24	14,5	5	3,0	527	65	12,3	23	4,4	495	55	11,1	6	1,2	528	48	9,1	10	1,9	538	53	9,9	4	0,7					
										400	51	12,8	8	2,0											634	46	7,3	2	0,3					
5	39	10,7	5	1,4	359	40	11,1	4	1,1	353	44	12,5	4	1,1	347	38	11,0	7	2,0	369	36	9,8	6	1,6	442	56	12,7	4	0,9					
7	21	5,4	1	0,3	502	25	5,0	7	1,4	515	31	6,0	11	2,1	481	39	8,1	12	2,5	473	31	6,6	5	1,1	457	24	5,3	5	1,1					
					3.612	266	7,4	31	0,9	4.176	302	7,2	37	0,9	4.050	304	7,5	49	1,2	4.367	323	7,4	44	1,0	4.800	341	7,1	39	0,8					
					926	153	16,5	45	4,9																						930	154	16,6	41	
					1.677	290	17,3	49	2,9																						1.344	278	20,7	86	6,4
6	79	10,3	8	1,0	770	76	9,9	12	1,6	712	62	8,7	12	1,7	784	89	11,4	7	0,9	787	68	8,6	12	1,5	808	82	10,1	12	1,5					
					1.487	525	35,3	192	12,9																										
6	449	12,2	56	1,5	3.639	394	10,8	46	1,3																4.350	477	11,0	41	0,9					
3	1	2,3	1	2,3	47	3	6,4	3	6,4	47	2	4,3	2	4,3																				
										3.122	338	10,8	60	1,9																				
	1	1,6	0	0,0	6	1	16,7	0	0,0	10	0	0,0	0	0,0	1	0	0,0	0	0,0						5	1	20,0	0	0,0					
3	36	14,5	1	0,4	294	33	11,2	0	0,0	272	36	13,2	3	1,1	322	45	14,0	2	0,6	289	46	15,9	3	1,0	261	37	14,2	4	1,5	266	27	10,2	1	0,4
										0	0		0		0	0		0		0	0		0		0	0		0						
															1.970	340	17,3	113	5,7	2.914	398	13,7	110	3,8										
					949	56	5,9	5	0,5	920	57	6,2	4	0,4	984	74	7,5	5	0,5	955	50	5,2	2	0,2	1.000	69	6,9	3	0,3					
																														1.826	619	33,9	84	4,6

133

ANTI-TB DRUG RESISTANCE IN THE WORLD   ANNEXES

Annex 8: Estimates of MDR-TB among new cases

Country	No. of New TB cases	No. of MDR cases	Low 95% CL	High 95% CL	% MDR TB	Low 95% CL	High 95% CL
Afghanistan	42.078	1.415	201	7.885	3,4	0,5	18,3
Albania	598	9	1	60	1,5	0,3	10,0
Algeria	18.699	217	60	437	1,2	0,4	2,5
Andorra	14	0	0	4	0,0	0,0	28,3
Angola	47.231	930	149	5.962	2,0	0,3	12,1
Antigua & Barbuda	5	0	0	0	1,3	0,2	8,2
Argentina	15.231	335	154	563	2,2	1,2	3,0
Armenia	2.236	211	125	310	9,4	7,1	12,2
Austria	1.046	20	8	36	1,9	1,0	3,
Azerbaijan	6.660	1.487	926	2.090	22,3	18,9	26,
Bahamas	126	1	0	10	1,2	0,2	7,
Bahrain	304	7	1	41	2,2	0,3	12,9
Bangladesh	350.641	12.562	1.829	70.022	3,6	0,6	19,
Belarus	5.989	695	115	2.906	11,6	2,0	46,
Belgium	1.389	17	5	32	1,2	0,5	2,
Belize	137	2	0	13	1,5	0,2	9,
Benin	7.878	24	0	83	0,3	0,0	1,
Bhutan	621	20	3	108	3,2	0,5	17,
Bolivia	18.562	224	61	455	1,2	0,4	2,
Bosnia & Herzegovina	2.005	8	2	17	0,4	0,1	1,
Botswana	10.230	87	33	159	0,8	0,4	1,
Brazil	93.933	852	414	1.401	0,9	0,5	1,
Brunei Darussalam	317	7	1	44	2,3	0,4	13,
Bulgaria	3.101	332	53	1.454	10,7	1,8	44,
Burkina Faso	35.678	732	117	4.593	2,1	0,3	12,
Burundi	30.052	722	114	4.479	2,4	0,4	14,
Cambodia	70.949	0	0	332	0,0	0,0	0,
Cameroon	34.905	601	93	3.863	1,7	0,3	10,
Canada	1.678	14	5	27	0,8	0,4	1,
Cape Verde	873	14	2	92	1,6	0,3	10,
Central African Republic	14.744	159	32	338	1,1	0,4	2
Chad	31.329	641	95	4.251	2,0	0,3	13,
Chile	2.417	17	5	34	0,7	0,3	1,
China	1.311.184	65.853	41.883	90.663	5,0	4,6	5,
China, Hong Kong SAR	4.433	38	21	59	0,9	0,6	1,
China, Macao SAR	283	6	2	13	2,3	0,8	4,
Colombia	20.514	302	144	509	1,5	0,8	2,
Comoros	358	7	1	44	1,8	0,3	11,
Congo	14.901	256	40	1.657	1,7	0,3	11
Costa Rica	620	9	2	21	1,5	0,4	3
Côte d'Ivoire	79.686	1.992	709	3.775	2,5	1,1	4
Croatia	1.832	9	0	23	0,5	0,1	1,
Cuba	1.018	0	0	18	0,0	0,0	1
Cyprus	42	0	0	3	1,1	0,2	7
Czech Republic	1.007	13	4	24	1,2	0,5	2
Denmark	444	7	2	15	1,6	0,5	3
Djibouti	6.622	220	32	1.185	3,3	0,5	17
Dominica	11	0	0	1	1,5	0,2	9
Dominican Republic	8.534	563	290	913	6,6	4,1	10
DPR Korea	42.147	1.538	233	8.450	3,7	0,6	19
DR Congo	237.985	5.657	878	34.850	2,4	0,4	14
Ecuador	16.958	835	477	1.266	4,9	3,5	6
Egypt	17.821	395	177	682	2,2	1,2	3
El Salvador	3.385	11	0	30	0,3	0,0	1
Eritrea	4.402	99	16	628	2,3	0,4	14
Estonia	519	69	40	104	13,3	9,7	17
Ethiopia	306.990	4.964	2.135	8.697	1,6	0,9	2
Finland	287	3	0	8	1,0	0,1	3
France	8.630	94	43	162	1,1	0,6	1
French Polynesia	68	1	0	9	2,1	0,3	12
Gabon	4.635	63	10	421	1,4	0,2	9
Gambia	4.278	20	0	72	0,5	0,0	2

Country	No. of New TB cases	No. of MDR cases	Low 95% CL	High 95% CL	% MDR TB	Low 95% CL	High 95% CL
Georgia	3.834	259	153	383	6,8	5,1	8,7
Germany	5.370	99	58	146	1,8	1,4	2,4
Ghana	46.693	898	143	5.534	1,9	0,3	12,0
Greece	2.009	22	3	149	1,1	0,2	7,4
Guatemala	10.277	308	155	503	3,0	1,8	4,6
Guinea	24.321	135	0	328	0,6	0,1	1,6
Guinea-Bissau	3.602	81	13	528	2,3	0,4	14,0
Guyana	1.215	21	3	140	1,7	0,3	11,2
Haiti	28.289	537	86	3.520	1,9	0,3	12,0
Honduras	5.322	93	33	176	1,8	0,8	3,4
Hungary	1.904	25	4	169	1,3	0,2	8,7
Iceland	13	0	0	4	0,0	0,0	34,8
India	1.932.852	54.806	33.723	78.291	2,8	2,3	3,4
Indonesia	534.439	10.583	0	28.811	2,0	0,2	7,0
Iran	15.678	777	428	1.204	5,0	3,4	6,9
Iraq	15.968	478	68	2.729	3,0	0,5	16,6
Ireland	555	3	0	10	0,5	0,0	2,8
Israel	521	30	13	52	5,7	3,0	9,7
Italy	4.393	72	25	137	1,6	0,7	3,2
Jamaica	197	3	0	19	1,4	0,2	9,1
Japan	28.330	199	99	328	0,7	0,4	1,1
Jordan	306	17	5	33	5,4	2,0	11,4
Kazakhstan	19.961	2.836	1.681	4.158	14,2	10,8	18,3
Kenya	132.578	0	0	890	0,0	0,0	0,7
Kiribati	348	11	2	61	3,2	0,5	17,6
Kuwait	667	13	2	79	1,9	0,3	11,5
Kyrgyzstan	6.454	949	154	3.580	14,7	2,6	53,4
Lao PDR	8.779	322	46	1.791	3,7	0,6	19,9
Latvia	1.312	141	87	201	10,8	8,8	13,0
Lebanon	452	5	0	13	1,1	0,1	3,8
Lesotho	12.670	115	0	278	0,9	0,2	2,6
Libyan Arab Jamahiriya	1.062	28	4	159	2,6	0,4	14,4
Lithuania	2.102	206	128	292	9,8	8,3	11,6
Luxembourg	57	0	0	5	0,0	0,0	8,0
Madagascar	47.469	234	45	517	0,5	0,1	1,3
Malawi	51.172	1.203	195	7.455	2,4	0,4	14,7
Malaysia	26.877	27	0	96	0,1	0,0	0,6
Maldives	136	4	1	21	2,9	0,4	15,6
Mali	33.460	680	108	4.413	2,0	0,3	12,7
Malta	25	0	0	6	0,0	0,0	25,9
Marshall Islands	127	4	1	21	2,9	0,4	16,1
Mauritius	284	4	1	25	1,3	0,2	8,7
Mexico	22.473	538	187	1.018	2,4	1,0	4,7
Micronesia	112	3	0	19	3,0	0,4	16,4
Mongolia	4.893	48	9	107	1,0	0,3	2,5
Morocco	28.776	137	28	288	0,5	0,2	1,1
Mozambique	92.971	3.256	1.829	5.018	3,5	2,5	4,8
Myanmar	82.687	3.271	1.797	5.065	4,0	2,7	5,6
Namibia	15.723	241	38	1.536	1,5	0,3	9,8
Nepal	48.772	1.401	736	2.239	2,9	1,8	4,3
Netherlands	1.249	9	2	18	0,7	0,2	1,6
New Zealand	352	1	0	5	0,4	0,0	2,2
Nicaragua	3.203	20	0	54	0,6	0,1	2,2
Niger	23.845	519	82	3.207	2,2	0,4	13,1
Nigeria	450.527	8.559	1.319	55.698	1,9	0,3	11,9
Norway	263	4	0	10	1,6	0,3	4,5
Oman	336	4	0	12	1,3	0,2	4,7
Pakistan	291.743	9.880	1.454	53.653	3,4	0,5	18,4
Palau	10	0	0	1	2,4	0,4	13,9
Panama	1.463	21	3	135	1,4	0,2	9,3
Papua New Guinea	15.473	563	82	3.142	3,6	0,6	20,0
Paraguay	4.267	91	19	193	2,1	0,7	4,9

Annex 8

Country	No. of New TB cases	No. of MDR cases	Low 95% CL	High 95% CL	% MDR TB	Low 95% CL	High 95% CL
Peru	44.815	2.353	1.446	3.375	5,3	4,3	6,
Philippines	247.740	10.012	5.676	15.135	4,0	2,9	5,
Poland	9.462	28	9	54	0,3	0,1	0,
Portugal	3.382	29	12	50	0,9	0,4	1,
Rep. Korea	42.359	1.141	686	1.655	2,7	2,1	3,
Republic of Moldova	5.551	1.077	684	1.504	19,4	16,7	22,
Romania	27.533	778	416	1.242	2,8	1,8	4,
Russian Federation	152.797	19.845	12.376	27.566	13,0	11,3	14,
Rwanda	37.644	1.467	768	2.324	3,9	2,5	5,
Saint Lucia	28	0	0	3	1,5	0,2	9,
Samoa	36	1	0	6	3,0	0,5	16,
Saudi Arabia	10.631	232	33	1.362	2,2	0,3	12,
Senegal	32.638	689	141	1.452	2,1	0,7	4,
Serbia	3.183	11	2	26	0,4	0,1	0,
Seychelles	28	0	0	3	1,3	0,2	8,
Sierra Leone	29.690	254	0	886	0,9	0,0	4,
Singapore	1.128	3	0	7	0,2	0,0	0,
Slovakia	829	13	3	30	1,6	0,4	4,
Slovenia	261	0	0	4	0,0	0,0	1,
Somalia	18.444	328	52	2.118	1,8	0,3	11,
South Africa	453.929	8.238	4.952	11.848	1,8	1,4	2,
Spain	13.180	17	0	62	0,1	0,0	0,
Sri Lanka	11.620	21	0	75	0,2	0,0	1,
St Vincent & Grenadines	35	1	0	4	1,7	0,3	10,
Sudan	91.331	1.696	265	10.681	1,9	0,3	11,
Swaziland	13.097	118	0	281	0,9	0,2	2,
Sweden	549	3	0	7	0,5	0,1	1,
Switzerland	500	3	0	8	0,6	0,1	2,
Syrian Arab Republic	6.251	192	27	1.050	3,1	0,5	16,
Tajikistan	13.532	2.164	359	7.855	16,0	2,8	55,
TFYR Macedonia	596	9	1	61	1,6	0,3	9,
Thailand	90.252	1.491	752	2.423	1,7	1,0	2
Timor-Leste	6.187	211	31	1.186	3,4	0,5	18
Togo	24.922	506	79	3.295	2,0	0,3	12
Tonga	24	1	0	4	3,1	0,5	17
Tunisia	2.520	68	10	382	2,7	0,4	15
Turkey	21.752	303	48	2.026	1,4	0,2	9,
Turkmenistan	3.175	121	24	269	3,8	1,1	9
Uganda	106.037	567	0	1.547	0,5	0,1	1
Ukraine	49.308	7.866	4.948	11.029	16,0	13,7	18
United Arab Emirates	681	16	2	91	2,3	0,4	12
United Kingdom	9.358	63	33	101	0,7	0,4	1
UR Tanzania	123.140	1.335	256	2.997	1,1	0,3	2
Uruguay	910	0	0	8	0,0	0,0	0
Uzbekistan	32.778	4.844	2.707	7.477	14,8	10,2	20
Venezuela	11.271	59	11	130	0,5	0,1	1
Viet Nam	148.918	4.047	2.341	6.056	2,7	2,0	3
West Bank and Gaza Strip	790	25	4	137	3,1	0,5	17
Yemen	16.985	500	234	850	2,9	1,7	4
Zambia	64.632	1.162	388	2.199	1,8	0,8	3
Zimbabwe	85.015	1.635	722	2.828	1,9	1,0	3

Annex 9: Estimates of MDR-TB among previously treated cases

Country	No. of previously treated TB cases	No. of MDR cases	Low 95% CL	High 95% CL	% MDR TB	Low 95% CL	High 95% CL
Afghanistan	1.957	724	159	1.619	37,0	8,7	76,2
Albania	45	5	1	18	10,3	2,0	39,5
Algeria	617	60	11	242	9,8	1,9	37,7
Andorra	1	0	0	1	10,4	2,1	40,5
Angola	5.463	735	142	2.643	13,5	2,6	46,5
Antigua & Barbuda	0	0	0	0	10,6	2,1	40,7
Argentina	829	128	67	206	15,4	9,8	22,6
Armenia	394	170	109	235	43,2	37,9	48,7
Austria	22	3	0	7	12,5	1,6	38,3
Azerbaijan	1.631	910	588	1.245	55,8	51,5	60,0
Bahamas	13	1	0	5	9,4	1,9	37,6
Bahrain	12	4	1	10	36,5	8,8	75,0
Bangladesh	10.492	2.022	407	6.266	19,3	4,2	57,8
Belarus	997	401	95	847	40,2	10,2	78,4
Belgium	112	8	0	19	7,3	1,5	19,9
Belize	16	2	0	6	9,8	2,0	39,0
Benin	719	66	12	269	9,2	1,8	37,2
Bhutan	41	8	2	25	19,9	4,3	58,6
Bolivia	1.514	71	15	147	4,7	1,5	10,6
Bosnia & Herzegovina	134	9	3	17	6,6	2,7	13,1
Botswana	428	44	18	79	10,4	5,3	17,8
Brazil	11.287	612	355	921	5,4	4,0	7,2
Brunei Darussalam	20	4	1	12	19,5	4,3	57,4
Bulgaria	316	119	28	262	37,8	9,2	76,6
Burkina Faso	4.566	439	80	1.852	9,6	1,8	38,4
Burundi	1.042	94	17	384	9,0	1,8	36,2
Cambodia	2.956	92	0	221	3,1	0,6	8,9
Cameroon	2.182	185	32	757	8,5	1,6	34,6
Canada	150	11	3	22	7,5	2,8	15,6
Cape Verde	83	8	2	33	10,2	2,0	39,0
Central African Republic	1.409	256	79	487	18,2	7,0	35,5
Chad	1.731	167	31	676	9,6	1,9	38,5
Chile	182	7	3	12	3,8	1,9	6,7
China	252.863	64.694	41.304	88.232	25,6	23,7	27,5
China, Hong Kong SAR	540	43	19	75	8,0	4,3	13,3
China, Macao SAR	27	4	0	10	15,8	3,4	39,6
Colombia	825	80	15	334	9,7	1,9	38,9
Comoros	23	2	0	9	10,1	1,9	39,2
Congo	733	64	12	268	8,8	1,7	36,1
Costa Rica	53	3	0	9	4,8	0,1	23,8
Côte d'Ivoire	4.761	411	76	1.722	8,6	1,7	35,2
Croatia	189	9	0	22	4,9	1,0	13,7
Cuba	70	4	0	13	5,3	0,1	26,0
Cyprus	1	0	0	0	9,6	1,9	37,7
Czech Republic	34	10	3	19	30,0	11,9	54,3
Denmark	46	0	0	7	0,0	0,0	15,3
Djibouti	648	229	51	526	35,4	8,8	74,5
Dominica	1	0	0	0	10,6	2,1	40,3
Dominican Republic	1.204	237	126	372	19,7	12,9	28,0
DPR Korea	8.634	1.933	391	5.611	22,4	4,8	61,4
DR Congo	15.195	1.387	268	5.594	9,1	1,9	36,1
Ecuador	2.661	647	380	955	24,3	18,3	31,2
Egypt	1.483	567	358	800	38,2	31,8	45,1
El Salvador	298	21	6	41	7,0	2,9	13,9
Eritrea	284	27	5	113	9,7	1,9	38,1
Estonia	114	59	36	86	52,1	39,9	64,1
Ethiopia	7.271	861	342	1.576	11,8	5,6	21,3
Finland	19	1	0	3	4,5	0,1	22,8
France	625	45	16	83	7,1	3,1	13,6
French Polynesia	8	2	0	5	18,8	3,9	57,5

Annex 9

Country	No. of previously treated TB cases	No. of MDR cases	Low 95% CL	High 95% CL	% MDR TB	Low 95% CL	High 95% CL
Gabon	426	35	6	147	8,2	1,5	33,2
Gambia	248	0	0	45	0,0	0,0	18,1
Georgia	1.435	393	247	551	27,4	23,6	31,4
Germany	456	56	32	87	12,4	8,5	17,1
Ghana	2.094	192	34	770	9,2	1,7	36,3
Greece	218	22	4	91	10,3	2,1	40,1
Guatemala	471	125	74	185	26,5	19,7	34,1
Guinea	1.648	464	193	806	28,1	13,7	46,7
Guinea-Bissau	282	27	5	112	9,7	2,0	38,3
Guyana	110	10	2	44	9,4	1,9	38,1
Haiti	638	57	10	237	9,0	1,7	36,0
Honduras	304	37	15	69	12,3	5,8	22,1
Hungary	386	45	8	172	11,6	2,3	42,5
Iceland	1	0	0	1	0,0	0,0	95,0
India	321.200	55.326	34.714	77.769	17,2	15,0	19,2
Indonesia	8.264	1.559	315	4.898	18,9	4,2	56,6
Iran	833	402	236	593	48,2	34,7	62,0
Iraq	1.295	492	112	1.074	38,0	9,5	77,0
Ireland	28	3	0	10	10,0	0,3	44,5
Israel	4	0	0	3	0,0	0,0	63,2
Italy	256	45	21	76	17,7	10,0	27,5
Jamaica	11	1	0	4	8,1	1,6	34,1
Japan	1.253	123	70	186	9,8	7,1	13,
Jordan	8	3	2	5	40,0	22,7	59,
Kazakhstan	6.686	3.773	2.388	5.225	56,4	50,8	61,
Kenya	13.012	0	0	820	0,0	0,0	6,
Kiribati	5	1	0	3	18,9	4,0	56,
Kuwait	9	3	1	7	36,5	8,8	75,
Kyrgyzstan	1.048	419	99	872	40,0	9,9	78,
Lao PDR	393	76	16	241	19,4	4,0	58,
Latvia	211	77	47	108	36,3	29,3	43,
Lebanon	10	6	3	10	62,5	35,4	84,
Lesotho	1.859	105	0	246	5,7	1,2	15,
Libyan Arab Jamahiriya	14	5	1	12	38,7	9,7	77,
Lithuania	461	219	139	301	47,5	42,8	52,
Luxembourg	3	0	0	1	9,8	2,0	39,
Madagascar	3.921	154	0	421	3,9	0,5	13,
Malawi	2.829	160	28	786	5,6	1,1	25,
Malaysia	1.707	0	0	291	0,0	0,0	17,
Maldives	7	1	0	4	19,3	4,1	57,
Mali	768	76	14	301	9,9	2,0	38,
Malta	1	0	0	1	9,8	1,9	38
Marshall Islands	8	2	0	5	21,3	4,7	60
Mauritius	10	1	0	4	9,5	1,9	37
Mexico	4.640	1.041	571	1.612	22,4	14,9	31
Micronesia	13	3	1	8	21,0	4,6	60
Mongolia	332	68	13	204	20,5	4,3	59
Morocco	1.101	134	70	214	12,2	7,8	17
Mozambique	4.975	163	31	356	3,3	0,9	8
Myanmar	6.312	979	499	1.573	15,5	9,5	23
Namibia	1.432	101	18	457	7,1	1,3	30
Nepal	4.439	521	260	848	11,7	7,2	17
Netherlands	46	2	0	5	3,3	0,1	17
New Zealand	21	0	0	4	0,0	0,0	17
Nicaragua	403	31	11	58	7,8	3,4	14
Niger	2.260	231	43	914	10,2	2,1	38
Nigeria	28.209	2.612	456	11.193	9,3	1,7	36
Norway	16	0	0	5	0,0	0,0	31
Oman	5	2	1	3	35,7	12,8	64

Country	No. of previously treated TB cases	No. of MDR cases	Low 95% CL	High 95% CL	% MDR TB	Low 95% CL	High 95% CL
Pakistan	14.675	5.353	1.136	11.803	36,5	8,7	75,3
Palau	2	0	0	1	20,3	4,5	59,8
Panama	252	26	5	102	10,2	2,0	39,6
Papua New Guinea	1.804	352	66	1.082	19,5	4,1	58,6
Paraguay	452	18	0	48	3,9	0,5	13,5
Peru	6.855	1.619	996	2.321	23,6	19,3	28,3
Philippines	8.771	1.836	1.007	2.810	20,9	14,3	29,0
Poland	1.198	99	56	148	8,2	6,0	10,9
Portugal	380	35	17	59	9,3	5,4	14,7
Rep. Korea	7.471	1.048	605	1.559	14,0	10,2	18,7
Republic of Moldova	1.886	959	611	1.298	50,8	48,6	53,0
Romania	6.985	768	440	1.158	11,0	8,0	14,6
Russian Federation	33.283	16.192	10.265	22.900	48,6	41,2	56,1
Rwanda	2.719	256	91	473	9,4	4,2	17,7
Saint Lucia	4	0	0	2	11,1	2,2	42,1
Samoa	5	1	0	3	21,1	4,6	60,4
Saudi Arabia	393	143	33	320	36,4	8,5	75,9
Senegal	3.723	621	214	1.182	16,7	7,0	31,4
Serbia	351	15	3	30	4,1	1,4	9,4
Seychelles	2	0	0	1	11,5	2,3	42,8
Sierra Leone	1.204	278	0	605	23,1	5,0	53,8
Singapore	149	1	0	5	1,0	0,0	5,2
Slovakia	113	8	2	18	7,1	2,0	17,3
Slovenia	17	1	0	2	3,6	0,1	18,3
Somalia	859	84	16	330	9,8	1,9	38,3
South Africa	86.642	5.796	3.542	8.303	6,7	5,5	8,1
Spain	715	30	6	69	4,3	1,2	10,5
Sri Lanka	610	0	0	53	0,0	0,0	8,7
St Vincent & Grenadines	4	1	0	2	14,7	3,0	49,5
Sudan	6.972	681	120	2.736	9,8	1,9	37,5
Swaziland	1.438	131	27	282	9,1	2,5	21,7
Sweden	12	1	0	4	11,8	1,5	36,4
Switzerland	50	3	0	9	6,7	0,8	22,1
Syrian Arab Republic	259	95	23	209	36,8	9,1	76,0
Tajikistan	2.454	1.040	254	2.127	42,4	11,0	80,1
TFYR Macedonia	84	10	2	37	11,4	2,3	42,3
Thailand	3.887	1.342	839	1.916	34,5	27,9	41,7
Timor-Leste	73	14	3	43	18,8	3,9	55,7
Togo	1.781	162	28	665	9,1	1,7	36,8
Tonga	2	0	0	1	20,3	4,3	59,1
Tunisia	43	16	4	35	36,1	8,8	74,9
Turkey	5.520	586	108	2.428	10,6	2,1	41,5
Turkmenistan	715	131	65	211	18,4	11,3	27,5
Uganda	6.061	269	0	713	4,4	0,5	15,1
Ukraine	12.549	5.563	3.547	7.697	44,3	39,9	48,8
United Arab Emirates	32	12	3	26	36,7	8,9	75,4
United Kingdom	418	11	3	21	2,6	1,0	5,2
UR Tanzania	9.932	0	0	589	0,0	0,0	5,9
Uruguay	76	5	0	12	6,1	0,7	20,2
Uzbekistan	8.309	4.985	3.094	7.059	60,0	48,8	70,5
Venezuela	683	92	44	157	13,5	7,6	21,6
Viet Nam	12.287	2.374	1.378	3.535	19,3	14,2	25,4
West Bank and Gaza Strip	30	11	3	25	36,8	10,2	77,1
Yemen	648	73	22	145	11,3	4,3	23,0
Zambia	7.394	168	0	586	2,3	0,1	12,0
Zimbabwe	9.906	826	0	1.966	8,3	1,8	22,5

Annex 10: Estimates of MDR-TB among all TB cases

Country	No. of All TB cases	No. of MDR cases	Low 95% CL	High 95% CL	% MDR TB	Low 95% CL	High 95% CL
Afghanistan	44.035	2.139	671	8.802	4,9	1,6	19,5
Albania	643	14	4	67	2,1	0,7	10,3
Algeria	19.316	277	105	561	1,4	0,6	2,8
Andorra	15	0	0	0	0,7	0,1	3,4
Angola	52.694	1.665	547	7.144	3,2	1,1	13,1
Antigua & Barbuda	5	0	0	0	1,3	0,7	9,1
Argentina	16.060	463	267	699	2,9	1,8	4,1
Armenia	2.630	381	273	501	14,5	11,6	18,0
Australia	1.414	21	11	36	1,5	0,8	2,6
Austria	1.068	23	10	39	2,1	1,0	3,4
Azerbaijan	8.291	2.397	1.744	3.074	28,9	25,1	33,2
Bahamas	139	3	1	12	1,9	0,7	8,5
Bahrain	316	11	4	43	3,5	1,1	13,4
Bangladesh	361.133	14.583	3.566	72.744	4,0	1,0	19,3
Belarus	6.986	1.096	371	3.272	15,7	5,4	46,5
Belgium	1.501	25	10	43	1,6	0,7	2,8
Belize	153	4	1	15	2,3	0,8	10,2
Benin	8.597	90	18	304	1,0	0,2	3,7
Bhutan	662	28	8	119	4,2	1,3	17,5
Bolivia	20.076	294	117	526	1,5	0,6	2,5
Bosnia & Herzegovina	2.139	17	7	29	0,8	0,3	1,4
Botswana	10.658	131	69	206	1,2	0,7	1,9
Brazil	105.220	1.464	945	2.077	1,4	1,0	1,9
Brunei Darussalam	337	11	3	47	3,3	1,1	13,8
Bulgaria	3.417	451	143	1.563	13,2	4,2	44,
Burkina Faso	40.244	1.170	369	5.402	2,9	1,0	13,
Burundi	31.094	815	199	4.725	2,6	0,7	15,
Cambodia	73.905	92	0	221	0,1	0,0	0,
Cameroon	37.087	786	227	4.036	2,1	0,6	11,
Canada	1.828	25	12	42	1,4	0,7	2,
Cape Verde	956	22	7	102	2,3	0,8	10,
Central African Republic	16.153	415	188	703	2,6	1,2	4,
Chad	33.060	807	230	4.297	2,4	0,7	13,
Chile	2.599	24	10	42	0,9	0,4	1,
China	1.564.047	130.548	97.633	164.900	8,3	7,0	10,
China, Hong Kong SAR	4.973	81	51	117	1,6	1,1	2,
China, Macao SAR	310	11	4	19	3,4	1,4	6,
Colombia	21.339	382	202	690	1,8	1,1	3,
Comoros	381	9	3	45	2,3	0,7	11,
Congo	15.634	321	90	1.737	2,1	0,6	11,
Costa Rica	673	12	2	25	1,8	0,4	3,
Côte d'Ivoire	84.447	2.403	1.033	4.574	2,8	1,3	5,
Croatia	2.021	19	5	36	0,9	0,3	1,
Cuba	1.088	4	0	13	0,3	0,0	1,
Cyprus	43	1	0	3	1,3	0,4	7,
Czech Republic	1.041	23	11	37	2,2	1,1	3,
Denmark	490	7	1	15	1,5	0,3	2,
Djibouti	7.270	449	150	1.489	6,2	2,1	20,
Dominica	12	0	0	1	2,2	0,8	10
Dominican Republic	9.738	800	496	1.162	8,2	5,7	11,
DPR Korea	50.781	3.472	1.136	11.248	6,8	2,3	21
DR Congo	253.180	7.044	2.030	36.534	2,8	0,8	14
Ecuador	19.619	1.483	1.034	1.998	7,6	5,8	9
Egypt	19.304	962	646	1.315	5,0	3,4	7
El Salvador	3.683	32	12	58	0,9	0,3	1
Eritrea	4.686	127	36	681	2,7	0,8	14
Estonia	633	128	91	172	20,3	15,9	25
Ethiopia	314.261	5.825	2.992	9.689	1,9	1,0	2
Fiji	186	0	0	17	0,0	0,0	9
Finland	306	4	0	9	1,2	0,0	2
France	9.255	138	76	214	1,5	0,9	2
French Polynesia	76	3	1	10	3,9	1,3	13

Country	No. of All TB cases	No. of MDR cases	Low 95% CL	High 95% CL	% MDR TB	Low 95% CL	High 95% CL
Gabon	5.061	98	31	460	1,9	0,6	9,1
Gambia	4.526	20	0	72	0,5	0,0	1,4
Georgia	5.269	652	467	847	12,4	9,9	15,4
Germany	5.826	155	107	210	2,7	2,1	3,5
Ghana	48.787	1.090	288	6.169	2,2	0,6	12,1
Greece	2.227	45	15	186	2,0	0,7	8,5
Guam	69	3	0	10	4,3	0,5	14,5
Guatemala	10.748	432	269	633	4,0	2,7	5,5
Guinea	25.969	599	287	978	2,3	1,1	4,1
Guinea-Bissau	3.884	109	32	545	2,8	0,8	13,9
Guyana	1.325	31	10	152	2,4	0,8	11,3
Haiti	28.927	594	139	3.515	2,1	0,5	11,9
Honduras	5.626	131	63	218	2,3	1,2	3,6
Hungary	2.290	69	23	258	3,0	1,0	11,1
Iceland	14	0	0	0	0,0	0,0	0,0
India	2.254.052	110.132	79.975	142.386	4,9	3,9	6,2
Indonesia	542.703	12.142	753	30.388	2,2	0,1	5,3
Iran	16.511	1.178	788	1.642	7,1	5,3	9,5
Iraq	17.263	969	334	3.246	5,6	2,0	18,6
Ireland	583	6	0	15	1,0	0,0	2,5
Israel	525	30	13	52	5,6	2,8	8,9
Italy	4.649	118	62	188	2,5	1,4	3,9
Jamaica	208	4	1	20	1,8	0,5	9,4
Japan	29.583	322	206	462	1,1	0,7	1,5
Jordan	314	20	8	36	6,3	2,6	10,8
Kazakhstan	26.647	6.608	4.806	8.534	24,8	20,0	30,4
Kenya	145.590	0	0	0	0,0	0,0	0,0
Kiribati	353	12	2	66	3,4	0,7	18,1
Kuwait	676	16	4	79	2,4	0,7	11,6
Kyrgyzstan	7.502	1.368	443	4.026	18,2	6,2	51,5
Lao PDR	9.172	398	106	1.837	4,3	1,2	19,8
Latvia	1.523	218	156	284	14,3	11,9	17,3
Lebanon	462	11	5	20	2,4	1,0	4,3
Lesotho	14.529	220	66	427	1,5	0,5	2,9
Libyan Arab Jamahiriya	1.076	33	8	166	3,1	0,8	15,2
Lithuania	2.563	425	313	545	16,6	13,6	20,5
Luxembourg	60	0	0	1	0,5	0,1	2,3
Madagascar	51.390	388	104	740	0,8	0,2	1,5
Malawi	54.001	1.362	341	7.663	2,5	0,7	14,4
Malaysia	28.584	27	0	95	0,1	0,0	0,3
Maldives	143	5	2	24	3,7	1,1	16,4
Mali	34.228	756	177	4.363	2,2	0,5	12,8
Malta	26	0	0	1	0,4	0,1	2,3
Marshall Islands	135	5	2	24	4,0	1,3	16,7
Mauritius	294	5	1	26	1,6	0,5	8,6
Mexico	27.113	1.579	960	2.301	5,8	3,6	8,7
Micronesia	125	6	2	22	4,8	1,7	17,7
Mongolia	5.225	116	42	263	2,2	0,8	5,3
Morocco	29.877	271	141	446	0,9	0,5	1,5
Mozambique	97.946	3.419	1.987	5.168	3,5	2,5	4,6
Myanmar	88.999	4.251	2.648	6.187	4,8	3,4	6,3
Namibia	17.155	342	103	1.716	2,0	0,6	9,8
Nepal	53.211	1.921	1.195	2.822	3,6	2,4	4,9
Netherlands	1.295	10	3	21	0,8	0,3	1,5
New Caledonia	74	0	0	39	0,0	0,0	52,2
New Zealand	373	1	0	5	0,4	0,0	1,1
Nicaragua	3.606	51	19	93	1,4	0,5	2,6
Niger	26.105	750	233	3.667	2,9	0,9	13,5
Nigeria	478.736	11.171	3.254	58.081	2,3	0,7	12,0
Northern Mariana Is	66	3	0	0	4,5	0,0	0,0
Norway	279	4	0	10	1,5	0,0	3,4
Oman	341	6	1	14	1,8	0,3	4,0

Annex 10

Country	No. of All TB cases	No. of MDR cases	Low 95% CL	High 95% CL	% MDR TB	Low 95% CL	High 95% CL
Pakistan	306.418	15.233	4.752	59.884	5,0	1,6	19,4
Palau	12	1	0	2	5,4	1,7	16,5
Panama	1.715	47	16	188	2,7	0,9	11,0
Papua New Guinea	17.277	915	285	3.560	5,3	1,7	20,1
Paraguay	4.719	109	34	212	2,3	0,8	4,2
Peru	51.670	3.972	2.842	5.192	7,7	6,3	9,4
Philippines	256.511	11.848	7.428	17.106	4,6	3,4	5,9
Poland	10.660	127	81	181	1,2	0,8	1,8
Portugal	3.762	64	38	96	1,7	1,1	2,5
Puerto Rico	206	0	0	0	0,0	0,0	0,0
Qatar	493	5	1	15	1,1	0,2	3,1
Rep. Korea	49.830	2.189	1.541	2.914	4,4	3,4	5,7
Republic of Moldova	7.437	2.035	1.504	2.581	27,4	23,8	31,4
Romania	34.518	1.546	1.047	2.138	4,5	3,3	5,9
Russian Federation	186.080	36.037	28.992	50.258	19,4	17,1	24,6
Rwanda	40.363	1.723	1.000	2.617	4,3	2,8	5,8
Saint Lucia	32	1	0	4	2,7	0,9	11,1
Samoa	41	2	1	8	5,2	1,8	18,6
Saudi Arabia	11.024	375	124	1.540	3,4	1,1	13,6
Senegal	36.361	1.309	587	2.225	3,6	1,6	6,0
Serbia	3.534	26	10	47	0,7	0,3	1,3
Seychelles	30	1	0	3	2,0	0,6	9,2
Sierra Leone	30.894	532	81	1.228	1,7	0,3	3,9
Singapore	1.277	4	0	9	0,3	0,0	0,7
Slovakia	942	21	7	40	2,3	0,8	4,1
Slovenia	278	1	0	2	0,2	0,0	0,8
Solomon Islands	664	0	0	29	0,0	0,0	4,3
Somalia	19.303	412	113	2.229	2,1	0,6	11,3
South Africa	540.571	14.034	10.019	18.409	2,6	2,1	3,2
Spain	13.895	48	8	102	0,3	0,1	0,7
Sri Lanka	12.230	21	0	75	0,2	0,0	0,6
St Vincent & Grenadines	39	1	0	5	3,1	1,1	12,2
Sudan	98.303	2.377	752	12.040	2,4	0,8	11,9
Swaziland	14.535	248	79	462	1,7	0,5	3,2
Sweden	561	4	1	9	0,7	0,1	1,
Switzerland	550	6	1	14	1,2	0,3	2,
Syrian Arab Republic	6.510	287	90	1.195	4,4	1,4	17,8
Tajikistan	15.986	3.204	1.072	8.916	20,0	6,8	53,
TFYR Macedonia	680	19	6	79	2,8	0,9	11,
Thailand	94.139	2.834	1.920	3.926	3,0	2,1	4,
Timor-Leste	6.260	225	46	1.192	3,6	0,7	18,
Togo	26.703	667	190	3.449	2,5	0,7	12,
Tonga	26	1	0	5	4,5	1,4	17,
Tunisia	2.563	84	22	413	3,3	0,9	15,
Turkey	27.272	889	284	3.320	3,3	1,1	12,
Turkmenistan	3.890	252	125	411	6,5	3,3	10,
Uganda	112.098	836	120	1.858	0,7	0,1	1,
Ukraine	61.857	13.429	9.810	17.150	21,7	18,8	25,
United Arab Emirates	713	27	9	104	3,8	1,3	14,
United Kingdom	9.776	74	42	113	0,8	0,5	1
UR Tanzania	133.072	1.335	240	2.942	1,0	0,2	2
Uruguay	986	5	0	13	0,5	0,0	1,
USA	13.616	159	133	190	1,2	1,0	1
Uzbekistan	41.087	9.829	6.891	13.073	23,9	18,4	30
Vanuatu	130	0	0	0	0,0	0,0	0
Venezuela	11.954	151	76	244	1,3	0,6	2
Viet Nam	161.205	6.421	4.402	8.760	4,0	3,0	5
West Bank and Gaza Strip	820	36	11	151	4,3	1,4	18
Yemen	17.633	573	299	923	3,2	1,9	4
Zambia	72.026	1.330	494	2.442	1,8	0,8	3
Zimbabwe	94.921	2.460	1.190	4.053	2,6	1,4	4

Annex 11: Estimates of MDR-TB by epidemiological region

Regions	No. of All TB cases	No. of MDR cases	Low 95% CL	High 95% CL	% MDR TB	Low 95% CL	High 95% CL
Established market economies	85.729	724	573	942	0,8	0,7	1,1
Central Europe	42.464	416	166	2.170	1,0	0,4	5,0
Eastern Europe	336.842	43.878	35.881	54.877	13,0	11,8	15,3
Latin America	315.216	7.196	5.850	10.360	2,3	1,9	3,3
Eastern Mediterranean Region	569.446	16.430	8.137	64.077	2,9	1,5	11,1
Africa, low HIV incidence	350.671	5.311	3.705	14.948	1,5	1,1	4,3
Africa, high HIV incidence	2.440.270	43.767	33.907	102.418	1,8	1,4	4,2
South-East Asia	3.100.354	85.908	58.085	148.884	2,8	2,1	4,7
Western Pacific Region	1.882.930	82.087	57.531	107.804	4,4	3,9	4,8
Surveyed countries (n=105)	7.029.716	228.367	190.128	267.943	3,2	2,9	3,6
Non surveyed countries (n=70)	2.094.206	57.351	45.599	164.828	2,7	2,2	7,7
All countries (n=175)	9.123.922	285.718	256.072	399.224	3,1	2,9	4,3

Regions	No. of All TB cases	No. of MDR cases	Low 95% CL	High 95% CL	% MDR TB	Low 95% CL	High 95% CL
Established market economies	5.036	413	330	528	8,2	6,8	10,2
Central Europe	8.038	785	303	2.625	9,8	3,9	31,3
Eastern Europe	79.474	36.179	29.216	43.769	45,5	41,8	49,4
Latin America	33.856	4.873	4.001	5.937	14,4	12,4	16,9
Eastern Mediterranean Region	31.286	9.040	4.733	15.901	28,9	15,5	48,9
Africa, low HIV incidence	25.130	3.105	2.169	5.527	12,4	8,9	21,4
Africa, high HIV incidence	216.152	14.528	11.004	24.886	6,7	5,4	11,4
South-East Asia	363.959	63.707	43.416	87.495	17,5	15,4	20,2
Western Pacific Region	289.214	70.601	47.134	94.543	24,4	22,7	26,1
Surveyed countries (n=96)	906.968	179.767	146.915	212.012	19,8	18,4	21,3
Non surveyed countries (n=79)	145.177	23.463	19.117	39.326	16,2	13,1	26,3
All countries (n=175)	1.052.145	203.230	172.935	242.177	19,3	18,2	21,3

Regions	No. of All TB cases	No. of MDR cases	Low 95% CL	High 95% CL	% MDR TB	Low 95% CL	High 95% CL
Established market economies	105.795	1.317	1.147	1.557	1,2	1,1	1,5
Central Europe	50.502	1.201	623	3.694	2,4	1,3	7,2
Eastern Europe	416.316	80.057	71.893	97.623	19,2	18,0	22,2
Latin America	349.278	12.070	10.523	15.526	3,5	3,0	4,4
Eastern Mediterranean Region	601.225	25.475	15.737	73.132	4,2	2,6	11,9
Africa, low HIV incidence	375.801	8.415	6.889	18.758	2,2	1,9	5,0
Africa, high HIV incidence	2.656.422	58.296	48.718	118.506	2,2	1,9	4,5
South-East Asia	3.464.313	149.615	114.780	217.921	4,3	3,5	6,2
Western Pacific Region	2.173.333	152.694	119.886	188.014	7,0	6,1	8,1
Surveyed countries	7.953.603	408.325	361.264	464.069	5,1	4,7	5,7
Non surveyed countries	2.239.383	80.814	71.684	188.605	3,6	3,2	8,4
All countries (n=185)	10.192.986	489.139	455.093	614.215	4,8	4,6	6,0

ANTI-TB DRUG RESISTANCE IN THE WORLD   ANNEXES

Global Project Coverage 1994–2007

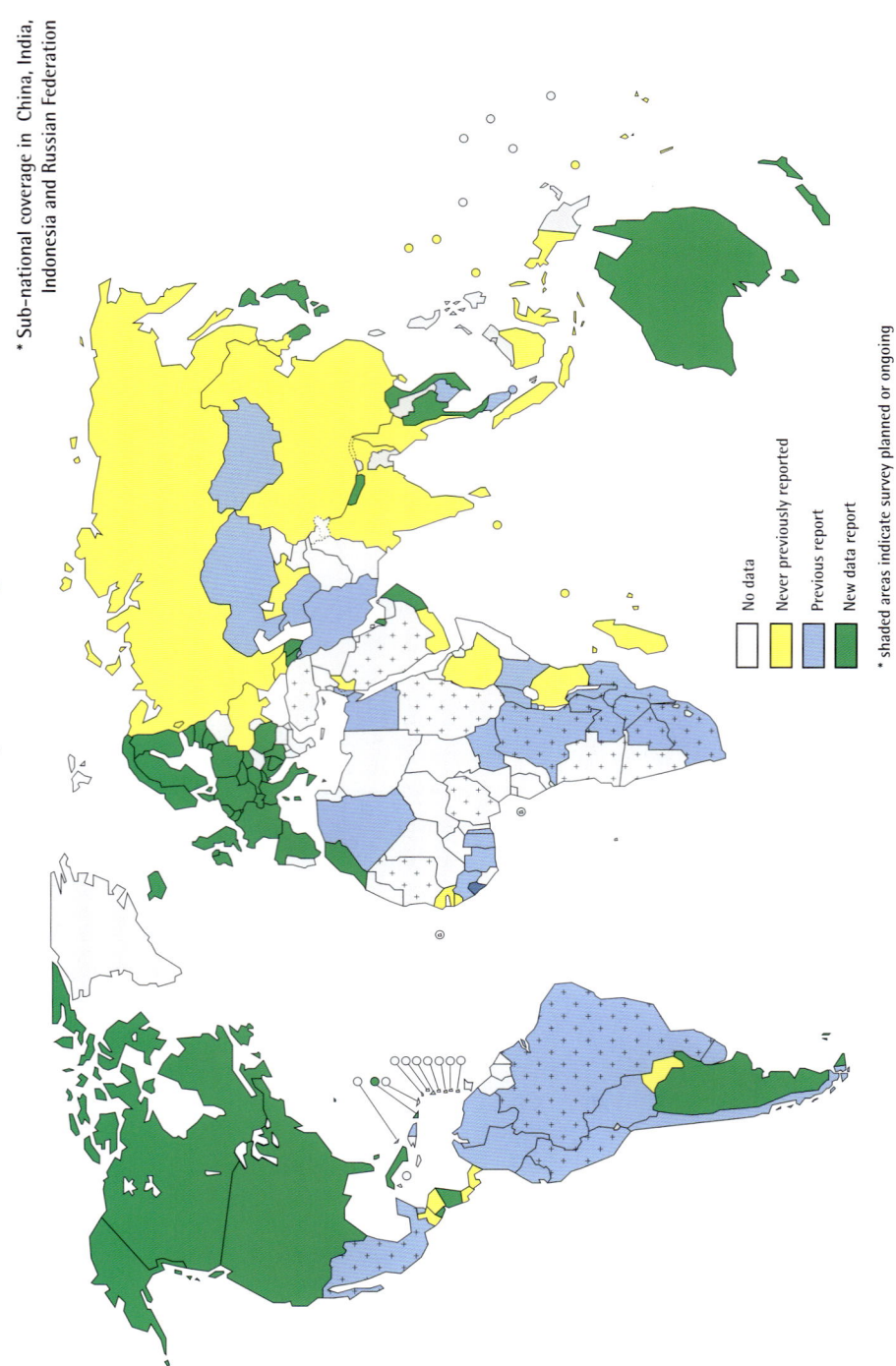

* Sub-national coverage in China, India, Indonesia and Russian Federation

- No data
- Never previously reported
- Previous report
- New data report

* shaded areas indicate survey planned or ongoing

The designations employed and the presentation of material on this map do not imply the expression of any opinion whatsoever on the part of the World Health Organization concerning the legal status of any country, territory, city or area of its authorities, or concerning the delimitation of its frontiers or boundaries. Dashed lines represent approximate border lines for which there may not be full agreement

Available trend data 1994–2007

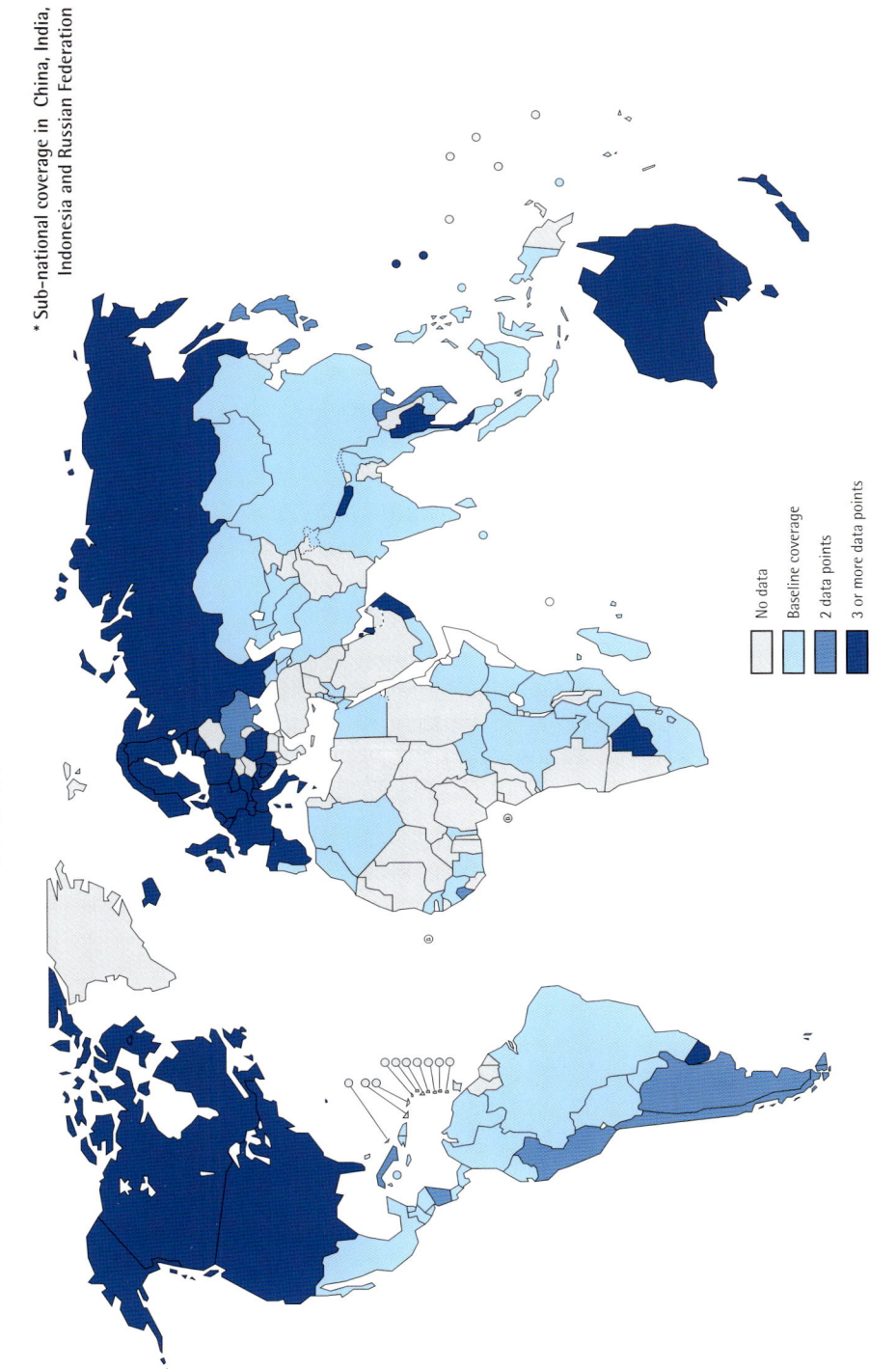

* Sub-national coverage in China, India, Indonesia and Russian Federation

Legend:
- No data
- Baseline coverage
- 2 data points
- 3 or more data points

The designations employed and the presentation of material on this map do not imply the expression of any opinion whatsoever on the part of the World Health Organization concerning the legal status of any country, territory, city or area or of its authorities, or concerning the delimitation of its frontiers or boundaries. Dashed lines represent approximate border lines for which there may not be full agreement

ANTI-TB DRUG RESISTANCE IN THE WORLD   ANNEXES

Any resistance among new cases 1994–2007

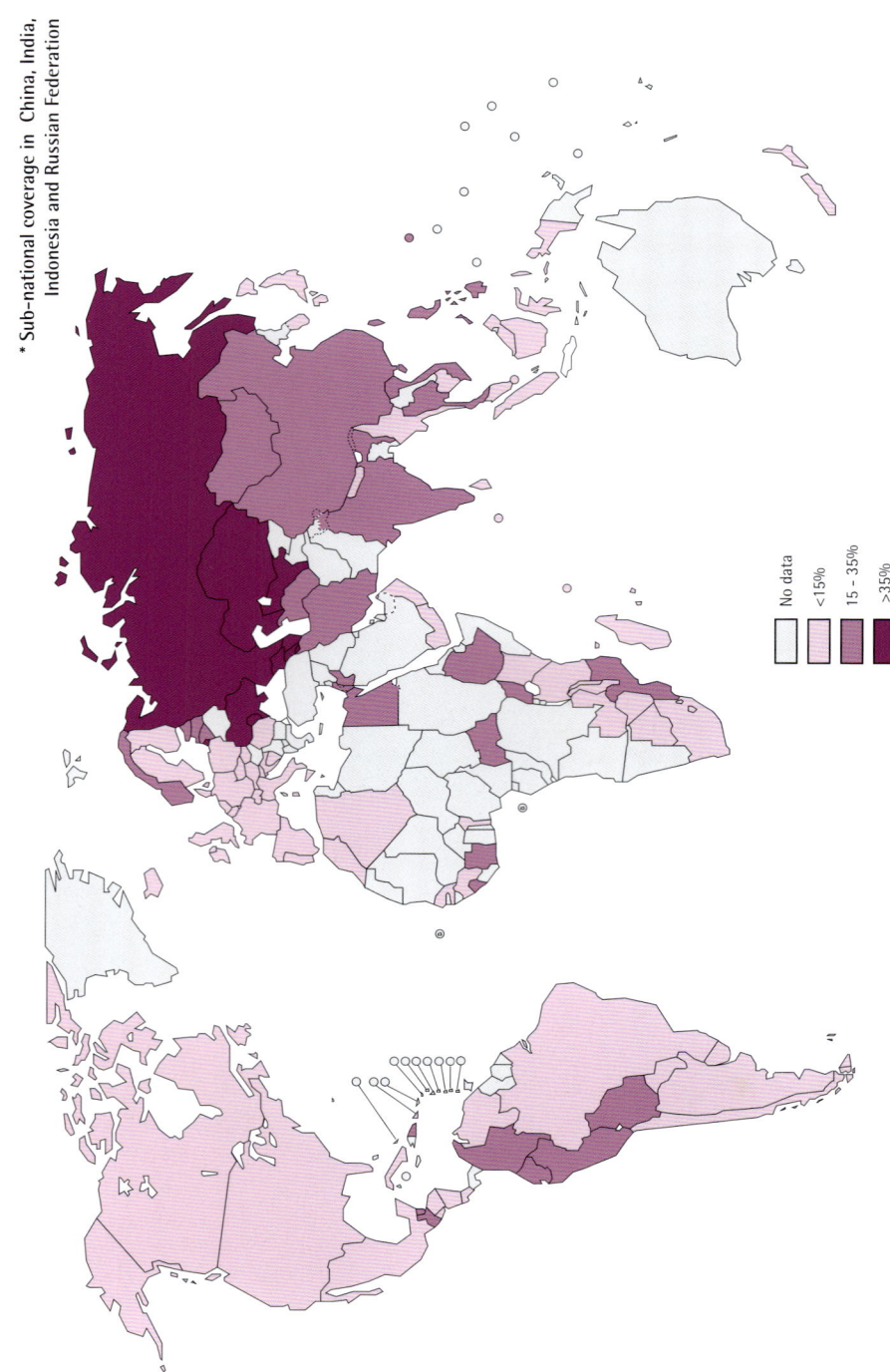

* Sub-national coverage in China, India, Indonesia and Russian Federation

- No data
- <15%
- 15 – 35%
- >35%

The designations employed and the presentation of material on this map do not imply the expression of any opinion whatsoever on the part of the World Health Organization concerning the legal status of any country, territory, city or area of its authorities, or concerning the delimitation of its frontiers or boundaries. Dashed lines represent approximate border lines for which there may not be full agreement

ANTI-TB DRUG RESISTANCE IN THE WORLD ANNEXES

MDR-TB among new cases 1994–2007

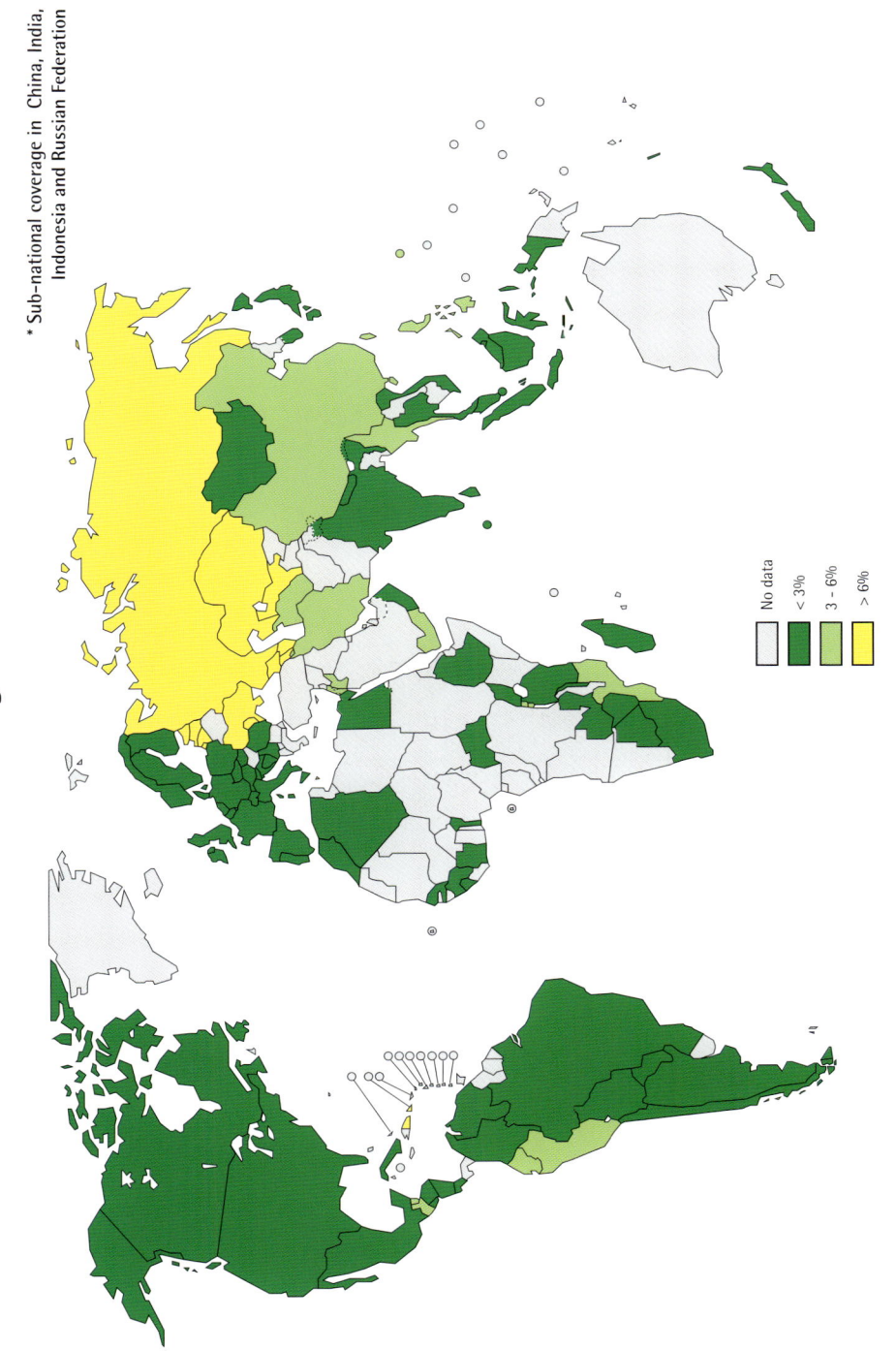

* Sub-national coverage in China, India, Indonesia and Russian Federation

No data
< 3%
3 – 6%
> 6%

The designations employed and the presentation of material on this map do not imply the expression of any opinion whatsoever on the part of the World Health Organization concerning the legal status of any country, territory, city or area of its authorities, or concerning the delimitation of its frontiers or boundaries. Dashed lines represent approximate border lines for which there may not be full agreement

ANTI-TB DRUG RESISTANCE IN THE WORLD   ANNEXES

Any resistance among previously treated cases 1994–2007

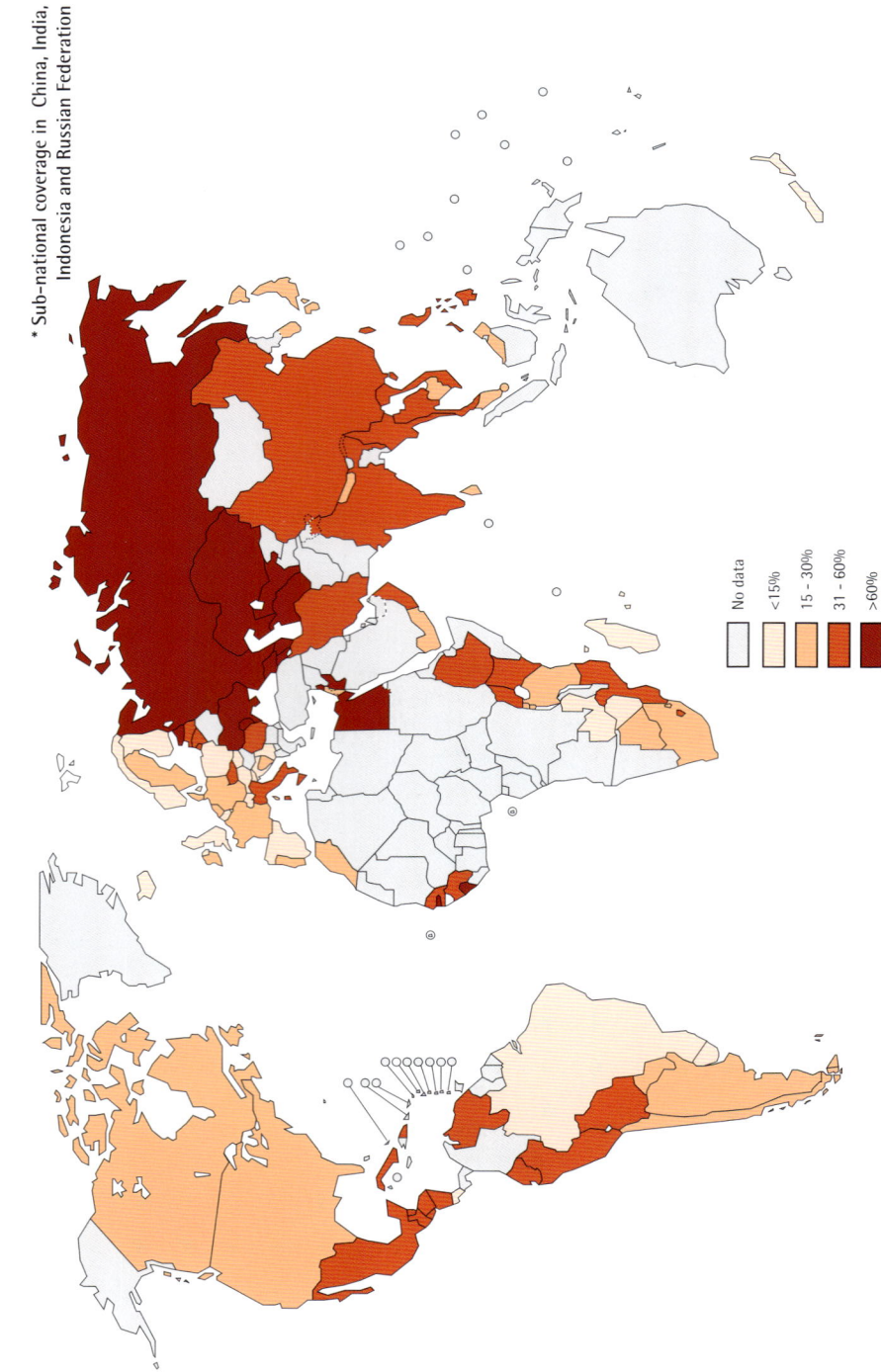

*Sub-national coverage in China, India, Indonesia and Russian Federation

- No data
- <15%
- 15 - 30%
- 31 - 60%
- >60%

The designations employed and the presentation of material on this map do not imply the expression of any opinion whatsoever on the part of the World Health Organization concerning the legal status of any country, territory, city or area of its authorities, or concerning the delimitation of its frontiers or boundaries. Dashed lines represent approximate border lines for which there may not be full agreement

ANTI-TB DRUG RESISTANCE IN THE WORLD ANNEXES

148

MDR-TB among previously treated cases 1994–2007

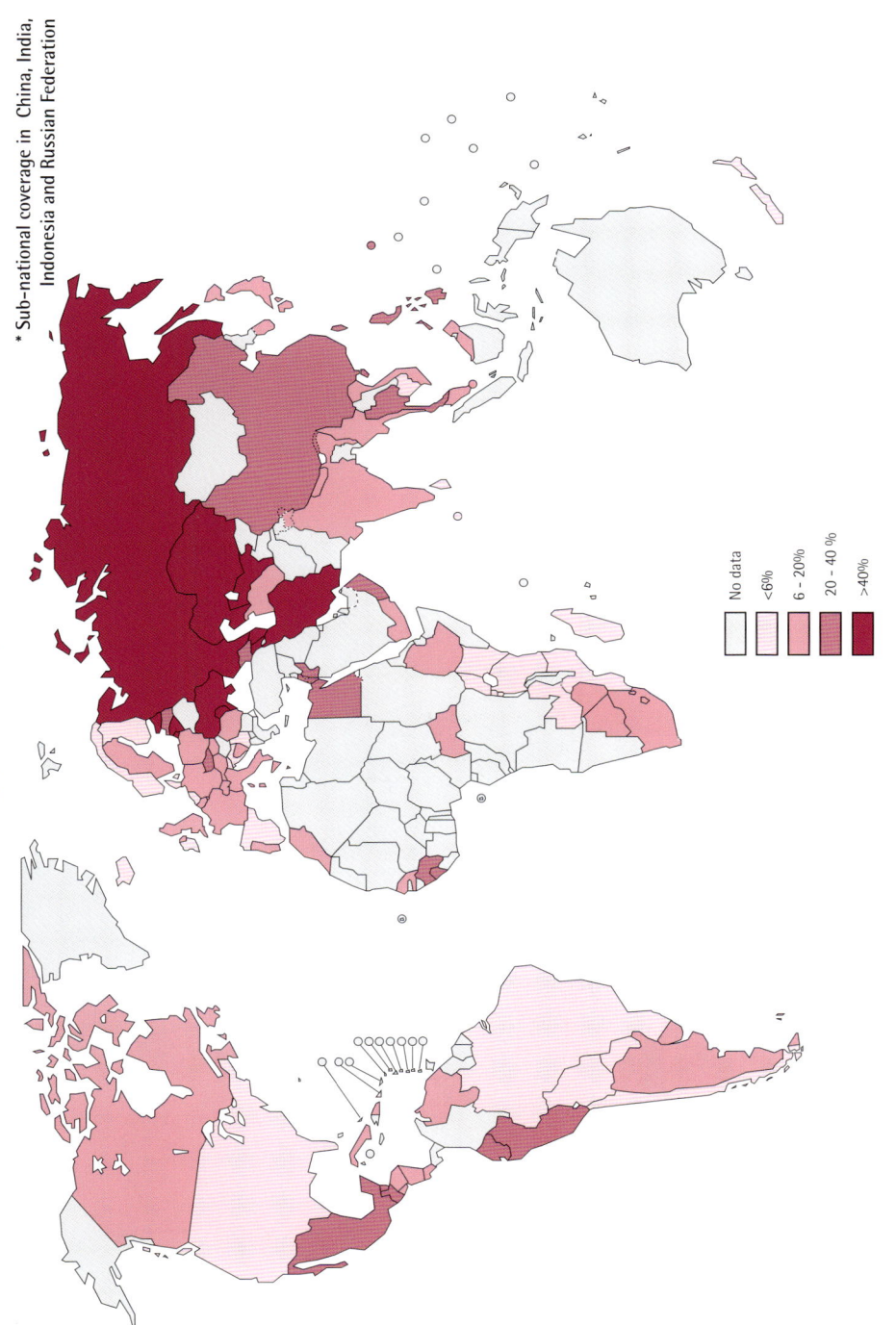

* Sub-national coverage in China, India, Indonesia and Russian Federation

No data
<6%
6 – 20%
20 – 40 %
>40%

The designations employed and the presentation of material on this map do not imply the expression of any opinion whatsoever on the part of the World Health Organization concerning the legal status of any country, territory, city or area of its authorities, or concerning the delimitation of its frontiers or boundaries. Dashed lines represent approximate border lines for which there may not be full agreement

ANTI-TB DRUG RESISTANCE IN THE WORLD   ANNEXES

ANTI-TB DRUG RESISTANCE IN THE WORLD ANNEXES

The Supranational Laboratory Network

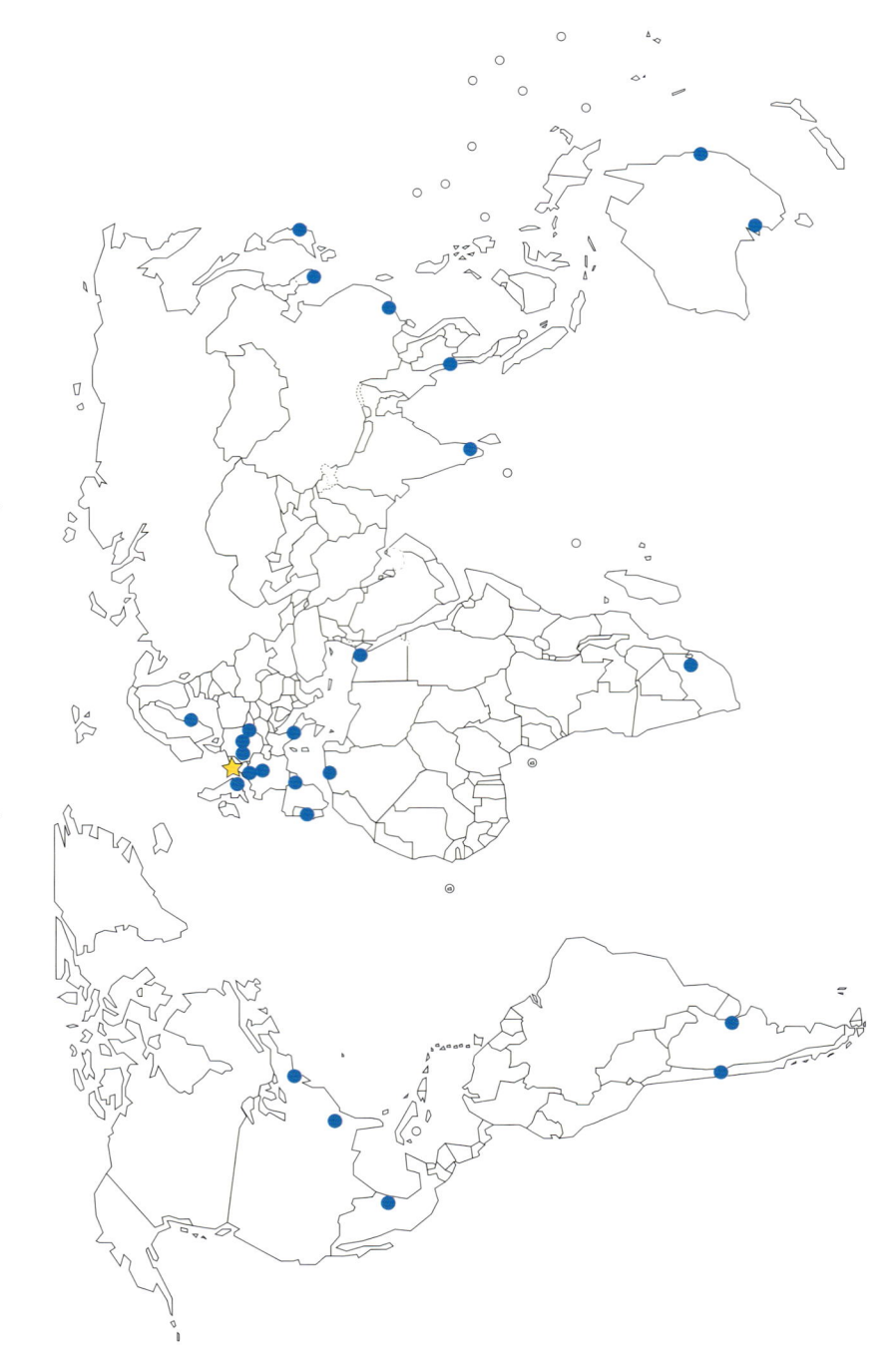

The designations employed and the presentation of material on this map do not imply the expression of any opinion whatsoever on the part of the World Health Organization concerning the legal status of any country, territory, city or area of its authorities, or concerning the delimitation of its frontiers or boundaries. Dashed lines represent approximate border lines for which there may not be full agreement

150

XDR-TB among MDR-TB cases 2002–2007

*Sub-national averages applied to the Russian Federation

- No data
- >3% or less than 3 cases in one year of surveillance
- 3–10%
- Report of at least one case
- >10%

The designations employed and the presentation of material on this map do not imply the expression of any opinion whatsoever on the part of the World Health Organization concerning the legal status of any country, territory, city or area of its authorities, or concerning the delimitation of its frontiers or boundaries. Dashed lines represent approximate border lines for which there may not be full agreement

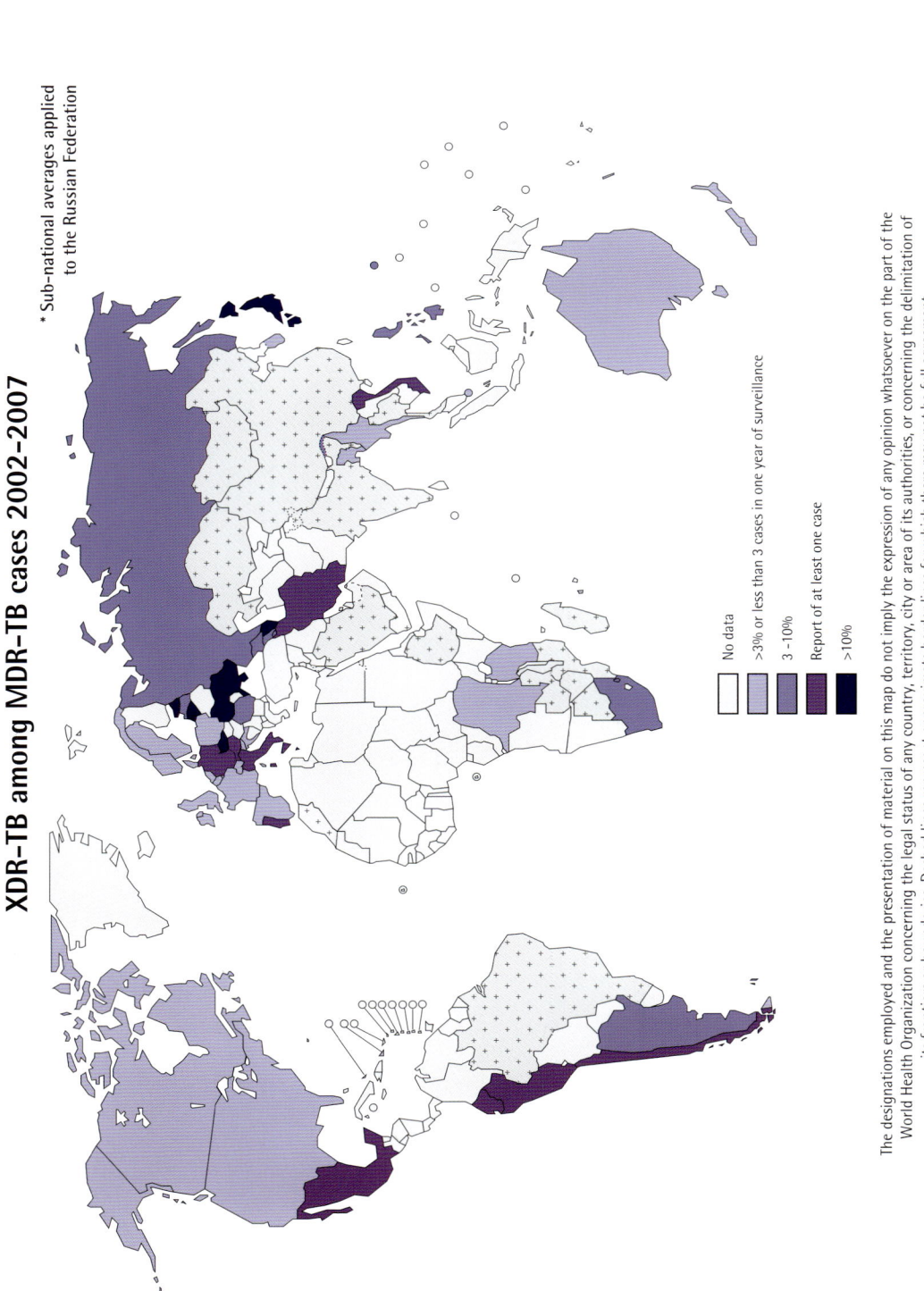

ANTI-TB DRUG RESISTANCE IN THE WORLD   ANNEXES